Children in Difficulty

A guide to understanding and helping

Third edition

Julian Elliott and Maurice Place

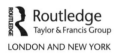

Routledge
Taylor & Francis Group

LONDON AND NEW YORK

First published 1998
by Routledge

This edition published 2012
by Routledge
2 Park Square, Milton Park, Abingdon, Oxon OX14 4RN

Simultaneously published in the USA and Canada
by Routledge
711 Third Avenue, New York, NY 10017

Routledge is an imprint of the Taylor & Francis Group, an informa business

British Library Cataloguing in Publication Data
A catalogue record for this book is available from the British Library

Library of Congress Cataloging in Publication Data
Elliott, Julian, 1955–
   Children in difficulty : a guide to understanding and helping / Authored by Julian
   Elliott and Maurice Place. — 3rd ed.
      p. cm.
      Includes bibliographical references and index.
   1. Child psychotherapy. 2. Child psychopathology. 3. Adolescent psychotherapy.
   4. Adolescent psychopathology. I. Place, Maurice. II. Title.
   RJ504.E43 2012
   618.92'8914—dc23   2011026288

ISBN: 978–0–415–67255–9 (hbk)
ISBN: 978–0–415–67263–4 (pbk)
ISBN: 978–0–203–14480–0 (ebk)

Typeset in Bembo
by Keystroke, Station Road, Codsall, Wolverhampton

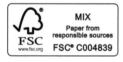

MIX
Paper from
responsible sources
FSC® C004839
www.fsc.org

Printed and bound in Great Britain by
TJ International Ltd, Padstow, Cornwall

Contents

Figures

Chapter 1

Introduction

There are few issues which can raise stronger feelings in the average person than those which relate to children. Be it outrage at their challenging behaviour, or distress at injury or neglect, adults quickly become moved by issues which involve children. Even more fascinating is the way that each person 'knows' how the situation or behaviour should be handled – and usually this means that the delinquent needs more punishment, or the hurt child needs more care. While such emotional responses are very understandable, they are not always the correct way to intervene in a situation to ensure that matters will be improved. A child's functioning and development are influenced by many (at times, competing) influences, and any efforts to help must be informed by an understanding of these.

Influences upon development

Genetics and epigenetics

The genetic make-up inherited from their parents is increasingly seen as a significant influence on many diverse aspects of the child's growth, development and ultimate functioning. The belief that problems located within the parents can be passed on to their children has been persuasive since biblical times. The advent of scientific study, and the work of Gregor Mendel, the Augustinian monk, gave a clear understanding of the principles of heredity, and prompted research into DNA and the chromosomes that are made from it.

Research into conditions such as Down syndrome has clearly shown that changes to the chromosomes can be responsible for some major, and sometimes profound, changes in functioning and development. However, research has also begun focusing upon the mechanisms and chemicals that take the information held in the DNA and translate it into the cell's structure and function.

Studies of how interventions bring about their effect have shown that experiences influence the translation machinery of the gene, changing in some instances the expression of the gene and the genome itself. This is the essence of a gene x environment interaction. Trying to understand this process is the science of epigenetics.

Experience modifies the gene's actions, creating changes in behaviour, and this is achieved by changing the mechanisms that translate the DNA information into the cell's activity. One of the main mechanisms by which this is achieved is by altering the chemical make-up of the surface of the DNA. For instance, the phenomenon of cytosine methylation tends to silence that part of the gene (Jaenisch and Bird 2003), while a process called histone modification tends to activate it (Jenuwein and Allis 2001). A third epigenetic system has been identified, and this interferes with the chemical that transfers the gene's instructions to the cell (messenger RNA) (Hamilton *et al.* 2002).

These epigenetic processes are tissue-specific and can be inherited, but they are also very prone to change by environmental experiences and factors. They appear to be particularly vulnerable to being altered at a number of key developmental points in the infant's early development (Waterland and Michels 2007). For instance, early in life, diet is important in order to provide sufficient nutrients to permit the usual epigenetic processes to proceed. Of particular importance in this regard is folate, vitamin B12 and vitamin B6, with deficiencies being linked to impaired central nervous system development and a number of psychiatric conditions, including behavioural disturbances in childhood (Reynolds 2006).

Such changes can persist for the remainder of the cell's life and may last for multiple generations, but this is achieved without any alteration to the original DNA sequence (Bird 2007). In some instances these changes can be transmitted through to subsequent generations. As we shall see when considering attachment (Chapter 4), this process is viewed as increasingly important in regulating maternal behaviour, and transmitting emotional states to the child. It is also implicated in the origin and persistence of numerous behavioural difficulties and psychiatric conditions (Tsankova *et al.* 2007).

However these changes need to be triggered, and it is environmental factors, and life events, which moderate or mediate these genetic influences on behaviour and functioning. Interestingly, although much of the focus has been upon the difficulties and problems that can result from the effect of the environment x gene interaction upon the developing brain, it is important to remember that these processes also make children susceptible to influence from positive experiences (Belsky and Pluess 2009). Indeed it is through such mechanisms that therapeutic interventions exert their effect, as they also alter the mechanisms of brain cell functioning (Meaney 2010).

Changes to specific brain cell functioning exert their influence through changes to the complex chemical and hormonal structures which control all of our bodily systems, and which in turn alter our emotions and behaviour. The detail and complexity of such elements make them beyond the scope of this text, but by way of illustration we can look at one particular body chemical: serotonin (or 5-HT). Work over the years has highlighted that this chemical plays a role in moderating emotional responses to adverse experiences throughout the animal kingdom (Steiner *et al.* 1997). Thus if there is any dysfunction in serotonin's action then emotional problems are likely to arise. From this research has sprung a new family of medications to treat depression, the serotonin specific reuptake inhibitors (SSRI's), which are discussed in Chapter 10.

The other aspects of brain development that need to be borne in mind are those of sensitive periods and brain plasticity. Sensitive periods of development are well recognised in many animals as points early in life when certain skills or abilities need to be acquired. If they are not acquired at this 'critical period', then it is more difficult, and perhaps impossible, to develop them later in life. So for instance, eyes need to receive light to develop the correct optical nerve networks (Weisel and Hubel 1965), and this is true for many other neural pathways as well. These critical periods have been highlighted as significant for human development (Bischof 2007), and are, for instance, especially significant in the development of attachment capacity (see Chapter 4).

Brain plasticity is the ability of the brain to adapt and change in response to experience. It appears to be at its greatest during early phases of development (Rueda *et al.* 2005) and may be associated with specific gene variations. The most promising of these is a variation of one of the genes which manages dopamine in the brain (DRD4 7-repeat allele), because this appears to make individuals more responsive to both positive and negative environmental influences (Belsky *et al.* 2009). There is a growing view that these two mechanisms make a powerful argument for seeking to recognise and intervene with difficulties at the earliest of ages, even if the difficulties are quite mild at that time (Dawson 2008).

Family functioning and dynamics

Although there is a major research focus upon genetic and biochemical mechanisms, and how they change function, their influence is dependent upon life experiences. The most significant of these for children is of course the environment in which they grow, and particularly the nature and quality of their family life. The general rules of positive family life can be easily stated with the four 'C's:

- Care and warmth;
- Consistency and predictability;
- Control and maintaining appropriate boundaries;
- Commitment.

For any chance of success, all four elements must be present in significant measure, but specific circumstances may require emphasis upon one strand for a period, e.g. a sick child tends to need more care, a wayward child more control. However although life's events may require these changes of emphasis it is important to remember that even at such times all the elements need to be tangibly present, and the balance between the four needs to be present in reasonable degree if problems are to be managed or prevented.

Louise was 15 years of age and was having difficulties in school. When challenged by her teachers over trivial matters she would become angry and storm from the classroom. Her parents said that she had behaved like this at home ever since being a toddler. They added that when these episodes occurred at home they either gave in to her wishes or tried to calm her down by offering treats or rewards. The parents adopted this placating style when Louise was 18 months of age, because it was then that she was diagnosed as having a major hormonal problem, and the doctors said it would be dangerous for her if she became upset. Over the years the parents had continued to believe that Louise's life would be in danger if she became too upset and so made every effort to avoid such situations ever arising.

Situations like these are not common. Too much control, which is not tempered by caring warmth, creates angry, and at times violent, children. Too little control, and the young person will live to the limit of that control, quickly exceeding it and usually only being pulled up by the limits which society imposes in the form of laws. Lack of parental commitment perhaps exerts the most detrimental effects for it removes the child's sense of being claimed, and there is clear evidence that harsh, inconsistent and unresponsive parenting can continue to exert a very negative influence into their adult life (Hoeve et al. 2009).

As discussed in Chapter 4, the younger the child the more significant the impact of any negative parenting might be, and in this regard the first three years of life are seen as critical. With early care being so important it is pertinent to ask what the impact of working parents and early child care arrangements might have upon the child. Frequent separations from the primary parent weaken the sense of attachment, but positive engagement with a persistent and predictable adult helps mitigate the effects of the separations, although there is some evidence that such arrangements continue to exert a negative effect upon the child's ultimate functioning (Bernal 2008).

However, we should not forget that family functioning is an interactive process. It is clear that difficult and challenging behaviour from a child increases a parent's sense of stress, which places a significant demand upon their ability to cope. Stressed parents are, in turn, more likely to respond to their children in ways that increase or reinforce problem behaviour (Plant and Sanders 2007), further exacerbating the problem. As discussed in Chapter 6, issues such as parental separation and divorce can also exert a very negative effect upon a child's current and future functioning.

Peer group influence

As all parents know, a child's friendships exert considerable influence upon their functioning as they become older. Healthy peer relationships are important to a child's development because they provide a context within which they learn social skills and develop coping mechanisms. Peer relationships also promote psychological well-being and a sense of positive self-esteem, and offer protection against negative comments by other peers. Positive peer relationships have also been shown to be associated with higher achievement and a cooperative rather than competitive style of functioning (Roseth *et al.* 2008).

However if the child is rejected or bullied by their peers, they are at risk of emotional and behavioural difficulties, both at the time and later in life. To reduce the sense of isolation, children who are bullied by peers will typically seek out others who are equally marginalised, which often puts them in a group of troubled and troublesome young people (Card and Hodges 2008).

Peer group influence is but one specific example of the impact which subculture can have upon the behaviour or emotional state of a child. A further example is the influence that specific school environments can exert upon children (Rutter *et al.* 1979). The school's ethos exerts an effect upon the pupils' behaviour – as well as the level of issues such as vandalism and graffiti – that is irrespective of the type of area from which the pupils are drawn.

Life experiences

As we have already seen, life experiences play a crucial role in shaping and developing a child's make-up and nature. Exposure to adverse, stressful events, such as marital conflict, maternal depression and financial stress, have all been linked to emotional and behavioural problems, as well as cognitive deficits (Masten and Obradović 2006). Similarly, physical illnesses or disorders can exert direct effects upon emotional well-being. For instance, it is well known that children with epilepsy experience a significantly greater level of emotional disturbance than children without this condition (Meltzer *et al.* 2000), and similar increases are also noted in conditions such as asthma (Mrazek *et al.* 1998).

Children have less well developed mechanisms of coping with adverse events and so depend quite heavily on the adults around them for support and help. Thus the history of the child's life often contains important clues about what influences have helped shape their present pattern of behaviour. The death of a parent, serious illness in brothers or sisters, being the victim of abuse or neglectful parenting – such themes are very powerful in prompting behavioural and emotional reactions. Sometimes the history is more a family myth than actual events – but if powerful enough it may still establish patterns of maladaptive behaviour.

John was 7 years of age and lived with his mother in a quiet part of town. He was seen in the neighbourhood as a helpful and pleasant boy, and school had only praise for his work there. John's mother presented to the adult mental health services because she was miserable. She explained that since her husband had left she had found it hard to manage her son's behaviour. John's father had been the main disciplinarian because she had never been able to control John's outbursts. She explained that as a teenager she had been expected to look after her older brother, who had also been called John. He had often been violent towards her and seemed to take particular delight in tormenting her. On the night of her son's birth her brother John had been killed while committing a robbery, and she was convinced that her son had taken on this malevolent spirit. The family's wish to have her child named after her dead brother compounded this belief.

The important theme here is not the veracity of John's mother's belief but rather the strength with which she believed it. Growing up with a parent who expects you to be difficult and violent towards her is very likely to encourage such behaviour to surface.

There are other events and issues which shape life experiences. For instance, there is clear evidence that poverty, especially in the early years of life, exerts a strong, and long-term, negative influence on a child's health and well-being (Cohen *et al*. 2010). The difficulties do not only stem from the curtailed life experiences which poverty brings, but also the extra stress which it places upon parents, and its resultant impact upon parenting practices.

Nevertheless, not all children are equally susceptible to adverse environmental influences. There has been significant research interest into why some children cope so well with adversity – the study of resilience. Black and Lobo (2008) described ten qualities of the family which were likely to promote resilience within the children. These were:

1 a positive outlook, confidence and optimism;
2 spirituality;
3 cohesion and family member accord;
4 flexibility;
5 successful family communication;
6 good financial management;
7 family time;
8 shared recreation;
9 routines and rituals;
10 support network.

A similar list of qualities could be drawn up for the individual child, and programmes which seek to develop, enhance, and strengthen such qualities in the vulnerable child and their family appear to be beneficial (Brownrigg *et al*. 2004).

Lifestyle issues

Issues such as diet and lifestyle can also play a significant part in the emergence and maintenance of emotional or behavioural difficulties. Children's leisure activities are changing, and with the increasing amount of time spent with television, computers and various other forms of electronic media there is a reduction in exercise and physical activities, as well as direct social interaction. These changes have been shown to have an association with psychological difficulties (Page et al. 2010). Perhaps more directly there is clear evidence that exposure to violent or inappropriate images can influence behaviour in a negative way whether that be from television or from video games (Anderson et al. 2010).

Developmental themes

In the first few years of life, the brain grows rapidly. As each neuron matures, it sends out multiple branches, each of which has thousands of connections to other neurons (synapses). At birth, each neuron in the cerebral cortex has approximately 2,500 synapses. By the time an infant is two or three years old, the number of synapses is approximately 15,000 synapses per neuron (Gopnic *et al.* 1999). This amount is about twice that of the average adult brain, and there is strong evidence that the quality of maternal care in the first month of life is associated with structural brain changes (Kim *et al.* 2010).

As the child grows, synaptic pruning eliminates weaker synaptic contacts while stronger connections are kept and strengthened. It is also clear that sophisticated brain circuits become 'stronger' through use (Shatz 1997). Thus, experience determines which connections will be strengthened and which will be pruned. Connections that have been activated most frequently are preserved. Ineffective or weak connections are 'pruned' in much the same way a gardener would prune a tree or bush, giving the plant the desired shape. It is this process that allows the brain to adapt itself to its environment. This process occurs at different times in different parts of the brain and reaches its peak in early adolescence, with sensory and perceptual regions of the brain experiencing these reductions early in life, while they occur later in areas of the brain involved in higher cognition (Huttenlocher 1984).

Thus children exposed to traumatic and abusive experiences may well have negative brain pathways stimulated as opposed to positive ones, leaving a troubling legacy when the pruning process begins (Passamonti *et al.* 2010).

This is not absolute, however, because the brain retains the capacity to change the organisation and properties of the brain's make-up in response to need – the capacity to show plasticity. Thus, neuronal changes can be moderated by positive life experiences, and favourable environmental experiences – especially those embedded within early caregiving relationships – have a positive impact on brain development (Schore 2001). It is however clear that the degree of recovery from abusive early childhood experiences is linked to the amount of exposure, and how early in life it occurred (Perry *et al.* 2002).

As the child moves through the developmental phases it becomes important for the adults around them to give clear guidance as to appropriate behaviour and positive rules around living. This provides the scaffolding upon which the child's personality and ultimately their unique identity will be built. The provision of such scaffolding is a key aspect of allowing the child to develop autonomy, and has also been found to have a positive impact upon other aspects of child cognitive development, such as language and problem-solving competence (Bernier *et al.* 2010).

These qualities are important to allow the child to learn how to manage their world, and the mechanisms used are grouped together under the heading of 'executive functioning'. It is a crucial control mechanism which regulates a wide range of the child's intellectual activities, for instance their proficiency in mathematics and reading ability. Executive functioning is developing from a very young age, and the quality of parenting helps to shape its nature and make-up, adding an additional dimension to the importance of appropriate parenting during the early years of life.

As well as these elements of influence it is important to remember that children are also developing organisms. This means that each child has to proceed through various stages of development, with each stage exerting influence upon their future life as an adult. There have been many suggestions as to how to conceptualise these processes, focusing on many different aspects of development, but in the context of this text the psychological/social sequence described by Erikson (1959) is perhaps the most helpful (Figure 1.1). This developmental process illustrates some of the elements that are most influential in a child's life. For example, in the

Trust v. Mistrust Birth to 1 year	Infants must learn to trust others. There must be minimal uncertainty, and with each demand satisfied the infant grows in trust. Maternal care fosters the child's sense of self-identity. Insufficient warmth and care and the infant views the world as a dangerous place and can become mistrustful of adults. The mother-figure is the primary agent.
Autonomy v. Shame and Doubt 1 to 3 years	The child's self-will emerges usually focused upon demanding to be able to control and order events. These strivings need to be matched by parental determination to maintain a clear sense of boundaries but combined with explicit care and security to safeguard the child's developing sense of self-esteem. Parental figures are paramount.
Initiative v. Guilt 3 to 6 years	Children at this age attempt to act grown up and project having some self-control. They seek to broaden their world and strive to achieve physical independence from their parents. They begin to notice sex and role differences, and explore them through play. The members of the family are key agents.
Industry v. Inferiority 6 to 12 years	Relates to parents and other adults on an equal basis. The child compares self to peers. Teachers and peers have the greatest influence.
Identity v. Confusion Adolescence	The teenager is seeking a path through the maze of life options to establish his or her own unique identity. Striving for emotional independence from parents. Key influences are peers, significant adults and society (but not parents).

Figure 1.1 Erikson's developmental process

Industry phase it is teachers and peers who exert the most influence. All parents will have experienced this when trying to help a child with homework, and the child becomes distressed because 'it is not the way my teacher said to do it'. The possibility that there may be other methods is not something the child can recognise easily at this age, but, more importantly, the way teachers demonstrated the task must be right because of their importance in the young person's world.

These stages should not be seen as gateways. The completion of the tasks in each stage is not a prerequisite to moving on to the next stage, but they do equip the child to cope with the next stage better and in a more robust fashion. This means that problems encountered during any stage do not prevent development, but they do make it more difficult for the child since important knowledge and skills may be lacking. For example, a child who has not fully developed social skills during the Industry phase will find negotiating the process of dating in adolescence especially difficult. Of course the earlier that difficulties occur the more profound the disruption might be, and as described in Chapter 4, one of the more significant areas of influence that can be disrupted by difficulties in infancy is that of attachment capacity.

A key factor, therefore, in trying to predict how a particular issue or event might be dealt with is to consider the child's age. After 18 months of age, infants begin to understand that they are independent entities separate from their parents. Self-regulation becomes increasingly important, but to achieve this the child has to learn frustration tolerance. Marked tantrums are common as this is developed, but if the relationship with parents has been solid and secure up to this point, then the infant feels free to express negative feelings directly, confident that the parents will be supportive through times of distress.

Play is important to young children because it is the medium they use to try to understand the world around them. This is because although young children can recognise that events have occurred, their sense of the world is not sufficiently developed for them to set the events in any context. By about two years of age toddlers' sense of self provides them with sufficient differentiation to begin to recreate experiences in play. It is interesting to note that children who have been abused at this young age find it difficult to develop all the skills of this stage, and so they engage in less symbolic play, find it difficult to play with peers, and are generally more aggressive (Alessandri 1991).

By 4 years of age the child can repress one view in preference to another and so there is the beginning of a recognition that there can be alternative origins for problems other than the child's own actions. Their play takes on a richer content as the roles of others in making things happen are gradually explored. By 6 years of age this ability is fully developed and the child is able to relate the cause of events to origins which the child recognises they can't influence. They also begin to evaluate their competence by comparing themselves with others, and with this comes the start of seeing peer approval as important, an influence which reaches its peak in adolescence. The areas of this influence tend, however, to be different for boys and girls; while boys seek approval for their actions, it is a girl's view of herself that is most strongly influenced by the views of others (Cole *et al.* 1997).

The significance of this developing awareness is that if traumatic events should occur early in a child's life it is likely they will believe themselves responsible. The help offered to children has therefore not only to take account of what the child may have experienced but at what age it has occurred, so that the correct emphasis can be given to the therapeutic help.

A structured assessment

When confronted with any type of problem, the first impulse may be one of bewilderment: where to start? It is nearly always best in such situations to recognise that there is no danger in silence. A quiet and reflective style will probably start the information flowing, and if all that is happening is weeping and distress then silent support is equally comforting. Although there is a need to know in order to be able to understand, the first response should be one of availability and support. From this basis the immediate issues can usually be clarified, and together these two themes give an excellent platform from which to begin to obtain the detail upon which decisions can be based.

The way forward

Armed with the detail of the situation it is then possible to formulate the next steps. There may be a clear recognition that more specialised help is needed, and the task then becomes one of helping the child, and the family, to see how important such assistance may be.

In most cases, however, the information is used to inform the process of assistance being offered by the concerned adult. For most situations, being clear and decisive can prove very beneficial. The young person feels less confused because an adult is bringing clarity, and if they are responsive to the help, they are likely to feel less frightened and alone. Not all young people want to be helped, and sadly there are a few who are set on a self-destructive path from which they will not be deviated. Knowing one's personal and professional limitations, while not underestimating innate skills, is the starting point for deciding what a particular individual's role should be. If the problem is one detailed in the following pages then the themes described will help to clarify how best to proceed.

Sources of further help

www.brightfutures.org/publications/index
www.rcpsych.ac.uk/mentalhealthinfoforall.aspx
www.aacap.org/cs/root/facts_for_families/facts_for_families
www.nimh.nih.gov/health/topics/child-and-adolescent-mental-health/index.shtml

References

Alessandri, S.M. (1991). Play and social behaviours in maltreated pre-schoolers. *Developmental Psychopathology* 3: 191–206.

Anderson, C.A., Shibuya, A., Ihori, N. *et al.* (2010). Violent video game effects on aggression, empathy, and prosocial behavior in Eastern and Western countries: A meta-analytic review. *Psychological Bulletin* 136: 151–73.

Belsky, J. and Pluess, M. (2009). The nature (and nurture?) of plasticity in early human development. *Perspectives on Psychological Science* 4: 345–51.

Belsky, J., Jonassaint, C., Pluess, M. *et al.* (2009). Vulnerability genes or plasticity genes? *Molecular Psychiatry* 14: 746–54.

Bernal, R. (2008). The effect of maternal employment and child care on children's cognitive development. *International Economic Review* 49: 1173–209.

Bernier, A., Carlson, S.M. and Whipple, N. (2010). From external regulation to self-regulation: Early parenting precursors of young children's executive functioning child development. *Child Development* 81: 326–39.

Bird, A. (2007). Perceptions of epigenetics. *Nature* 447: 396–8.

Bischof, H.J. (2007). Behavioral and neuronal aspects of developmental sensitive periods. *Neuroreport* 18: 461–5.

Black, K. and Lobo, M. (2008). A conceptual review of family resilience factors. *Journal of Family Nursing* 14: 33–55.

Bowlby, J. (1969) *Attachment and Loss.* London: Basic Books.

Brownrigg, A, Soulsby, A. and Place, M. (2004). Helping vulnerable children to become more resilient. *International Journal of Child and Family Welfare* 7: 14–25.

Card, N.A. and Hodges, E.V.E. (2008). Peer victimization among schoolchildren: Correlations, causes, consequences, and considerations in assessment and intervention. *School Psychology Quarterly* 23: 451–61.

Cohen, S., Janicki-Deverts, D., Chen, E. *et al.* (2010) Childhood socioeconomic status and adult health. *Annals of the New York Academy of Sciences* 1186: 37–55.

Cole, D.A., Martin, J.M. and Powers, B. (1997). A competency-based model of child depression: A longitudinal study of peer, parent, teacher, and self–evaluations. *Journal of Child Psychology and Psychiatry* 38: 505–14.

Dawson, G. (2008). Early behavioral intervention, brain plasticity, and the prevention of autism spectrum disorder. *Development and Psychopathology*, 20: 775–803.

Erikson, E. (1959). *Identity and the Life Cycle.* New York: International University Press.

Gopnik, A., Meltzoff, A.N. and Kuhl, P.K. (1999). *The Scientist in the Crib: Minds, Brains and How Children Learn.* New York: HarperCollins.

Hamilton, A., Voinnet, O., Chappell, L. *et al.* (2002). Two classes of short interfering RNA in RNA silencing. *The EMBO Journal* 21: 4671–9.

Hoeve, M., Dubas, J.S., Eichelsheim, V.I. *et al.* (2009) The relationship between parenting and delinquency: A meta-analysis. *Journal of Abnormal Child Psychology* 37: 749–75.

Huttenlocher, P.R. (1984). Synapse elimination and plasticity in developing human cerebral cortex. *American Journal of Mental Deficiency* 88: 488–96.

Jaenisch, R. and Bird, A. (2003). Epigenetic regulation of gene expression: How the genome integrates intrinsic and environmental signals. *Nature Genetics* 33: 245–54.

Jenuwein, T. and Allis, C.D. (2001). Translating the histone code. *Science* 293: 1074–80.

Reynolds, E. (2006). Vitamin B12, folic acid, and the nervous system. *Lancet Neurology* 5: 949–60.

Kim, P., Leckman, J.F., Mayes, L.C. *et al.* (2010) Perceived quality of maternal care in childhood and structure and function of mothers' brain. *Developmental Science* 13: 662–73.

Masten, A.S. and Obradović, J. (2006). Competence and resilience in development. *Annals of the New York Academy of Sciences* 1094: 13–27.

Meaney, M.J. (2010). Epigenetics and the biological definition of gene–environment interactions. *Child Development* 81: 41–79.

Meltzer, H., Gatward, R., Goodman, R. *et al.* (2000). *Mental Health of Children and Adolescents in Great Britain.* London: Stationery Office.

Mrazek, D.A., Schuman, W. and Klinnert, M. (1998). Early asthma onset: Risk of emotional and behavioural difficulties. *Journal of Child Psychology and Psychiatry* 39: 247–54.

Obradović, J., Bush, N.R., Stamperdahl, J. *et al.* (2010). Biological sensitivity to context: The interactive effects of stress reactivity and family adversity on socio-emotional behavior and school readiness. *Child Development* 81: 270–89.

Page, A.S., Cooper, A.R., Griew, P. *et al.* (2010). Children's screen viewing is related to psychological difficulties irrespective of physical activity. *Pediatrics* 126: 1011–17.

Passamonti, L., Fairchild, G., Goodyer, I.M. *et al.* (2010). Neural abnormalities in early-onset and adolescence-onset conduct disorder. *Archives of General Psychiatry* 67: 729–38.

Perry, B.D. (2002) Childhood experience and the expression of genetic potential: What childhood neglect tells us about nature and nurture. *Brain and Mind* 3: 79–100.

Plant, K.M. and Sanders, M.R. (2007) Predictors of care-giver stress in families of preschool-aged children with developmental disabilities. *Journal of Intellectual Disabilities* 51: 109–24.

Roseth, C.J., Johnson, D.W. and Johnson, R.T. (2008). Promoting early adolescents' achievement and peer relationships: The effects of cooperative, competitive, and individualistic goal structures. *Psychological Bulletin* 134: 223–46.

Rueda, M.R., Rothbart, M.K., McCandliss, B.D. *et al.* (2005). Training, maturation, and genetic influences on the development of executive attention. *Proceedings of the National Academy of Sciences of the United States of America* 102: 14931–6.

Rutter, M., Maughan, B., Mortimore, P. *et al.* (1979). *Fifteen Thousand Hours: Secondary Schools and their Effects on Children.* London: Open Books.

Schore, A.N. (2001). Effects of a secure attachment relationship on right brain development, affect regulation, and infant mental health. *Infant Mental Health Journal* 22: 7–66.

Shatz, C.J. (1997) Neurotrophins and visual system plasticity. In M. Cowan, T.M. Jessell and L. Zipursky (eds) *Molecular and Cellular Approaches to Neural Development.* New York: Oxford University Press.

Steiner, M., LePage, P. and Dunn, E.J. (1997). Serotonin and gender specific psychiatric disorders. *International Journal of Psychiatric Clinical Practice* 1: 3–13.

Tsankova, N., Renthal, W., Kumar, A. *et al.* (2007). Epigenetic regulation in psychiatric disorders. *Nature Review of Neuroscience* 8: 355–67.

Waterland, R.A., Dolinoy, D.C., Lin, J.R., *et al.* (2006). Maternal methyl supplements increase offspring DNA methylation at Axin Fused. *Genesis* 44: 401–6.

Wiesel, T.N. and Hubel, D.H. (1965). Extent of recovery from the effects of visual deprivation in kittens. *Journal of Neurophysiology* 28: 1060–72.

Chapter 2

The basics of being helpful

Introduction

Perhaps the most important distinction between the child and the adult client is that children with difficulties rarely seek help themselves. Rather, they are typically referred for help by concerned others, usually the child's family or teachers. It should not be assumed that because the child is deeply unhappy about his or her circumstances and strongly desires change to take place that professional intervention will be welcomed or accepted. Many forms of therapy, particularly the psycho-therapies, are based upon an assumption that the client is a willing participant who actively wishes to change. The reality is that many children come unwillingly to the therapist and respond only because they have been brought. Furthermore, successful work with children is likely to involve direct support and intervention from others, such as parents, teachers, social workers and peers.

This chapter cannot provide an exhaustive account of the many differing forms of therapy. Where this is required the reader is advised to examine the specialised texts referred to in each section.

The talking therapies

Talking with others, outlining the difficulties we are experiencing and receiving advice on how to remedy a difficult situation is a natural, effective and everyday way of tackling problems. The old adage, 'a problem shared is a problem halved' reflects the fact that merely by unburdening ourselves to others our difficulties may often appear less arduous, our sense of confusion and powerlessness less overwhelming. In a world where communication is often brief or misunderstood, where there often appears to be insufficient time for one another, the availability of another person who, in a non-judgemental fashion, will try to understand your problems, concerns and frustrations, who will provide a sounding board for your own, often confused understandings, and who may suggest ways forward is often rare.

Despite the effectiveness of a problem-solving discussion between a child and a concerned adult in everyday situations, the types of problem outlined in this book are unlikely to be resolved solely by such means. The problems of the highly anxious, depressed, aggressive or defiant child are likely to require a more specific and therapeutically focused approach.

A term increasingly used to describe supportive forms of talking is counselling. The use of this as a description of the process of discussing problems has now become so widespread as to render the term virtually meaningless; parents counsel their children, teachers their students, police counsel potential lawbreakers, financial brokers their clients. With regard to children, counselling is frequently used to describe the process of listening to problems, advising on action and explaining the constraints within which the child should operate. Indeed, counselling is misguidedly used as a euphemism for controlling behaviour – the headteacher who asked one of the present authors to 'severely counsel' a wayward 5-year-old was by no means exceptional. As is shown in Chapter 8, counselling is often misunderstood and misused.

Such a criticism, however, does not imply that counselling, undertaken appropriately and skilfully, is of little therapeutic value. Indeed, the basic elements of counselling and psychotherapy have shown a tendency to converge over the years, with much cross-fertilisation of approach and technique resulting. Counselling uses a variety of techniques to help people, but often involves assistance to help them express emotion over painful events (Lindemann 1944), communicate their feelings more accurately, and develop problem-solving behaviour. The core technique demands engagement with the client, showing empathy and displaying concern, interactions which help to increase the client's self-esteem (Rogers 1951, 1961). In contrast to the psychotherapies, there is, perhaps, less reliance on a theory of development to which themes are referenced, and this makes it very suitable, for instance, as a way of helping people come to terms with traumatic events that are still troubling them (see Chapter 6). In recent years there has also been a rapid growth of pre-emptive counselling: offering assistance to people in the immediate aftermath of an incident. This approach assumes that early intervention, and the rapid ventilation of feelings in a controlled way will prevent problems later. Although this has some theoretical attraction, the results of such processes suggest that this is not totally successful (Roberts et al. 2010).

The psychotherapies have tended to emerge as a way of applying a theoretical model about individual or family functioning. While these theoretical models vary greatly, they have several elements in common. At the heart of this commonality is the establishment of a therapeutic relationship. The sense of regard and concern shown by the therapist for the client is a foundation point from which other elements can emerge, and as can be seen with motivational interviewing, this in itself may be an agent of change. A second key theme common to most psychotherapies is facilitating the emergence of emotional arousal. The linking of emotions with recalled events or memories provides the basic material from which therapy proceeds because being able to tolerate such emotions and then recognising their associations is a key element of working through the areas of difficulty.

At the heart of each psychotherapy model, however, is the aim of giving the person insight into their problems, and their origins, on the assumption that from such self-knowledge they will begin to change and the difficulties will be eased.

This is perhaps seen at its clearest when dealing with someone who has experienced a traumatic early life and now has difficulties that the therapist believes are occurring as a consequence of those experiences. By helping the person see these links their growing understanding modifies their sense of inevitability and helps them to find new ways of behaving.

The specific theoretical model gives the therapist a framework in which to understand the client's difficulties, and guides the therapeutic responses towards the model's goal. For example, in psychoanalytical psychotherapy (Freud 1976) the model is based around psychosexual development, and the way that basic drives (id) and the higher morality of conscience (superego) interacted with each other to influence behaviour. Such theories offer the child a context within which the issues and difficulties can be understood because there is a framework from which to analyse beliefs, feelings and reactions. These theoretical frameworks also have common elements: for example, the offering of a predictable space and time dedicated to exploring the themes. Within each session information is gathered which helps the therapist to refine the understanding of the specific difficulties, and these hypotheses are tested by subsequent information. Therapists will then use their specific understanding and the theoretical base to reflect upon the origins of specific behaviours, feelings or beliefs. Most of these therapies also depend upon using the emotion generated within sessions to inform the process. So, for instance, a passage in which the client becomes upset may be specifically noted – because people sometimes experience emotions but have no name for them or, more commonly, may display emotions without realising they are doing so. 'I notice you become angry whenever you mention your father' could be the starting point for a young person to realise such a link. On other occasions the therapist may use an emotion that arises within themselves to highlight the unspoken emotions and feelings of the client. This is described as transference and can arise in many situations. For example, when a mother's death is spoken of by a child, it is possible that the therapist also feels a personal sense of sadness. Commenting on such feelings is seen in some therapeutic styles (particularly psychoanalytical psychotherapy) as a key element of the process. It is also important to recognise that within such therapies silence is equally important as a form of emotional communication (Lane et al. 2002).

Although there is evidence that psychoanalytical psychotherapy is an effective treatment (Kennedy and Midgley 2007), most psychotherapy offered today is less frequent and far less lengthy than that offered by Freud and his followers. Known as short-term dynamic (Davanloo 1980) or brief dynamic psychotherapy (Malan 1963) this work uses similar principles to the longer-term analyses, but there is a greater emphasis upon specific issues, and indeed most brief dynamic therapies depend upon finding a focus from which themes can be explored. Although in such approaches it is still seen as important to make the client aware of unconscious fantasies, the most fundamental therapeutic lever is seen as helping the client to re-work relationship patterns that have been damaging. This is achieved through the relationship they develop with the therapist, a process that has been described as the 'corrective emotional experience' (Alexander and French 1946). Because of this emphasis, transference is perhaps of even greater importance in these types of approach, as is the need to establish a good therapeutic relationship quickly.

The effectiveness of psychotherapy has been examined in over 250 studies. The results from these indicate that about 79% of children will show some benefit from psychotherapy (Weisz *et al.* 1987), although on average children show only a small improvement in their functioning (Weiss and Jensen 2001). Work with adults suggests that no one type of psychotherapy is more effective than another (Andrews 1993), although techniques which focus upon observable behaviour may be particularly valuable for work with children (Kazdin 1990).

Play therapy

Play is the medium by which a child gains an understanding of the world. When confronted by difficult or poorly understood situations the child's natural reaction is to incorporate these into play, and by regular repetition there emerges an explanation and understanding which the child can adopt. The accuracy of this explanation is, however, dependent on many factors, not least of which is the child's limited understanding of the world and its complexities. It is not surprising then that play should be seen as the obvious medium by which to work therapeutically with a young child. The therapeutic approaches are broadly similar to the talking therapies, but the emphasis is shifted to using play as the medium of communication. It can operate on several levels. The play can be used as a method of communicating inner world feelings and so becomes the exact equivalent of the psychotherapy used in adults. Such work is again rooted in a theoretical model of child development, the most well-known being those described by Anna Freud (1966) and Melanie Klein (Segal 1964).

The client-centred non-directive approach described by Rogers (1951, 1961) also has its equivalent in play therapy. The leading exponent of this type of approach is Virginia Axline (1947), whose description of play therapy is the foundation for many therapists' practice. She outlined eight rules:

1   Quickly develop a warm, and friendly relationship.
2   Accept the children as they present themselves, not as they should be.
3   The relationship should be permissive, allowing children to express their feelings freely.
4   Recognise and reflect feelings so that the child gains insight.
5   The responsibility for making changes is the child's.
6   The child's wishes give direction.
7   Sessions are at the child's pace.
8   The only limitations are those of safety and responsibility within the therapeutic relationship.

Allan was referred at 8 years of age because of the aggressive and hostile behaviour he was showing both at home and school. He had been adopted by his present family when he was 5 years of age, his life with his birth family having been one characterised by violence and neglect from early infancy. Allan had no explanation for his behaviour other than to say that he became angry when people 'bugged' him.

A regular sequence of play sessions was established which quickly became dominated by themes of tragedy (people being killed or seriously injured; rescue attempts being sabotaged). Gradually the therapist became a participant in the play and verbalised that it seemed that there was no way to help the characters of the games. Some three months into the work an additional theme began to emerge from the play. When the models and toys had been injured or hurt they would seek revenge, and would let nothing stand in the way of it being achieved.

Later, these elements faded somewhat and there were several sessions which focused upon being small and helpless in large, complex and confusing worlds. When the therapist reflected on how small and vulnerable that must feel the tempo of the play increased, as did its chaotic quality. Almost immediately after commencing the sessions Allan's aggressive behaviour at school faded, but became more evident at home. Seven months after commencing therapy his behaviour at home began to moderate, but when therapy stopped after a year he was still seen by the family as more difficult than his siblings.

This description illustrates how play can be used by a child to portray his or her inner world. It also shows how recognising the link between apparently distinct play activities is often the key to understanding this portrayal. This example also illustrates a key factor that must be considered when deciding if therapy is appropriate. Effective therapy reduces the defences which the child is using to cope with the world, and this can be a very frightening experience. As a result, in the early stages of therapy there is often a deterioration rather than an improvement. Similarly, if the child is not in an environment in which he or she feels safe and secure the ability to take risks in therapy evaporates and little meaningful work is achieved. With the potential for so much emotion to arise within the sessions, and the possibility that the child does not feel secure enough to share, it is crucial that the pace of any work done within the sessions is set by the child.

As well as being a medium through which psychotherapy is pursued, play therapy can also be used more directly. As the child works through a difficulty or a painful experience, the play is usually transparent enough for an acute observer to see the underlying themes. This can be used as a basis for exploring such issues in more detail, and can also be used to offer alternative views and explanations. As with all psychotherapies, the sharing of emotions becomes an important element of healing, although within a play context it is easy to transfer such feelings on to other elements of the activity – for example, 'the doll is naughty and must be smacked'.

Brief (solution-focused) therapy

As is discussed below, it is a fundamental tenet in the management of all animal behaviour that more is achieved by reward than by punishment. It is, however, only very recently that this has seen its expression in a dynamic (i.e. interpersonal) therapy. Brief solution-focused therapy is an approach which can be seen as using this position as a starting point, underpinned by the assumption that successful work depends upon knowing where the client wants to get to. From this flows the principles that understanding the problem is not necessary, and indeed focusing on the problem more than is needed for the client to feel heard is probably counter-productive. The philosophy here is that successful work depends upon taking the positive path, which means determining what the client is trying to achieve, working out the quickest way of achieving this goal, and detailing what they are already doing that might start them on this path (de Shazer 1991). This philosophy has become summarised in three rules:

1 If it ain't broke, don't fix it.
2 Once you know what works, do more of it.
3 If it doesn't work, then do something else.

Work usually, therefore, begins by identifying 'exceptions to the rule' of the problem, in other words identifying what is already working, even if this is only in very small pockets. The drive towards emphasising the positive means that even small acknowledgements that things are moving in a positive direction can be the start of a cascade of change which gathers momentum, carrying the client towards their desired goals.

There are several aspects to this type of approach which harness these basic themes. For example, a question like 'If a miracle has occurred and the problem has been solved what will be the first thing you notice?' (usually described as 'the miracle question') may begin the process of clarifying the desired goals, and identifying the first steps that need to be taken to achieve them. These are then built upon by asking what might be the first small step they need to take to progress towards their goal. As with any therapy, the client will frequently doubt the progress made and, in so doing, will often highlight times when things have not gone as expected. However, these exceptions can also feed the therapeutic process, because subsequent questions can continue to emphasise the positive – 'Tell me about times it doesn't happen' or, if the statement is that it never stops, then the question might be, 'When does it happen least?' It is also important to realise that any pattern of improvement will consist of both forward and backward steps. When such situations occur the therapist can help the client to identify what resources, skills and techniques have been used to prevent slipping too far backwards, and through this recognition, additional strengths are acknowledged.

The content of a therapeutic session in this therapeutic approach is flexible, the goal for each often being established by simple questions such as, 'How will you know at the end of the session that it was useful to come today?' The general aim of every session, however, is always to follow the basic behavioural principle of emphasising the positive, and to identify with the client those exceptions when the problem was stopped or did not occur. Techniques such as rating the occurrence and intensity of good spells can be used to demonstrate progress, but these can also be valuable in identifying the next step towards the full solution. The framing of the questions around such elements adds to the overall emphasis upon the positive. For example, examining the most recent scores on the rating scale could prompt the question 'What will be happening when you are just one point higher on the scale?', a question which contains an implicit assumption that the next point will be achieved.

There is evidence that such an approach, albeit brief, is effective (Lethem 2002), with outcome evaluations showing that, for instance, 60% of cases report improvement (Macdonald 1997), and on average this is achieved by a three-session intervention (Berg and de Jong 1996). It is sometimes used within a family context, and here again the results are positive (Kim 2008). However, for children with behavioural problems this may not be an appropriate form of intervention, because although the child may appear to engage with the treatment programme there is no evidence that it leads to improved behaviour (Corcoran 2006).

Group therapy

Dynamic group therapy is useful for broadly the same type of person as the individual approach. It adds the extra dimension of sharing difficulties with others and tends to reduce the sense of isolation, and thoughts that 'I'm the only one'. However, it does require the group members to be able to tolerate the frustrations which arise in sharing relationships, although for some this can have a therapeutic benefit in its own right. In addition to this tolerance, the group process usually seeks to encourage group members to give feedback to others, which includes expressing their own feelings about what someone says or does (Yalom 1995). Such interaction among group members gives each person an opportunity to try out new ways of behaving and provides members with an opportunity to learn more about the way they interact with others. They may sometimes recreate the difficulties that brought them to group therapy in the first place. This is valuable as one of the main goals of process is always to gently confront the person with an unconscious difficulty so it can be resolved.

These elements tend to result in groups being run for children, or parents, who have a shared experience or difficulty. In child abuse, for instance, this type of intervention is commonly used because the sense of personal isolation is reduced. In addition, if the group is working well there can be a tremendous sense of support which allows participants to share far more than they might have done in other circumstances. For instance, group therapy has been found to be helpful in preventing the recurrence of self-harming behaviour in adolescents who have deliberately harmed themselves, but it has proved difficult to show specific value in other settings (Hazell et al. 2009), though this may be because the full benefits may emerge well after the work is complete (Kolvin et al. 1988).

Family therapy

Children grow up not in isolation but with myriad influences operating upon them. These influences shape, alter and colour the child's evolving feelings and beliefs so that each adult becomes a unique individual, made up of the way that these developmental experiences interact with the person's genetic make-up and life events. Recognising the importance of these influences opens a major branch of potential intervention, for if these influences can be changed in a helpful way, a lasting impact upon the adult that is to come may be achieved. In the 1960s many centres began to explore the potential for bringing about such change, and the main focus of this work was the family, for as Erikson has pointed out (see Chapter 4) it is the family which exerts the most powerful influence in the formative years.

Some therapy styles seek to detail the family's belief system, and acknowledging with them its content can help the family to explore new ways of relating (Byng-Hall 1995). This may involve working with the family in the construction of their family tree (known as a genogram), not only to record linkage, but more especially to recognise family traits and similarities (Lieberman 1979).

In its early development, there were two broad schools of theory applied to this work. Structural therapy recognises that certain family patterns and make-ups are more helpful than others and seeks to set tasks and goals that move families towards these patterns. For instance, a child may be acting as a parent, with the new step-parent marginalised and prevented from taking any role within the family. The stepfather's complaint that the child will not go to sleep except in the parental bed has to be seen in this context. Helping the parents develop an equal relationship, to which the children are subordinate, and recognising that there is a boundary around the adults which children have to respect become key in resolving such problems (Mann *et al.* 1990). It is, of course, not always possible to help families achieve such change, but any movement along the path may be deemed to be helpful.

For some time, the most common style of family therapy has been that based upon systems theory (Carr 2009). The approach is less rooted in family history, concentrating instead upon day-to-day interactions and the impact each family member has upon the others. These interactions have often become established over time. When presented with specific situations each member of the family can be expected to respond in a specific way. This reaction in turn prompts other family members to behave in predictable ways. This creates a pattern of predictable behaviours within the family, which gives a sense of balance in the family system, albeit dysfunctional. For example, Paul's parents are arguing and he fears that, like some of his friends at school, they are going to separate. Paul begins to refuse to attend school to try to stop the arguments, and finds that the parents put their differences aside to try to get him to school. As long as Paul has difficulties attending school his parents appear more settled. This creates a sense of equilibrium for the family, but Paul is not attending school. If the significance of the wider family issues is not identified and dealt with, then Paul will not be able to return to school. In this type of approach it is assumed that the symptoms that are presented are in fact an unsatisfactory solution to the family's difficulties, and that by making the present symptoms even less successful at reducing the underlying difficulties a new pattern of family functioning will emerge.

In recent years the use of narrative, an approach which focuses upon understanding the central themes in a family's life story, has emerged as a powerful style of family therapy (Epston and White 1990). This therapy seeks to understand the way people view themselves, their family, and the world in which they live. The family members are regarded as the experts on their story, and the therapist is regarded as someone who can comment and observe, but has no special knowledge that makes their view correct (Legg and Stagaki 2002). The therapy starts by listening to and acknowledging the family's stories. The therapist must listen with no preconceptions, and there is great effort made not to 'take sides' or offer any judgement about individual family member actions. This allows the family members to explore their own personal experiences and explanations, and by listening to each other a gradual shift in perceptions can occur.

Research into family therapy has shown that such work, no matter what its style, can bring about major changes in a child's environment and presenting problems (Cottrell and Boston 2002; Carr 2009). What is also becoming clear is that whatever the style of therapy, establishing trust and a positive rapport with the family is the starting point for an effective intervention (Hogue *et al.* 2006) though adhering to the chosen therapeutic model ensures gains are maximised (Sexton and Turner 2010).

Brief solution-focused family therapy

As was described above, there has been increasing interest in using this type of therapy, and this enthusiasm has also been evident within family therapy work. This is not surprising since the therapy was largely developed from a systemic perspective (de Shazer et al. 1986), the techniques are easily transferred into the family context, and the approach is proving to be equally effective when used with families (Kim 2008). As its name implies, the task of the therapist within sessions is continually to guide the conversation in the session towards solution talk. To do this the therapist fits in with the family process while highlighting exceptions to the rule that 'the problem is always there', the potential solutions they have already found, and the individual or family strengths which they themselves identify.

Sarah was 12 years of age when she was brought by her mother and grandmother because of their concern about the difficult behaviour she was displaying. Problems had begun after her grandfather's death a year ago. Since that time she had been stealing, lying and avoiding school at every opportunity. Both mother and grandmother clearly found Sarah's behaviour very annoying, and although they had identified the onset as coinciding with Sarah's grandfather's death, they found it difficult to understand why she was behaving like this.

The 'miracle question' was used to clarify that Sarah wanted to feel as she had before her grandfather's death, and that the adults wished she would behave as she did then. With this goal in mind, questions were asked which focused upon what they would notice about themselves after they had reached this goal, and by using scaling questions they clarified for themselves how close they were to achieving it. The first session showed they had already moved three points from the low ebb they had been at immediately after Sarah's grandfather died, recognising how this had been achieved and identifying strengths and resources which the family possessed and which they could use to move further forward.

Over the next three sessions each small positive change was highlighted and emphasised. When talk about problems began, exceptions were sought and so the focus was persistently kept upon encouraging solution talk. The homework at the end of each session was to record when each family member saw signs that her goal was being achieved. As this task highlighted the genuine affection which they had for each other, the irritation of the adults towards Sarah dissipated and the problem behaviour stopped. The last session was dominated by descriptions of how much they were now enjoying their time together, and how helpful Sarah had become once more.

Motivational interviewing

A very consistent finding throughout all of the therapeutic approaches is the degree to which emotional connection and engagement that occurs with the therapist is a marker of positive therapeutic outcome. Focusing on this element in its own right proved more significant in bringing about improvement with problem drinkers than a behavioural therapy programme (Miller and Baca 1983) and over time this has evolved into motivational interviewing (Miller 1983). This approach has many similarities to that advocated by Rogers (1951) because it seeks to use empathy to encourage the client to identify helpful changes, while the therapist avoids any elements of challenge or confrontation. Its main use has remained in substance misuse areas, where it has often proven to be a helpful way forward (Macgowan and Engle 2010).

Behavioural approaches and therapies

In contrast with the talking therapies, behavioural therapies place less emphasis upon helping the client to achieve insight into why he or she is exhibiting problem behaviour. Rather than dwelling upon the past or considering hypothetical underlying causes of problems, behaviourists are primarily concerned with observable, measurable behaviour in the here and now. In most cases the goal of therapy is to assist the client to change specific problem behaviour in ways which are predetermined.

Behavioural techniques have their origins in experimental studies of animal learning where it was found that behaviour could be systematically changed (conditioned) by modifying its consequences (reinforcement). Behavioural therapies are based upon the principle that all behaviour (adaptive and maladaptive) is learned and can thus be unlearned or replaced by alternative behaviours. Therapy consists of altering the client's environment in such a way that desirable behaviour replaces that which was giving rise to problems.

Behaviour therapies draw upon two major types of learning: classical and operant conditioning. Classical conditioning refers to the process by which a naturally occurring, largely involuntary, behaviour becomes linked with a neutral object or event (a stimulus) in such a way that the two become associated. As a result, the presence of the stimulus results in the behaviour's occurrence. This phenomenon was identified by the Russian psychologist, Pavlov, in studies with animals, and was subsequently applied to human behaviour. In a highly influential study, Watson and Rayner (1920) demonstrated the effectiveness of classical conditioning with an eleven-month-old child, Albert. When initially presented with a white rat, Albert showed no fear; when, subsequently, the rat's presentation was accompanied by a sudden, very loud noise, Albert became highly anxious and fearful. After several presentations of the rat and the noise together, the child became intensely fearful of the rat alone. In essence a previously neutral object, the rat had become the source of a conditioned fear response.

Drawing upon these early studies of classical conditioning, many sophisticated techniques for treating problem behaviours have been developed. Perhaps the simplest example is the bell and pad treatment for nocturnal enuresis (bedwetting). When the sleeping child begins to urinate a bell awakens the child and further urination is inhibited. This process is repeated nightly and, over time, the child associates the sensations from the bladder as it fills with the exercise of sphincter control. Eventually the bladder's contents are contained all night without waking.

As Albert's case might suggest, classical conditioning underpins many treatments for phobias and other forms of emotional disorder. Techniques such as systematic desensitisation and emotive imagery, for example, through the process of association, involve the gradual substitution of a pleasant, relaxed state for the unpleasant anxiety or fearfulness previously experienced.

Operant conditioning, based upon the pioneering work of B.F. Skinner, is a rather different behavioural technique which emphasises the importance of consequences in maintaining and shaping an individual's behaviour. Where a behaviour is followed by a positive consequence, it is more likely to recur (i.e. it can be said to have been reinforced). Where behaviour is not reinforced, it is less likely to be repeated.

Reinforcement is a key conceptual tool for analysing why people behave as they do and is of particular value for understanding and treating problem behaviour. Frequently, one finds that undesirable behaviour is reinforced in ways that are not always obvious.

Samantha, aged 4, was a member of a class of children who were listening to the teacher read from a giant-sized book full of colourful illustrations. She was bored, restless and kept fidgeting. This was beginning to disturb the other children. As a means of deflecting her behaviour, Samantha's teacher asked her to come to the front of the class and help her hold up the book for the other children to see.

While the reactions of the teacher are likely to have resolved the immediate problem caused by Samantha's disruptiveness, a behavioural analysis would suggest that, in the long term, her reaction may have made things worse. The child's undesirable behaviour was rewarded by attention and the allocation of a 'high-status job'. If such situations were repeated, Samantha would be likely to associate 'being a nuisance' with desirable outcomes and, as a consequence, the undesirable behaviour would be 'reinforced', that is, it would become stronger and be exhibited more frequently (see Chapter 8 for further case studies).

In contrast, there are many situations where desirable behaviours are not reinforced as frequently or as strongly as they should be. For some adults, because children are expected to behave appropriately, they are rarely rewarded by thanks, praise or more tangible rewards when exhibiting desired behaviour. Over time, the child finds that 'good' behaviour goes unrewarded while 'bad' behaviour often gains adult attention and can alleviate boredom.

It is exceedingly rare for any human behaviour to be reinforced each time it is exhibited and the term 'intermittent reinforcement' describes situations where behaviour is reinforced in an unpredictable fashion. In such situations one can never be certain when rewards will follow behaviour. When reinforcement is stopped completely, the individual will tend to persist in the undesired behaviour for a much greater period of time than in other situations where behaviour had consistently been reinforced. The principle of intermittent reinforcement helps to explain the immense hold which fruit machines exert over people, for the customer always hopes that reinforcement will take place next time!

Allan, aged 9, was allowed one chocolate biscuit a day by his mother, although he continually pestered for more. His mother would usually refuse his requests for a second biscuit and, invariably, this would result in scenes where the boy would become highly demanding, either by pleading and coaxing or by becoming verbally aggressive.

On some occasions, his mother's resolve was strong and, however poor Allan's behaviour, her determination to 'stick to her guns' meant that he could not get his own way. On other days, however, her son's temper tantrums and pleading often became too much for her and on such occasions she would give in 'for a quiet life'.

The above case study represents a classic illustration of intermittent reinforcement. Because Allan can never be certain whether prolonging his undesirable behaviour will eventually result in the achievement of his desires, he is likely to persevere with demanding behaviour even when it is not being reinforced. The expectation that his goal will eventually be met is often so strong that parental resolve to resist is unlikely to modify the child's behaviour in the short term. Given such a scenario, it is hardly surprising that parents who decide to 'stand up to their child' often come to believe that their new stance is not working and are tempted to give up. Where this happens, the pattern of intermittent reinforcement is continued and future attempts to take charge are likely to be met by even greater resistance.

In work with challenging children, the selection and effective use of reinforcement to shape behaviour is often more difficult than it might first appear. Children vary greatly in what is reinforcing for them; for example, some may respond to stars and stickers, others may see these as childish and prefer more tangible rewards. While many parents perceive yelling and scolding to be a form of punishment, for some children, receiving parental attention – in whatever form – is highly reinforcing.

It is also often difficult to control reinforcement. The range of possible reinforcers is usually limited and these may be insufficient to counter the perceived rewards which are associated with the problem behaviour. The child may find peer admiration when disrupting a class, the excitement and emotional rush from stealing a car, or the satisfaction obtained from baiting a family member to be far more attractive outcomes than any rewards which parents or teachers might be able to offer.

There are many behavioural techniques which are employed as parts of treatment programmes. Some of the most common forms of therapy are listed in Figure 2.1. Behaviour therapies have been shown to be among the most effective types of child therapy (Kazdin 1990), often being delivered as part of parenting programmes (Thomas et al. 2007). They have been the cornerstones of treatment for phobias and anxieties, though pure behavioural programmes have now largely given way to ones that contain cognitive elements.

Cognitive therapy

Cognitive therapy uses techniques from several sources to pursue its aim of helping people change the way they think about their problems, and their general functioning. As described in the context of treating depression (see Chapter 10), the basic principle upon which cognitive therapy is based is that moods and feelings are directly influenced by thoughts and ways of thinking – known as cognitions. These cognitions include the inner dialogue we use to understand events, and the template by which we always judge certain events. So, for example, a summons to the boss's office may always prompt the spontaneous thought 'What have I done wrong?' even though there is nothing to suggest that this is the reason for the request. Using such 'spontaneous' explanations is not usually a cause of problems, but if they become routinely negative and make the person permanently anxious, angry or depressed, they become a source of major difficulty. Cognitive therapy seeks to change such explanations, and so produce a more accurate, and hopefully healthier, view of the world for the individual to live by.

Positive reinforcement (e.g. praise, pocket money) Follows the occurrence of a desired response (e.g. making one's bed). Such behaviour should occur more frequently in future. A process where positive reinforcement is used to change behaviour over a number of gradual stages is known as shaping.

Negative reinforcement An undesirable situation (e.g. being kept in at playtime) is removed upon the occurrence of a desired response (e.g. classwork is completed). Such behaviour should occur more frequently in future.

Punishment An unpleasant situation (e.g. detention) follows the occurrence of an undesired response (e.g. failure to complete classwork). Such behaviour should occur less frequently in future.

Extinction Undesirable behaviour is not reinforced and, as a result, gradually disappears (e.g. the child exhibiting a tantrum is completely ignored until he or she exhibits acceptable behaviour).

Token economy Symbolic rewards (e.g. points, stars, tokens) are given in response to desirable behaviour. These can subsequently be exchanged for material items, such as money and sweets, or privileges, such as staying up to watch TV. In some programmes undesirable behaviour may result in a 'fine' where rewards are removed (sometimes known as 'response cost').

Contingency contracting An explicit agreement is drawn up between two or more parties which sets out desired and undesired behaviours and the rewards and sanctions which will be made contingent upon these.

Time out When specific, undesirable behaviours occur, the child is removed from all sources of positive reinforcement (e.g. the child is required to sit alone in the hall for a fixed period of time).

Systematic desensitisation Through relaxation training and a gradual exposure to a feared situation (via the imagination or in reality), a fearful or anxious state is gradually substituted by one of relaxation and calmness.

Emotive imagery Closely allied to systematic desensitisation, this involves developing an association between the feared object and a heroic figure with whom the child identifies. This association permits the child to confront and reduce the feared situation.

Flooding/implosive therapy Rather than introducing, through gradual exposure, that which is most feared (as in systematic desensitisation), the child is asked to imagine, or actually experience, this from the outset. Sometimes the feared object or situation is deliberately exaggerated to maximise its initial impact. The situation does not permit escape from the feared object or event and gradually the high level of anxiety lessens. The child comes to realise that the fear is unrealistic and that it can be controlled.

Modelling The child is asked to observe and imitate behaviour modelled by another (e.g. family member, therapist). Successful performance is subsequently reinforced. Modelling may be used in respect of phobias (e.g. holding a spider in one's hand) or conduct disorders (e.g. tidying up one's toys at bedtime).

Figure 2.1 Major forms of behavioural therapy

The first major description of this type of therapy was given by Aaron Beck (1963, 1964) who studied its use with people who had severe depression. Since that time the therapy has undergone major development, and is now seen as a cornerstone of treatment for a wide range of conditions from depression (Klein *et al.* 2007), to substance misuse (Waldron and Turner 2008). This value is especially evident in children where, for instance, drug treatment is less often used, though there is evidence that with some conditions, such as depression, combining cognitive behaviour therapy with medication gives the best outcome (Vitello 2009).

With children, there may be an advantage in the work being done within a family context because there is some evidence that having a focus upon the family may give the added benefit of improving general family functioning (Wood *et al.* 2009). As discussed in Chapter 1, successful therapies bring about physical brain changes, and this is true of cognitive behaviour therapy also, where for instance an effective programme which focused upon young people's sense of their own body resulted in changes to the activity in the brain centres involved in this process (Vocks *et al.* 2010). As the use of cognitive behaviour therapy has increased there has been a growing interest in delivering the therapy through other settings and mediums. Positive results have been reported when the sessions have been carried out in schools (Shirk *et al.* 2009), or delivered by an interactive computer programme (March *et al.* 2009).

Drug treatments

Drug treatments can only be prescribed by doctors, and so for many situations where problems are being addressed by other professionals, the role of drugs is not considered. In adults, drug treatments have been a significant part of the way that doctors try to help people with major mental health problems. It is not surprising, therefore, that similar endeavours have been seen when trying to assist with emotional and behavioural difficulties that arise in childhood. The efforts have, however, been more muted because of concern about the long-term effects of giving any drug to a child. In addition there is the ethical dilemma that since problems in childhood can be strongly influenced by many factors, is it right to subdue the symptom and not tackle the cause? This dilemma can be illustrated by the child who demonstrates aggressive behaviour primarily as a result of his or her parents' own marital violence. Should such a child be treated with drugs to minimise what is, in effect, a natural response to such behaviour in his or her caregivers?

Interestingly, the response to this question has tended to be different depending on which side of the Atlantic you live. In the UK the giving of drugs to children who do not have physical or demonstrable major psychiatric illness has, until quite recently, been rare. By contrast, American clinicians have been much more likely to explore drug regimes (Campbell and Cueva 1995). However, the growing number of studies which show that medication can have a positive impact upon young people's lives, for instance, by reducing their aggression (Nevels *et al.* 2010) is prompting a shift in prescribing in the UK. Major psychiatric illnesses, such as schizophrenia (Ardizzone *et al.* 2010) and obsessional compulsive disorder

(Ipser *et al.* 2009), do show a positive response to medication similar to that seen in adults, and in some disorders, drug therapy can play an important role in treatment (see Chapter 7). For some problems however, e.g. depression, the improvement achieved by medication appears less than in adults, but despite this, it may still be the most effective way of reducing the young person's distress when experiencing moderate to severe depression (Masi *et al.* 2010). However caution is always needed, because most of the medicines used with children and young people have only been officially approved (i.e. licenced by the Drugs Licensing Authority in the UK) for use with adults, and some may show unwanted effects when given to younger people.

Milieu therapy and intensive approaches

Residential units

It has been a traditional response when confronted with someone who has severe emotional or behavioural problems to look to place them in a residential setting which not only offers continuous assistance and treatment to the individual, but also removes them from the community where their problems may be prompting concern or distress. In psychiatry this residential setting has been a hospital, in education a residential school, and in the social services arena it may range from a residential family group home to a secure accommodation provision.

The vast majority of young people with behavioural or mental health problems never need admission to residential settings. However, a small number of children and adolescents do when, for instance, they are at high risk of harming themselves or others. These settings can offer an intensive intervention, and may permit specific treatment approaches to be implemented which would be impractical in the community. Each setting tends to have a quite distinct philosophy of care which can lead to very different experiences for young people in different units (Butler and McPherson 2007). For instance, some may operate a very traditional authoritarian model, while others may be set up as therapeutic communities where some of the treatment element comes from peer influence.

The programmes offered in residential settings have to take account of the developmental stage which the child has reached. Regimes that would be suitable for young children would clearly be inappropriate for adolescents, and offering a suitable range of responses, in what are usually quite small units, is one of the major challenges which residential settings typically face. As with any effective intervention its content must be tailored to the needs of the individual but usually there are elements of work with the child individually as well as group activities. One of the most powerful therapeutic elements in any treatment setting is its atmosphere or milieu. Because so much time is spent in residential settings, the power which this exerts is particularly important.

Milieu is difficult to define, and yet we all experience it several times a day. As human beings we are sensitive to the mood in a room, or the 'atmosphere' that exists in some meetings. Children are especially sensitive to ambience, and can be strongly influenced by it. Any therapeutic environment, therefore, is not only influencing the child by the stated treatment programme but by way the unit 'feels'. 'First impressions' and 'prevailing atmosphere' are indicators of the milieu which the unit is offering. This is partly to do with the physical environment, but is mostly made up of a blend of warmth and personal regard, combined with clear expectations about behaviour, and general conduct. A staff view that 'we care about you too much to let you do this' is an excellent foundation for a positive milieu, and once accepted by the child as genuine this can be far more powerful at bringing about change than a formal treatment strategy.

Removal of children from their families and their community is always a major step which carries with it potentially negative effects for the young person, which must be weighed against the potential advantages. Over recent years these issues, and the financial costs involved, have led to the role of residential settings being questioned, and their use has tended to dwindle, especially for younger children, despite the fact that there is often clear benefit for the children who are admitted (Garralda et al. 2008).

Overall, the provision of hospital places for children has reduced considerably, while the provision for teenagers continues to demand expansion. The decision to seek specialised residential schooling is now rarely made to meet a specific educational need of an academic nature, but rather, is a response to extreme social and behavioural difficulties. Indeed responding to children and young people whose behaviour is beyond the control of their families, and is disturbing to their community and society in general, represents the greatest challenge for the caring professions today. An effective residential regime for children with such difficulties is slowly emerging, but units providing such programmes are still few.

In general it appears that residential care offers little extra over intensive day provision (Barth et al. 2007), but there can still be benefits for certain young people to have periods of residential treatment (Bettmann and Jasperson 2009).

Day units

As mentioned above, one of the difficulties with residential treatment is the way that it separates the child from family and community. This has led to the emergence of day treatment programmes as a means of providing an intensity of care with the minimum of disruption to the day-to-day functioning of the child. As well as offering a greater intensity of involvement than can be achieved by outpatient appointments, such programmes allow the child to remain within the family, and this in turn produces issues and information that can be used to inform and progress family change. In addition, with careful planning it is possible to provide focused treatment packages which are age-specific, and use the continued attendance at school and so on as a positive lever for change (Place et al. 1990). By remaining within their community children may also develop support networks through friends, school, and so on. These become particularly important when the day programme comes to an end.

Confronting and challenging inappropriate behaviour is a key element of the programmes offered by many residential settings and day units. To achieve this they often use the interpretative style described by Redl (1959) which he called 'the life-space interview'. This seeks to use incidents not only to help the child recognise patterns and repetitions in their behaviour, but to assist them in developing new responses which are more appropriate.

The diversity of day unit programmes and the differing goals which they aspire to makes it difficult to offer a general view on their effectiveness. In units which deal with psychological difficulties about three-quarters of the children continue to have improved functioning two years after discharge (Place *et al.* 1990). These improvements are often not only in the presenting problem but also in the child's self-esteem and hopefulness about the future (Grizenko *et al.* 1993). Long-term follow-up studies show that, for both residential and day treatment programmes, two-thirds of the children have sustained their improvement after ten years (Erker *et al.* 1993).

Multisystemic therapy

A single therapeutic response that effectively reduces marked antisocial behaviour has proved difficult to find and this has led to programmes which combine elements of various approaches, and perhaps the most effective of these is the multisystemic therapy developed by Scott Henggeler and his colleagues (1998).

The approach is intensive, with each clinician having five or six families, and involves being available to them every day, and through the night. Family, behavioural and individual approaches are combined with school, peer and social network elements, with the exact make-up being determined by the needs of the specific family and young person. The input seeks to address the issues that the young person and family are facing, from improving parenting skills to addressing substance misuse and developing coping strategies. The duration of treatment usually ranges from four to five months, but can be longer especially if there are safety concerns for family members, or the wider community. There is a high level of supervision for each clinician and monitoring of progress is routine. It has been used in several countries to intervene with a variety of mainly delinquency-type problems, and the outcomes are generally good. It is especially encouraging that the programme is of value when trying to treat adolescent sexual offenders (Henggeler *et al.* 2009).

Parent training programmes

Efforts to respond to behavioural problems in children have increasingly widened from the presumption that therapy with the child is the most helpful approach. In parallel with the rise of interest in family dynamics there has been a rapid increase in programmes which seek to help parents manage their child's difficult behaviour. These are usually described as 'parent training programmes', although some are not teaching 'parenting', but quite advanced behavioural management. Their focus may range from preventing children's disruptive behaviour becoming criminal acts, to seeking to reduce the risk of the parent abusing their child. There has also been an extension of the approach to encompass parents of children who do not have challenging behaviours but more emotional ones, or specific health conditions.

Perhaps the best known of the programmes is Carolyn Webster-Stratton's 'Incredible Years' (Webster-Stratton 2006). In many of these programmes there tend to be two presenters and the programme is delivered over 12–20 two-hour sessions. The better programmes have a varied content which includes discussions, problem-solving exercises, skills training, role play practice, and DVD vignettes of parent–child interactions. The Incredible Years Parenting Programme seeks to promote positive parenting by helping the parents build positive and close relationships with their children through constructive play times, giving effective praise and rewards, and reducing criticism and unnecessary commands, while ensuring they can establish clear limits and boundaries. The more subtle aims are to help them to strengthen their children's problem-solving abilities and social competence as well as reducing aggression at home and in school (Webster-Stratton 1998).

There is clear evidence that such approaches can be helpful in families where the children are disruptive and challenging by changing parenting behaviour and reducing the severity of problems (Maughan et al. 2005; Thomas et al. 2007). When these programmes were examined to identify elements that predict success (Kaminski et al. 2008), teaching parents about child development had no impact on the success of the intervention, nor did the fact that it was a structured, manual-based programme. Indeed programmes that could offer innovation and adapt to the needs of the current group were the ones that tended to be more successful. The other slightly surprising finding was that offering additional services as well as the parent training programme seemed to result in the parents being less skilled than where the programme had been all that was offered.

Treatment foster care

When remaining with the family is not possible, alternative family placement is the usual response. Recently there has been a growing interest in whether children could be helped to overcome their difficulties by placing them in a substitute family whose purpose is to offer a therapeutic regime. For some children whose family of origin is limited in its parenting resources, moving to a family which offers good-quality care may be sufficient to bring about positive change. However, for more damaged children these substitute families have to offer a deliberately therapeutic regime.

The placements tend to operate a strict behavioural regime with each of the day's tasks being allocated points for completion. For instance, getting up on time, washing, and being on time for breakfast would each be rewarded with points that can be traded for pleasurable activities, CDs, etc. Interest in using treatment foster care has been increasing since its introduction in the USA (Clark et al. 1994) and the results are encouraging enough for programmes to be established around the UK. Treatment foster care has a relatively strong evidence base, with it showing a reduction in symptoms and lower rates of offending for mentally disordered and young offenders respectively compared to inpatient care groups (Chamberlain 2003).

Voluntary agencies

In any locality there is a variety of voluntary and charitable agencies which may be helpful in dealing with difficulties. For instance, in the UK:

- *Relate* is a voluntary agency that will help couples to explore, and hopefully resolve, relationship difficulties. Although the agency's workers are volunteers, as with other voluntary agencies, they are trained to ensure they can offer the appropriate skills necessary to help couples address their problems.
- *Cruise* is a voluntary service which helps both adults and children cope with bereavement.
- *Victim Support* gives practical advice and support to anyone who has been the victim of crime.
- *Rape Crisis* offers help and support to people who have been the victims of rape, though they usually only offer services to teenagers and adults.

In addition to such focused agencies children's charities, for example, NSPCC, Barnardo's, and National Children's Homes (NCH), are increasingly developing specialised sources of help for specific situations – such as the victims of sexual abuse, or supporting children from very damaging homes who have been adopted. Such services tend to be patchy, but local Social Services Departments will be able to provide details of their availability in each locality.

The place of diet and exercise

The concept that a healthy body is important for a healthy mind has been prevalent since ancient times. In recent years there has been growing emphasis upon maintaining a positive level of fitness and eating what is considered to be a healthy diet. There has also been an increased interest in considering whether diet could play a part in both the emergence of mental health difficulties, and their treatment. There is a growing encouragement for everyone to have a healthy balanced diet because of the wealth of data about diet's role in heart disease, cancer, and other major health issues (World Health Organization 2003). The role of diet in the emergence of behavioural and emotional problems is less robust, but associations have been been found (Oddy *et al.* 2009).

It has been known for some time that malnutrition in childhood can create both short- and long-term cognitive difficulties and be the source of behavioural problems. This is especially so if the deprivation occurs within the first two years of life when the brain is in the midst of its most rapid growth spurt (Georgieff 2007). However, more specific dietary deficits are also capable of causing major emotional and behavioural difficulties. For instance, iodine is important to ensure effective thyroid functioning as well as positive intellectual development. Iron deficiency can lead to problems with sustained attention, and zinc has been of particular interest in anorexia nervosa (Birmingham and Gritzner 2006) and attention deficit hyperactivity disorder (Arnold and DiSilvestro 2005). Finally, vitamins such as B and D play significant roles in brain development and so deficits are quite likely to increase the likelihood of emotional and behavioural difficulties both during childhood and into adulthood.

Attempting to treat difficulties by dietary means has involved the process of simply correcting such deficits, often through major public health initiatives. For instance, salt now contains iodine, and cereals have added B vitamins. Research that suggests that dietary intake can affect behaviour within school has prompted various studies to explore the impact of interventions such as breakfast clubs and carefully managed school meals, the results of which do suggest that these could assist some children (Ni Mhurchu et al. 2010).

As well as general programmes of this kind, there has also been a great interest in whether specific dietary elements could reduce symptoms of clinical disorders. An example of more specific treatment of disorders through diet is the focus upon omega-3 for the treatment of various conditions, for example attention deficit hyperactivity disorder. As discussed in Chapter 7, the value of this in reducing the symptoms is unclear, and this may in part be because the science suggests that it is only the long chain omega-3 that comes from fish that is helpful (Richardson 2007). Of more traditional supplements, perhaps only *Ginkgo biloba* has been shown to improve certain aspects of mood and attention in healthy subjects (Gorby et al. 2010).

Currently there is no real evidence as to the benefit of treating mental health and behavioural difficulties through dietary supplements alone, though if carefully chosen, addition to more established treatments may well bring additional benefit for the child. But it is important to draw a distinction between dietary changes which exert a positive benefit and potential allergic reactions to food substances, where their exclusion can bring about positive change. For instance, the potential role of an allergy to cow's milk in producing health and behavioural difficulties is well established (Vandenplas et al. 2007). In attention deficit hyperactivity disorder it has been known for some time that certain food items can provoke inattention and restless behaviour (Egger et al. 1985) and the relationship continues to be demonstrated (Pelsser et al. 2011).

There can be little doubt that children's day-to-day lifestyle has become more sedentary over recent years. Walking to school has been largely replaced by parent transport, or the school bus. Children's leisure time tends to have a high degree of computer-based activity, and so physical activity is increasingly becoming something that has to be deliberately undertaken rather than being a routine part of everyday life. There has also been growing interest about the potential value of exercise as part of the treatment for mental health difficulties such as depression (Teychenne et al. 2010). There are various potential explanations why this should be helpful – from establishing positive routines to making fundamental changes to the person's body and brain chemistry (Ströhle 2009).

Of course an obvious area where diet and exercise are important is the issue of childhood obesity. Research work looking at the impact of diet and physical activity upon childhood obesity (Oude Luttikhuis et al. 2009) found that such programmes are capable of making a positive impact upon these difficulties, but to be successful it is important that the diet and physical activity regimes are combined with more positive behavioural components which are focused upon changing lifestyle. Perhaps not surprisingly it is also clear that positive parental involvement is also crucial if such approaches are to prove successful (Munsch *et al.* 2008).

References

Alexander, F. and French, T. (1946). *Psychoanalytic Therapy: Principles and Application*. New York: Ronald Press.

Andrews, G. (1993). The essential psychotherapies. *British Journal of Psychiatry* 162: 447–51.

Ardizzone, I., Nardecchia, F, Marconi, A. *et al.* (2010). Antipsychotic medication in adolescents suffering from schizophrenia: A meta-analysis of randomized controlled trials. *Psychopharmacology Bulletin* 43: 45–66.

Arnold, L.E. and DiSilvestro, R.A. (2005). Zinc in attention deficit hyperactivity disorder. *Journal of Child and Adolescent Psychopharmacology* 15: 619–27.

Axline, V. (1947). *Play Therapy*. Boston: Houghton-Mifflin.

Barth, R.P., Greeson, J.K.P., Green, R.L. *et al.* (2007). Outcomes for youth receiving intensive in-home therapy or residential care: A comparison using propensity scores. *American Journal of Orthopsychiatry* 77: 497–505.

Beck, A.T. (1963). Thinking and depression: I. Idiosyncratic content and cognitive distortions. *Archives of General Psychiatry* 9: 324–33.

Beck, A.T. (1964). Thinking and depression: II. Theory and therapy. *Archives of General Psychiatry* 10: 561–71.

Berg, I.K. and de Jong, P. (1996). Solution-building conversations: Co-constructing a sense of competence with clients. *Families in Society* 2: 376–91.

Bettmann, J.E. and Jasperson, R.A. (2009). Adolescents in residential and inpatient treatment: A review of the outcome literature. *Child Youth Care Forum* 38: 161–83.

Birmingham, C.L. and Gritzner, S. (2006). How does zinc supplementation benefit anorexia nervosa? *Eating and Weight Disorders* 11: e109–11.

Butler, L.S. and McPherson, P.M. (2007). Is residential treatment misunderstood? *Journal of Child and Family Studies* 16: 465–72.

Byng-Hall, J. (1995). *Re-writing Family Scripts*. New York: Guilford Press.

Campbell, M. and Cueva, J.E. (1995). Psychopharmacology in child and adolescent psychiatry: A review of the past seven years, II. *Journal of the American Academy of Child and Adolescent Psychiatry* 34: 1262–72.

Carr, A. (2009). The effectiveness of family therapy and systemic interventions for child-focused problems. *Journal of Family Therapy* 31: 3–45.

Chamberlain P. (2003). *Treating Chronic Juvenile Offenders: Advances Made through the Oregon Multidimensional Treatment Foster Care Model*. Washington, DC: American Psychological Association.

Clark, H.B., Prange, M.E., Lee, B.L. *et al.* (1994). Improving adjustment outcomes for foster children with emotional and behavioral disorders: Early findings from a controlled study on individualized services. *Journal of Emotional and Behavioral Disorders* 2: 207–18.

Corcoran, J. (2006). A comparison group study of solution-focused therapy versus 'treatment-as-usual' for behavior problems in children. *Journal of Social Service Research* 33: 69–81.

Cottrell, D. and Boston, P. (2002). The effectiveness of systemic family therapy for children and adolescents. *Journal of Child Psychology Psychiatry* 43: 573–86.

Davanloo, H. (1980). *Short-term Dynamic Psychotherapy*. New York: Aronson.

de Shazer, S. (1991). *Putting Difference to Work*. New York: W.W. Norton.

de Shazer, S., Berg, I.K., Lipchik, E. *et al.*(1986). Brief therapy: Focused solution development. *Family Process* 25: 207–22.

Egger, J., Carter, C., Graham, P. *et al.* (1985). A controlled trial of oligoantigenic treatment in the hyperkinetic syndrome. *Lancet* 9 March, I: 540–5.

Epston, D. and White, M. (1990). *Narrative Means to Therapeutic Ends*. New York: Norton.

Erker, G.J., Searight, H.R., Amanat, E. *et al.* (1993). Residential versus day treatment for children: A long term follow-up study. *Child Psychiatry and Human Development* 24: 31–9.

Freud, A. (1966). *The Writings of Anna Freud. Vol. 2: The Ego and Mechanisms of Defense.* New York: International University Press.

Freud, S. (1976). *Introductory Lectures on Psychoanalysis*. Harmondsworth: Penguin.

Garralda, M.E., Rose, G. and Dawson, R. (2008). Measuring outcomes in a child psychiatry inpatient unit. *Journal of Children's Services* 3: 6–16.

Georgieff, M.K. (2007). Nutrition and the developing brain: Nutrient priorities and measurement. *American Journal of Clinical Nutrition* 85: 614S–20S.

Gorby, H.E, Brownawell, A.M. and Falk, M.C. (2010). Do specific dietary constituents and supplements affect mental energy? Review of the evidence. *Nutrition Review* 68: 697–718.

Grizenko, N., Papineau, D. and Sayegh, L. (1993). Effectiveness of a multimodal day treatment program for children with disruptive behavior problems. *Journal of the American Academy of Child and Adolescent Psychiatry* 32: 127–34.

Hartmann, A., Herzog, T. and Drinkman, A. (1992). Psychotherapy of bulimia nervosa: what is effective – a meta-analysis. *Journal of Psychosomatic Research* 36: 159–67.

Hazell, P.L., Martin, G., Mcgill, K. *et al.* (2009). Group therapy for repeated deliberate self-harm in adolescents: Failure of replication of a randomized trial. *Journal of American Academy of Child and Adolescent Psychiatry* 48: 662–70.

Henggeler, S.W., Schoenwald, S.K., Borduin, C.M. *et al.* (1998). *Multisystemic Treatment of Antisocial Behavior in Children and Adolescents*. New York: Guilford.

Henggeler, S.W., Letourneau, E.J., Chapman, J.E. *et al.* (2009). Mediators of change for multisystemic therapy with juvenile sexual offenders. *Journal of Consulting Clinical Psychology* 77: 451–62.

Hogue, A., Dauber, S., Stambaugh, L.F. *et al.* (2006). Early therapeutic alliance and treatment outcome in individual and family therapy for adolescent behavior problems. *Journal of Consulting and Clinical Psychology* 74: 121–9.

Ipser, J.C., Stein, D.J., Hawkridge, S. *et al.* (2009). Pharmacotherapy for anxiety disorders in children and adolescents. *Cochrane Database of Systematic Reviews*: CD005170.

Kaminski, J.W., Valle, L.A., Filene, J.H. *et al.* (2008). A meta-analytic review of components associated with parent training program effectiveness. *Journal of Abnormal Child Psychology* 36: 567–89.

Kazdin, A.E. (1990). Psychotherapy for children. *Annual Review of Psychology* 41: 21–54.

Kennedy, E. and Midgley, N. (2007). *Process and Outcome Research in Child, Adolescent and Parent-Infant Psychotherapy: A Thematic Review*. London: NHS London.

Kim, J.S. (2008) Examining the effectiveness of solution-focused brief therapy: A meta-analysis. *Research on Social Work Practice* 18: 107–16.

Klein, J.B., Jacobs, R.H. and Reinecke, M.A. (2008). Cognitive-behavioral therapy for adolescent depression: A meta-analytic investigation of changes in effect-size estimates. *Journal of American Academy of Child and Adolescent Psychiatry* 46: 1403–13.

Kolvin, I., Macmillan, I., Nicol, A.R. *et al.* (1988). Psychotherapy is effective. *Journal of the Royal Society of Medicine* 81: 261–6.

Lane, R.C., Koetting, M.G. and Bishop, J. (2002). Silence as communication in psychodynamic psychotherapy. *Clinical Psychology Review* 22: 1091–104.

Legg, C. and Stagaki. P. (2002). How to be a postmodernist: A user's guide to postmodern rhetorical practices. *Journal of Family Therapy* 24: 385–401.

Lethem, J. (2002). Brief solution focused therapy. *Child and Adolescent Mental Health* 7: 189–92.

Lieberman, S. (1979). *Transgenerational Family Therapy*. Guildford: Biddles.

Lindemann, E. (1944). Symptomatology and management of acute grief. *American Journal of Psychiatry* 101: 101–48.

Macdonald, A.J. (1997). Brief therapy in adult psychiatry: Further outcomes. *Journal of Family Therapy* 19: 213–22.

Macgowan, M.J. and Engle, B. (2010). Evidence for optimism: Behavior therapies and motivational interviewing in adolescent substance abuse treatment. *Child and Adolescent Psychiatric Clinics of North America* 19: 527–45.

Malan, D.H. (1963). *A Study of Brief Psychotherapy*. London: Social Science Paperbacks.

March, S., Spence, S.H. and Donovan, C.L. (2009). The efficacy of an internet-based cognitive-behavioral therapy intervention for child anxiety disorders. *Journal of Pediatric Psychology* 34: 474–87.

Masi, G., Liboni, F. and Brovedani, P. (2010). Pharmacotherapy of major depressive disorder in adolescents. *Expert Opinions in Pharmacotherapy* 11: 375–86.

Maughan, D.R., Christiansen, E., Jenson, W.R. *et al.* (2005). Behavioral parent training as a treatment for externalizing behaviors and disruptive behavior disorders: A meta-analysis. *School Psychology Review* 34: 267–86.

Miller, W.R. (1983). Motivational interviewing with problem drinkers. *Behavioural Psychotherapy* 11: 147–72.

Miller, W.R. and Baca, L.M. (1983). Two-year follow-up of bibliotherapy and therapist-directed controlled drinking training for problem drinkers. *Behavior Therapy* 14: 441–8.

Munsch, S., Roth, B., Michael, T. *et al.* (2008). Randomized controlled comparison of two cognitive behavioural therapies for obese children: Mother versus mother-child cognitive behaviour therapy. *Psychotherapy and Psychosomatics* 77: 235–46.

Nevels, R.M., Dehon, E.E., Alexander, K. *et al.* (2010). Psychopharmacology of aggression in children and adolescents with primary neuropsychiatric disorders: A review of current and potentially promising treatment options. *Experimental and Clinical Psychopharmacology* 18: 184–201.

Ni Mhurchu, C., Turley, M., Gorton, D. *et al.* (2010). Effects of a free school breakfast programme on school attendance, achievement, psychosocial function, and nutrition: A stepped wedge cluster randomised trial. *BMC Public Health* 10: 738.

Oddy, W.H., Robinson, M. and Ambrosini, G.L. (2009). Dietary patterns are associated with mental health in early adolescence. *Preventive Medicine* 49: 39–44.

Oude Luttikhuis, H., Baur, L., Jansen, H. *et al.* (2009). Interventions for treating obesity in children. *Evidence-Based Child Health* 4: 1571–729.

Pelsser, L.M., Frankena, K., Toorman, J. *et al.* (2011). Effects of a restricted elimination diet on the behaviour of children with attention-deficit hyperactivity disorder (INCA study): A randomised controlled trial. *The Lancet* 377: 494–503.

Place, M., Rajah, S. and Crake, T. (1990). Combining day patient treatment with family work in a child psychiatry clinic. *European Archives of Psychiatry and Neurological Sciences* 239: 373–8.

Redl, F. (1959). A strategy and technique of the life-space interview. *American Journal of Orthopsychiatry* 29, 1–15.

Richardson, A.J. (2007). N-3 fatty acids and mood: The devil is in the detail. *British Journal of Nutrition* 99: 221–3.

Roberts, N.P., Kitchiner, N.J., Kenardy, J. *et al.* 2010). Early psychological interventions to treat acute traumatic stress symptoms. *Cochrane Database of Systematic Reviews* (3): CD007944.

Rogers, C.R. (1951). *Client-centred Therapy*. London: Constable.

Rogers, C.R. (1961). *On Becoming a Person*. London: Constable.

Segal, H. (1964). *Introduction to the Work of Melanie Klein*. London: Heinemann.

Sexton, T. and Turner, C.W. (2010). The effectiveness of functional family therapy for youth with behavioral problems in a community practice setting. *Journal of Family Psychology* 24: 339–48.

Smyke, A.T., Zeanah, C.H., Fox, N.A. *et al.* (2010). Placement in foster care enhances quality of attachment among young institutionalized children. *Child Development* 81: 212–23.

Shirk, S.R., Kaplinski, H. and Gudmundsen, G. (2009). School-based cognitive-behavioral therapy for adolescent depression: A benchmarking study. *Journal of Emotional and Behavioral Disorders* 17: 106–17.

Ströhle, A. (2009). Physical activity, exercise, depression and anxiety disorders. *Journal of Neural Transmission* 116: 777–84.

Teychenne, M., Ball, K. and Salmon, J. (2010). Sedentary behavior and depression among adults: A review. *International Journal of Behavioral Medicine* 17: 246–54.

Thomas, R. and Zimmer-Gembeck, M.J. (2007). Behavioral outcomes of Parent-Child Interaction Therapy and Triple P-Positive Parenting Program: A review and meta-analysis. *Journal of Abnormal Child Psychology* 35: 475–95.

Vandenplas, Y., Brueton, M., Dupont, C. *et al.* (2007). Guidelines for the diagnosis and management of cow's milk protein allergy in infants. *Archives of Diseases in Childhood* 92: 902–8.

Vitiello, B. (2009) Combined cognitive-behavioral therapy and pharmacotherapy for adolescent depression: Does it improve outcomes compared with monotherapy? *CNS Drugs* 23: 271–80.

Vocks, S., Schulte, D., Busch, M. *et al.* (2010). Changes in neuronal correlates of body image processing by means of cognitive-behavioural body image therapy for eating disorders: A randomized controlled fMRI study. *Psychological Medicine* 16: 1–9.

Waldron, H.B. and Turner, C.W. (2008). Evidence-based psychosocial treatments for adolescent substance abuse. *Journal of Clinical Child and Adolescent Psychology* 37: 238–61.

Watson, J.B. and Rayner, R. (1920). Conditioned emotional reactions. *Journal of Experimental Psychology* 3: 1–14.

Webster-Stratton C. (1998). Preventing conduct problems in Head Start children: Strengthening parent competencies. *Journal of Consulting and Clinical Psychology* 66: 715–30.

Webster-Stratton, C. (2006). *The Incredible Years*. Washington, DC: The Incredible Years.

Weisz, J.R. and Jensen, A.L. (2001). Child and adolescent psychotherapy in research and practice contexts: Review of the evidence and suggestions for improving the field. *European Child Adolescent Psychiatry* 10, Suppl. 1: I12–18.

Weisz, J.R., Weiss, B., Alicke, M.D. *et al.* (1987). Effectiveness of psychotherapy with children and adolescents: A meta-analysis for clinicians. *Journal of Consulting and Clinical Psychology* 55: 542–9.

Weisz, J.R., Weiss, B. and Donenberg, G.R. (1992). The lab versus the clinic: Effects of child and adolescent psychotherapy. *American Psychology* 47: 1578–85.

Wood, J.J., McLeod, B.D., Piacentini, J.C. *et al.* (2009). One-year follow-up of family versus child CBT for anxiety disorders: Exploring the roles of child age and parental intrusiveness. *Child Psychiatry and Human Development* 40: 301–16.

World Health Organization. (2003). *Diet, Nutrition and the Prevention of Chronic Diseases: Report of the Joint WHO/FAO Expert Consultation.* WHO Technical Report Series, No. 916 (TRS 916). Geneva: World Health Organization.

Yalom, I.D. (1995). *The Theory and Practice of Group Psychotherapy,* New York: Basic Books.

Chapter 3

School refusal

Introduction

Children may not wish to attend school for many reasons ranging from boredom in class, to fear of classmates, to a reluctance to leave their parents. The list of reasons is long and applies to most children at some time during the 15,000 hours that they typically spend in school.

Most children are likely to miss occasional days from school at some stage during their childhood because of what may often appear to an onlooker to be trivial fears or anxieties. Perhaps a lesson has been misunderstood and a teacher's anger is feared, or a best friend has teamed up with someone else. Usually such problems are resolved or quickly forgotten and school attendance soon resumes. Some children maintain a strong dislike of school throughout their childhood but accept the requirement to attend regularly. A much smaller proportion cease to attend school for a prolonged period of time; these are the individuals who usually come into contact with helping agencies.

Truants or school refusers?

A major distinction is often drawn between truants and school phobics (the latter are now more commonly termed 'school refusers'). Although truants also choose not to attend school they are usually perceived as experiencing no major psychological difficulty in attending; rather they prefer not to. In contrast, school refusers may wish to attend but often find that they cannot. To some extent, then, one distinction between truancy and school refusal centres upon volition. Truancy is widely perceived as one variant of acting-out behaviour, often associated with delinquency and disruptiveness, whereas school refusal is typically perceived as a form of neurosis characterised by anxiety and fearfulness. This widely held distinction is complicated because some writers (e.g. Kearney 2008) include all those who refuse to attend school, both truants and those with school-related anxiety disorders, under the broader, all-encompassing heading of school refusal. This chapter, however, will maintain the generally accepted distinction between truants and school refusers.

In distinguishing school refusal from truancy, Berg *et al.* (1969) note that unlike truants, refusers tend to share the following features:

- severe difficulty in attending school, often amounting to prolonged absence;
- severe emotional upset, which may involve such symptoms as excessive fearfulness, temper tantrums, misery or complaints of feeling ill without obvious organic cause when faced with the prospect of going to school;
- during school hours, the child remains at home with the knowledge of the parents;
- absence of significant antisocial disorders such as juvenile delinquency, disruptiveness and sexual activity.

In contrast, truants are more likely to attend school on a sporadic basis. They are typically not excessively anxious or fearful about attending school, nor do they usually complain about physical discomfort. Truants are more likely to conceal their absence from their parents, often by wandering the streets during the day, and are more likely to engage in antisocial acts. In a comparative study of truants and school refusers (Galloway 1983) parental reports indicated that truants were more influenced by peers and had a greater history of lying, stealing and wandering from the home out of school hours. In contrast, school refusers were reported as having more concerns about academic matters, were more anxious about parental well-being and were reluctant to leave the home. There were, however, no significant differences in peer relationships, the frequency of eating and sleeping difficulties or the proportion of cases of enuresis.

It should be recognised, however, that truants and school refusers do not always fall into clear-cut groups and a relatively small proportion of absentees can show features of both truancy and school refusal (Kearney 2008; Steinhausen *et al.* 2008). In one study of one hundred chronic absentees, for example, Bools *et al.* (1990) found that approximately 10% of the sample demonstrated both emotional and antisocial conduct disorders. It has been suggested that the truant/school refuser distinction can be relatively arbitrary, reflect differential access to professional services, and lead to those from disadvantaged backgrounds being more likely to be treated in a punitive, rather than therapeutic fashion (Lyon and Cotler 2007).

Prevalence

Estimates of the prevalence of school refusal vary considerably, primarily because of the differing criteria that have been used to define the term. Where estimates of school refusal, not including truancy, are employed (consistent with the use of the term in this chapter) figures in the USA and UK generally range from 0.4% to 2% of the population.

Types of school refuser

Hersov outlines a common picture of school refusal immediately recognisable to those with experience of such difficulties:

> The problem often starts with vague complaints about school or reluctance to attend progressing to total refusal to go to school or to remain in school in the

face of persuasion, entreaty, recrimination and punishment by parents and pressures from teachers, family doctors and education welfare officers. The behaviour may be accompanied by overt signs of anxiety or even panic when the time comes to go to school and most children cannot even leave home to set out for school. Many who do return home halfway there and some children, once at school, rush home in a state of anxiety. Many children insist that they want to go to school and are prepared to do so but cannot manage it when the time comes.

(Hersov 1977: 458–9)

In addition to the psychological distress noted above, such children often complain of physical illness such as headaches, stomach aches, dizziness or vomiting for which there are no organic causes. In many cases these physical symptoms disappear once the child is allowed to remain at home. The high levels of anxiety may also be compounded by depression leading to tearfulness, sleeping difficulties, irritability and low self-esteem.

While such a picture is common, it is important to recognise that there is no single form of school refusal. Major areas of controversy centre on, first, the extent to which school refusal should be seen as a consequence of fear of being in school rather than of separating from parents and home, and, second, whether there is a difference between those children whose non-attendance is sudden, as opposed to developing over a long period. In both issues the influences of age and gender are seen as important mediating factors.

Although Broadwin (1932) is credited as being the first writer to describe a form of persistent school absence marked by fearfulness and prolonged refusal to attend, Johnson et al. (1941) coined the term 'school phobia' to describe this phenomenon. According to these early theorists, the school-refusing child had an excessively strong love attachment to the parent and fantasised about returning to the nour-ishing and protective maternal situation enjoyed in infancy. The mothers of such children were perceived as having similarly unfulfilled emotional needs and, as a result, became overprotective of their child and overdemanding of attention. It was thought that anger, resentment and hostility experienced by both mother and child in the resolution of the quest for independence/dependence resulted in anxiety about separation directly resulting in school refusal. This view became highly popular in the 1950s and 1960s to the extent that some writers (e.g. Johnson 1957) saw school phobia being replaced by separation anxiety as the key diagnostic criterion.

Separation anxiety is now seen by many practitioners as an inadequate explana-tion for all cases of school refusal. The theory does not explain why the peak age for school refusal is between the ages of 11 and 13 (Last et al. 1987) rather than in the early years of schooling as the theory would suggest. Furthermore, many school phobic children appear to have little difficulty in separating from their parents for other social/recreational activities. Given these weaknesses in the theory, many contemporary writers tend to place equal emphasis upon the school itself as the source of anxiety (Pilkington and Piersel 1991). For such reasons, Knollmann et al.

(2010), differentiate between school anxiety and school phobia, where the former largely concerns fear of the school context, and the latter is more closely related to separation anxiety.

In identifying differing types of school anxiety/phobia, a distinction is often drawn between acute and chronic school refusal, a factor that may be important in the devising of appropriate interventions. Berg *et al.* (1969) suggested that where absence had been preceded by at least three years' trouble-free attendance, irrespective of current duration, the school refusal should be considered as acute. Other cases should be considered as chronic. Studies comparing children falling into these two categories have repeatedly demonstrated that chronic refusal is associated with a greater dependency, a higher incidence of parental mental illness, less sociability and lower self-esteem. In contrast, acute refusal is associated with higher levels of depression.

Given the greater incidence of problems experienced by chronic cases and findings indicating that such children are often unlikely to be provided assistance by support services for several months, it is hardly surprising that the prognosis for chronic refusal is poorer than for acute cases (Berg 1970). Indeed, it is arguable that chronic cases are merely acute cases that have been allowed to persist over time.

Studies have been inconsistent and variable in determining both age and sex differences (Trueman 1984), although there is some evidence to suggest that separation anxiety is more a feature of younger female children while fear of school tends to be more prevalent in older male children (Last *et al.* 1987). There is some evidence, however (e.g. Smith 1970), that cases are high at the time of school entry and peak between the ages of eleven and thirteen (at a time when most children transfer from primary to secondary schooling). In general, studies suggest that older school refusers suffer from more severe disorders and have a poorer prognosis (Atkinson *et al.* 1985). Intellectual functioning in school refusers, contrary to earlier thinking, tends to mirror that of non-school refusers of comparable ages (Trueman 1984).

It is now widely accepted that school refusal is not a unitary syndrome but, rather, multicausal and heterogeneous. As such, rather than focusing upon simple school phobia/separation anxiety or acute/chronic onset distinctions, it may be more helpful for practitioners to examine the needs of the child that are met by non-school attendance (Kearney *et al.* 2006; Evans 2000). Understanding what the child gains by not attending school should help the practitioner derive the most effective forms of intervention. Kearney and Silverman's clinical and research work has led them to the conclusion that, for each individual, school refusal is maintained by one or more of four major categories (see Figure 3.1). Preferred modes of intervention for each of these categories can be outlined (see Chapter 2) and their effectiveness measured over time. It appears that focusing upon the functions of school refusal, rather than the problem behaviours themselves may be more helpful for clinical decision making (Kearney, 2007a).

Category 1	Avoidance of specific fearfulness or general overanxiousness related to the school setting. This includes cases where one or more particular features of school (a corridor, toilets, test situations, a particular teacher) are feared. It is often the case, however, that the child is unable to articulate the specific cause of their distress.
Category 2	Escape from aversive social situations. This focuses on situations where problems centre upon unsatisfying relationships with others (peers and/or teachers). Often this incorporates an evaluative element. Such difficulty is more common for older children or adolescents and is often associated with generalized and social anxiety disorder.
Category 3	Attention-getting or separation-anxious behaviour. This may be manifested by tantrums and/or somatic complaints where the child's intention is primarily to stay at home with a parent or important other.
Category 4	Rewarding experiences provided out of school. Children who fall into this category may wish to remain at home because this provides opportunities for engaging in preferred activities such as watching the television or associating with friends. This function may often be associated with conduct or oppositional defiance disorder.

Figure 3.1 Kearney and Silverman's functional categories for school refusal

Assessment

The heterogeneous nature of school refusal is such that a detailed assessment of the child is necessary in order to derive the most appropriate intervention. It is important that consideration is given to the child's affective, cognitive and behavioural functioning both generally and in relation to the specific context of the refusal. Most practitioners favour the employment of a range of procedures, including child interviews (in both one-to-one and whole-family settings), the employment of self-report questionnaires, ratings of the child by significant others (e.g. parents and teachers), self-monitoring by the child (e.g. the use of a diary to record feelings and behaviours), direct behavioural observation of the child in the home and school setting and an assessment of family dynamics.

At the initial stages, information about the child's general functioning at home and at school is sought. The precise nature of the refusal is explored in greater detail in order to ascertain the extent of the child's difficulty. Subsequently, consideration of specific aspects of the child's environment that induce fearfulness, together with examination of the responses of others to this, are examined. At this early stage, the practitioner may discover that school refusal is a secondary symptom of another, more pervasive problem. This may be a genuine physical illness, severe depression, agoraphobia, a complex learning difficulty, or more generally defiant or challenging behaviour.

Many practitioners advocate the use of self-report instruments that gauge children's perceptions of their feelings and emotions. Widely used measures include the Children's Manifest Anxiety Scale – Revised (Reynolds and Paget 1983), the Fear Survey Schedule for Children – Revised (Ollendick 1983), the Children's Depression Inventory (Kovacs and Beck 1977) and the Social Anxiety Scale for Children – Revised (La Greca and Stone 1993). Such scales typically ask children to respond to a variety of situations printed on a questionnaire. The Fear Survey Schedule for Children – Revised, for example, lists eighty situations that are potentially fearful (e.g. spiders, being in a fight, failing a test, having to go to hospital). For each, the child is asked to indicate whether he or she experiences no fear, some fear or a lot of fear. As a number of the situations relate to school contexts, this measure provides a useful means of differentiating between those whose difficulties relate specifically to one or more aspects of school life and those who experience a wider form of separation anxiety (Ollendick and Mayer 1984).

A self-report measure that specifically addresses school-refusal behaviour is the School Refusal Assessment Scale (Kearney and Silverman 1993) which attempts to ascertain what needs are served by the child's school-refusal behaviour. This scale, available in child, teacher and parent versions, originally contained sixteen items, whereby four questions each measure the relative influence of one of the four maintaining conditions (see Figure 3.1). Kearney (2002) has since produced revised student and parent versions, each now containing twenty-four (six per function) questions. Ideally, the scale should be used in conjunction with direct observation of the child at home, in particular at the beginning of the school day (Kearney 2001).

An important issue to assess in understanding what maintains any phobic behaviour is whether it is negatively or positively reinforced – that is, whether the 'reward' is escaping from something unpleasant (negative reinforcement) or achieving a pleasing experience (positive reinforcement). In relation to school refusal, such an analysis involves considering whether avoidance of school is maintained because:

1 it results in the reduction or elimination of unpleasant experiences, such as no longer being teased by schoolmates (negative reinforcement); or
2 it results in an increase in the experience of desirable outcomes, such as playing at home on one's computer (positive reinforcement).

Clearly, the intervention programme will differ greatly according to the nature of the factors that maintain the behaviour. An illustrative example is provided below.

Richard, a 14-year-old, was an only child living at home with his mother and her partner. Two years earlier his natural parents had separated, and shortly after his mother's new boyfriend moved in on a permanent basis. Richard spoke widely of his liking for his mother's new partner, though he readily admitted that he would like to see his parents reunited. The boy was referred to an educational psychologist on the grounds of his prolonged absence from school. His parents informed the psychologist that in order to persuade the boy to return to school they had bought him a motorcycle for use in the woods near his home. Richard, however, subsequently reneged on his promise to return to school and was now stating that he would only return to school if he were bought a more powerful machine. His mother informed the psychologist that she was prepared to accede to this request if it led to a return to school but she wasn't optimistic that this would be the case.

Detailed examination of Richard's situation resulted in the following observations:

1   There was little evidence of fearfulness and/or anxiety when Richard was in school (prior to the onset of the refusal and during a brief, ultimately unsuccessful, staged return trial programme).
2   Richard's day at home was undemanding and generally pleasurable. He got up late, watched the television or played with his computer. His mother and her partner were at work all day so he spent his time at home alone. Most evenings he met his schoolmates in the woods and rode his motorcycle. Occasional attempts to restrict his use of the motorcycle had been introduced but these appeared to make no impact upon his unwillingness to attend school. His mother had therefore ceased to use this threat as a means of persuasion.
3   Richard enjoyed good relations with most people with whom he came into contact. Apart from friction concerning his non-attendance at school, there was little conflict or hostility in the home. Richard appeared to have accepted his mother's partner and enjoyed going out with him to fish or to play sports. There was no indication of any specific difficulties at school (e.g. academic problems, bullying or harassment). His behaviour in class was good and his teachers were mystified by his unwillingness to attend.
4   From the outset, Richard was eager to establish a positive relationship with those professionals who were attempting to help him. His presentation of himself as relaxed and sociable was backed up by a rather jocular manner that appeared somewhat inappropriate.
5.   Richard could not articulate any reasons for not attending school other than to state that he 'couldn't face it'. When pressed, he would clam up and become silent. If another topic was raised he would immediately become communicative once more. When asked about his bargaining over the replacement motorcycle he replied that he wanted it so badly that he would force himself to attend school.
6   Richard's mother was meeting regularly with her husband in order to persuade him to exert influence over their son. Father was coming to the house on a regular basis but family discussions usually ended with Dad losing his temper with Richard.

The investigation of Richard's case indicated that his school refusal was maintained primarily by the fourth of Kearney and Silverman's (1993) categories, that is, his school refusal behaviour was being positively reinforced by his out-of-school experiences. His enjoyable daytimes, together with the power he was exerting over the adults in his life, appeared to combine in the maintenance of his school refusal. This power not only resulted in his bargaining for material things but gave him control over his parents, frequently bringing them together, possibly in the hope that they might ultimately be reunited. School refusal may be a powerful weapon for a child who feels generally powerless to control a break-up of the family.

There was no indication that the other three functional categories had any bearing on this case. The implications for intervention were clear: change the reinforcement schedules operating at home by relating access to enjoyable activities at home and in the evenings to school attendance and establishing a more appropriate daily routine (e.g. bedtimes, getting up in the morning); and engage the family in therapeutic work geared to the resolution of the family-based problems and tensions that were leading to the school refusal.

Intervention approaches

The many different conceptions and manifestations of school refusal, each with differing underlying causes and symptoms, have led to fierce debate about the most appropriate interventions and it has proven impossible to derive any one strategy that has proven effective or appropriate for all school refusers. What is clear is that if support agencies or the school fail to work collaboratively, and fail to understand the contribution that other professionals will be making, the chances of a successful return are greatly reduced. The following sections deal initially with types of clinical intervention and then go on to consider the central role which the school plays.

In treating school refusal, a distinction is often made between psychodynamic approaches, which are concerned with disturbances of thought, feeling and behaviour, and which are typically addressed by means of some form of individual, group or family therapy, and behaviour therapy approaches based upon the premise that disordered behaviour is learned and can thus be unlearned through the use of a variety of 'behavioural' techniques. With regard to school refusal, behavioural approaches usually involve a graduated weakening of the relationship of school attendance with associated negative emotions, and ensuring that rewards and sanctions in the child's life become contingent upon desired behaviour (i.e. school attendance).

A number of techniques are used to address school refusal. These are based upon applications of talking therapy, behavioural techniques and medication (see Chapter 2). The most widely advocated techniques are:

- systematic desensitisation through relaxation;
- emotive imagery;

- shaping and contingency management;
- modelling;
- social skills training;
- cognitive behavioural therapy (CBT);
- family therapy;
- medication.

Each of these will be briefly described below, although for a more detailed account of research studies, see Elliott (1999).

Systematic desensitisation through relaxation

Systematic desensitisation usually consists of a three-stage procedure (the reader is referred to Kratochwill and Morris (1991) for a more detailed account):

1 Teaching the client to become progressively relaxed. King *et al.* (1995) outline a helpful format of relaxation training that involves progressive muscle relaxation. The programme involves systematically tensing and relaxing muscle groups (e.g. arms and shoulders, legs and feet) with, for younger children, the assistance of associated mental imagery. It is suggested that no more than three muscle groups should be introduced in each 15- to 20-minute session.

2 Constructing a hierarchy of anxiety-evoking situations. The child and practitioner agree upon a target fear (such as attending school). The child is presented with a number of blank cards and is asked to write down briefly about each situation (e.g. undressing for PE) where that fear is evoked. The child is asked to outline situations where there are differing degrees of fearfulness or other forms of emotional discomfort. Cards are then ranked in order of fearfulness. Additional cards are completed as necessary in follow-up sessions until there is a hierarchy ranging from zero-level fearfulness to that which evokes the most extreme emotions.

3 Replacing anxiety by relaxation for each of these situations. Once the child has become skilled at practising relaxation techniques he or she is asked to imagine each of the situations on the cards, commencing in ascending order. Usually, three or four situations are considered in any one session. The intention is that the fearful situation becomes associated with being in a relaxed state and, as a result, anxiety is diminished.

Emotive imagery

Emotive imagery is another fear-reduction method that closely resembles systematic desensitisation. First employed by Lazarus and Abramovitz, it involves the association between each situation on the fear hierarchy with imagined scenes which 'arouse feelings of self-assertion, pride, affection, mirth and similar anxiety-inhibiting responses' (1962: 191). Typically, the child's usual hero images (e.g. a famous footballer) or activities that are greatly desired (e.g. driving a speedboat) are elicited, imagined and then related to items in the fear hierarchy by means of a narrative. As with systematic desensitisation, as anxiety is gradually inhibited in each of the lower-level items, the procedure is repeated until the highest item can be considered without undue anxiety.

More recently, computer technology, in the form of virtual reality, has been used to provide a new form of exposure, or imagery, for a variety of different forms of anxiety (Wiederhold and Wiederhold 2005; Bouchard 2011). While the use of this approach for school refusal is still in its infancy, there is some evidence that such an approach may help to reduce school-specific fears (Gutiérrez-Maldonado *et al.* 2009).

Although desensitisation and relaxation approaches are recommended widely by clinicians, particularly with primary-aged children whose refusal is marked by extreme phobic reactivity (King *et al.* 1995), these methods have yet to be supported by controlled research studies (Kratochwill and Morris 1991).

Shaping and contingency management

Contingency management procedures are based upon behavioural principles whereby the influence of events taking place before and after specific behaviours is highlighted and subsequently modified to effect desired behavioural change. For school refusal, this approach involves maximising rewarding experiences for being in school and minimising the rewards for remaining at home during the school day. Common elements include the reduction of parental or sibling attention when the child is at home, the removal of pleasures such as the use of television and computer during school time and during evenings and weekends.

Shaping refers to a procedure where the child's behaviour is gradually modified by means of contingent reinforcement, until a desired result is achieved. This may involve a number of steps: for example, rewards for undertaking homework at home, progressing to undertaking homework in a friend's house, undertaking homework in a classroom with a parent after school hours, attending school for one lesson each day, attending for half a day, and so on. At each step, the child's successful behaviour is reinforced by praise and attention and by those more tangible rewards that are deemed appropriate.

Modelling

This approach is based upon the premise that an individual may acquire behavioural dispositions as a result of the process of observing another individual. A popular approach for many child phobias, it involves the child observing a model (e.g. the therapist, peer or significant other) engaging in the behaviour that is feared. This may take place either by means of live modelling or through film and imagination. The child observes the model successfully handling the situation with no adverse consequences. Subsequently, the child is asked to imitate the performance of the model. As a result, the child's anxiety is reduced and appropriate skills acquired.

It is important to note, however, that many of the studies reported in the literature deal with less complex social situations than those relating to school attendance. Typically, these studies concern a fear of animals (often dogs) or dental or medical procedures. Although modelling techniques have also proven valuable in work with children who lack social skills/confidence (King *et al.* 1995), many fearful situations (e.g. showering in public, going to the toilet, performing in PE) are not easily modelled. Furthermore, controlled studies of the effectiveness of this technique for cases of school refusal are very few (Kratochwill and Morris 1991).

Social skills training

Closely allied to modelling approaches, social skills training involves assisting the child to perceive and understand the behaviour of others and to respond in a more appropriate and skilled fashion. In relation to school refusal, such training is geared to help the child manage interpersonal situations more effectively, so reducing anxiety about evaluation by peers and/or teachers. Social skills training typically includes such skills as listening, non-verbal and verbal expression, recognising the position of others and self-assertion.

Cognitive behavioural therapy (CBT)

Underlying many cognitive therapy approaches is the assumption that patterns of thinking and self-statements about one's ability to cope with potentially challenging situations result in the maintenance of adverse emotions and unpleasant physical sensations and inappropriate, maladaptive patterns of behaviour. A range of approaches has been designed to tackle such faulty thinking, among the most popular being rational-emotive therapy (Ellis 1984), cognitive therapy (Beck 1976) and self-instruction training (Meichenbaum and Goodman 1971). Cognitive behaviour therapy (CBT) involves combining such approaches with behavioural techniques and a plan of action.

With regard to school refusal, such approaches operate on the basis that the child perceives an aspect of school attendance as dangerous (usually because it is considered that harm may result to the child at school or to the caregiver at home). The child does not consider himself or herself to be capable of managing the situation and as a result anxiety/fearfulness increases. By remaining at home, the problem is avoided, anxiety is reduced and school refusal is reinforced.

CBT approaches involve the clinician and child in an investigation of unhelpful, inappropriate and unrealistic beliefs that are subsequently challenged and, hopefully, replaced by new understandings. During this process the child is helped to identify and monitor self-statements that lead to anxiety or fearfulness. Maladaptive thoughts (e.g. 'My classmates will laugh at me if I answer a question incorrectly') are contrasted with competing, more positive conceptions (e.g. 'Everyone makes mistakes from time to time; other children are unlikely to take much notice of me') and the child is shown how these may alternatively result in anxiety production or reduction. Subsequently, a plan of action detailing steps to be taken in achieving a return to school is drawn up.

Although CBT for children's anxiety disorders has become increasingly popular with clinicians (Weissman *et al.* 2009), research evaluations of its effectiveness with school refusers are few and, despite enthusiastic endorsement (e.g. Doobay 2008) it remains unclear whether such approaches are more effective than other forms of intervention. While King *et al.* (1998) found gains for the approach in comparison with a control group receiving no therapeutic input, Last *et al.* (1998) found an education support group to be equally as effective. A further study of children with social phobia, rather than a more specific fear of school, found that CBT, in conjunction with a social skills training programme, resulted in significant reduction of anxiety compared to those on a waiting list (Spence *et al.* 2000). Layne *et al.* (2003) found that a combination of CBT and imipramine led to a better response to treatment than when the therapy was provided in isolation. In a detailed study of eight students, Kearney and Silverman (1999) found that the four who received behavioural interventions, closely linked to the particular functions served by their refusal, made considerably greater gains than those receiving relaxation therapy and cognitive therapy. When this latter group were subsequently provided with prescriptive behavioural interventions, gains became evident.

There is increasing interest in the use of family-focused approaches to CBT for general childhood anxiety (Wood and McLeod 2008; Wood *et al.* 2006). Long-term outcomes for both child and family-focused CBT appear to be similar (Barmish and Kendall 2005) although, in one comparative study, the family-focused approach appeared to result in more positive parental perceptions of reduction in their child's anxiety in a follow-up assessment one year later (Wood *et al.* 2009). However, these studies are concerned with a range of anxiety disorders rather than school refusal in particular, and understandings about which components of child and family-focused CBT programmes are effective for which kinds of problems are still unclear (Silverman *et al.* 2008).

Helpful guidelines using a CBT approach are available for therapists and parents (Kearney 2007b; Kearney and Albano 2007a, 2007b)

Family therapy

This technique is outlined in greater detail in Chapter 2 so will be only briefly discussed here. In the case of school refusal, the problem is often not seen as merely residing in the child, or even in the mother–child relationship, but rather as a product of faulty family functioning. Kearney and Silverman (1995) describe five differing types of family of school refusers: enmeshed and overdependent; coercive and marked by conflict; detached with little interaction among family members; isolated, with little interaction with people outside of the family; healthy families with a child with an individualised psychopathology. According to these writers, each of these types of family will require different forms of therapeutic intervention. Such interventions will also be heavily influenced by the theoretical form of family therapy to which the therapist subscribes.

It should be noted that while assessment of family functioning and some form of family work are universally advocated, it is rare that family therapy, in isolation, is seen as the preferred mode of treatment. In a survey of treatment approaches operated by a large sample of American psychologists, Kearney and Beasley (1994) found that work with families tended to focus upon parent training and contingency management; family therapy did not register as a specific treatment. It is possible, however, that a rather different picture would have emerged if psychiatrists and social workers, rather than psychologists, had been canvassed. To date, however, no large-scale studies of the efficacy of family therapy for school refusers have been published.

Medication

The primary medical intervention for children and young people who are struggling to attend school has tended to focus upon treatments for anxiety-based difficulties (Kearney 2008) although evidence for their effectiveness is limited (Tyrrell 2005). Early studies using imipramine (a tricyclic antidepressant) reported mixed results, and there is little evidence that medication alone can offer significant benefits. More recently, interest has focused upon a combination of medication with behavioural approaches and these appear more promising (Beidel *et al.* 2007). In specific cases, the medication helps to moderate anxiety symptoms as the treatment programme progresses (Keeton and Ginburg 2008), with the newer antidepressants being the first choice as these medications have fewer side effects than older preparations (Fremont 2003).

Combining methods to create individual programmes

Kearney *et al.* (2006) argue that practitioners should assess the particular functions that are served by school refusal and suggest that these are usually typified by one of four categories (see Figure 3.1). Such an assessment can provide clear guidance as to appropriate intervention. Kearney (2008) offers the following treatment suggestions:

Where school refusal is predominantly the result of a strongly phobic reaction to being in school, intervention would normally involve the gradual reduction of anxiety or fear by means of some form of desensitisation. In essence, the goal is to assist the child to be able to think of, and subsequently attend, school with progressive reduction in emotional reaction.

Where school refusal is primarily a means of avoiding social and/or evaluative situations, modelling, role play and social skills training techniques are widely advocated. In addition, counselling which aims to change the nature of the child's perceptions, thoughts and beliefs (cognitive therapy) is advocated.

Where the problem results primarily from a desire to obtain caregiver attention, parent training focusing upon the contingent use of attention and the use of reward systems is advocated. The importance of establishing set daytime routines (particularly in the morning) is emphasised. In some cases, forced school attendance is appropriate.

Where school is refused because home and the local community have more attractions (for example, television, staying in bed, playing computer games, spending time with friends), family work and the systematic use of rewards and sanctions (contingency contracting) are suggested. In such situations, there may often be conflict between family members on the appropriate way of dealing with the problem (typically, one family member advocating a 'get tough' line, another arguing for a need to be sympathetic, or even indulgent). Such conflict often provides the child with attention and an inconsistent parenting regime. The systematic and contingent use of rewards may include the use of computer/TV, pocket money, outings, toys. Sanctions for non-attendance may involve the removal of such incentives and limitations placed upon evening and weekend activities. On occasions the young person may need to be escorted to school or classes and have their attendance closely monitored. There is some evidence to suggest that this particular function for school refusal is less susceptible to intervention, perhaps because it often involves several overlapping difficulties (Evans 2000).

It is important to recognise, however, that the above approaches should not be limited to particular categories and that in many cases school refusal may result from a combination of factors. As with all problems, interventions should be closely tailored to the needs and dispositions of the individual child in a flexible and sensitive fashion. Unfortunately, our understanding of which types of intervention are most efficacious for which children with differing forms of school refusal behaviour continue to be unclear (Pina *et al.* 2009).

The role of the school in intervention

The majority of published studies and reviews have been produced by American researchers (often with a medical background) who may have little expertise or professional involvement in educational matters. The focus for these writers is usually the child and family system, and school is often taken as a given to which the child should accommodate. It is perhaps for this reason that the literature makes little reference to examining the ways by which the school can help a child to overcome a reluctance to attend. It is clear, however, that school settings where bullying, truancy or disruption proliferate, where there is rigid streaming that can result in the child being placed in a class containing a significant proportion of disaffected, alienated peers, where teacher–pupil relationships are impersonal or generally hostile, where toilets and other public areas are not closely monitored by staff, are all likely to be important factors in contributing to school refusal. In such cases operating at the level of the child and the immediate family may prove insufficient for resolving non-attendance.

The role of teachers is crucial both in identifying difficulties at an early stage and in providing as supportive and as facilitative a school environment as possible. Early signs of persistent school refusal may include occasional absences, excessive anxiety and frequent complaints about feeling unwell. Some children may seem pre-occupied with concerns about home and the well-being of family members, others may seem hypersensitive to seemingly trivial incidents in school. Given widespread agreement that a swift return to school increases the likelihood of successful reintegration, it is essential that teachers are alert to possible present or future cases of school refusal and, where the child's needs cannot be catered for by school-based personnel, readily seek the assistance of support agencies at an early stage. Where teachers, particularly those in senior management, and education social workers have a sound understanding of school refusal and appropriate intervention techniques, however, much of the early diagnostic and treatment work can be undertaken before other services become involved. Thus, training teachers in skilled and effective management of school refusal can lead to a reduction in the referral rate of school refusers to psychologists and psychiatrists (Blagg and Yule 1984). Unlike truancy, the child's absence may be explained by parents on the grounds of minor medical ailments such as head or stomach aches. In such cases school registers will indicate absence on medical grounds and scrutiny of attendance patterns by education welfare services may not identify the existence of a problem until a later, and potentially more intransigent, stage. Here, the vigilance of the school nurse may also prove particularly valuable.

In cases of school refusal, teachers also have an important role to play in managing the school environment. This may involve making short-term modifications to the child's timetable, ensuring that opportunities for the child to be unsupported in threatening situations (e.g. break-times and lunchtimes) are avoided, that inquisition of the child about recent absences is minimised, and that the child has ready access to teachers should additional guidance, support or counselling be required (Kearney and Bates 2005).

Blagg (1987) outlines a number of school-based considerations that are important for an effective return to school:

1   *Academic-related concerns.* Does the child need help to catch up with work that has been missed? Will individual tutorials by specialist teachers be necessary? Does the child have learning difficulties that will need to be addressed? Will it be possible to set up a graduated reintegration package where, initially, only some lessons will be attended? Will the child remain in school at other times?
2   *Peer-related concerns.* Are measures necessary to ensure that victimisation, in the form of bullying or taunting, does not take place? Does the child require a means of avoiding potentially threatening break-time and lunchtime settings? Are teachers aware that the child may need to have a low profile in the classroom (e.g. by avoiding situations where they are required to read aloud or answer questions in front of their classmates)?
3   *Teacher-related concerns.* Does the child have a particular anxiety about one or more teachers? Is it appropriate to change the child's class in order to accommodate specific teacher-related (or peer-related) anxieties or can the problem be resolved through other means?

It is essential that the school can provide a suitably quiet area where the child can begin the school day and be based at other times when not in class. At the early stages of reintegration it is possible that the child may show signs of panic or anger and it is advisable that an area free from onlookers is reserved for dealing with such difficulties. A trusted teacher who greets the child at the beginning of the school day and prepares him or her for entry to the classroom can help to minimise potential difficulties, as can the involvement of close friends who are sympathetic to their classmate's dilemma. At an early stage, plans should be drawn up to prevent any slips or relapses once the child begins to attend regularly again (Kearney 2001). It is important that teachers recognise that children's seemingly irrational fears are meaningful rather than dismissing them as attention-seeking or fanciful. It should be recognised that even where a child's physical discomfort does result from psychological rather than organic causes, the adversity of the experience is no less real or unpleasant. Nevertheless, while demonstrating a sensitivity to the child's feelings, it is unwise to engage in lengthy and repeated discussion with the child about these symptoms as this may have a reinforcing effect.

Where school refusal is seen as genuine by teachers, school-based factors that contribute to the problem are often de-emphasised in favour of a focus upon the excessive child–parent dependency of separation anxiety theories (King *et al.* 1995). Some teachers may fail to recognise the effect their interpersonal style has upon the highly sensitive child and find references to this, however sensitively handled, by senior colleagues or support professionals to be demeaning or inaccurate.

It is also important to be sensitive to wider, whole-school influences. A number of practitioners (Hersov 1985; Blagg 1987; King *et al.* 1995) have noted that school refusal is associated with high staff and student absenteeism rates, low levels of achievement, large class sizes, high levels of indiscipline, low staff morale, a management style characterised by authoritarianism and rigidity, and teachers who are themselves authoritarian, anxious or eager to obtain student approval. Despite such considerations, it is rare that a change of school is recommended in the literature. In cases where children do change school, difficulties often recur but are now compounded by the child's unfamiliarity with teachers and peers. A change of school is usually only advisable where the child's school refusal is wholly related to a specific educational context that is unlikely to be successfully modified. Even then, anxiety may be displaced to the new setting (see case study, Stacey, below).

Stacey, a 13-year-old girl, had displayed anxiety about attending her local secondary school after a child in another class had been murdered in front of her schoolmates by an intruder. Concurrently, she had also been subject to bullying by other girls who had teased and tormented her. After periods of sporadic attendance, marked by frequent arguments, crying fits and somatic complaints, absence became almost total. Stacey's mother (a single parent with no other children), believing that school was not recognising the nature of her daughter's difficulties, arranged for her daughter to transfer to another secondary school several miles away. As there had been no difficulties in primary school, it was anticipated that Stacey's problems would be left behind her.

At first, Stacey settled happily into her new school and enjoyed good relations with her new schoolmates. There was no recurrence of the bullying and she liked her new teachers. After four months, however, she began to become increasingly anxious before school each morning and her sleep pattern became disturbed. After six months she stopped attending school totally. Investigation by the school's educational psychologist suggested that Stacey's difficulties did not relate to a specific feature of her new school; rather, the earlier trauma had continued to haunt her. A graduated return programme, involving attendance at some lessons and, at other times, the provision of work in a quiet room, was established and appeared initially to be succeeding. After a few weeks, however, this programme failed as Stacey's mother unexpectedly withdrew her daughter from school with the stated intention of educating her at home. Mother stated that she did not have the emotional strength to continue to insist that Stacey attend school each day and could no longer cope with the stress that was being experienced at home. She then declined to have any further involvement with clinical support services.

In the light of the discussion above, this case study illustrates two important points:

1   The unwillingness of the staff at the first secondary school to demonstrate a recognition of, and sympathy towards, Stacey's difficulties alienated the family, reduced the mother's commitment to seeking a school-based solution and delayed the involvement of appropriate support agencies.
2   A change of school may not resolve a problem even if its origins are clearly located in the original setting.

Immediate or gradual return to school?

A major issue in school refusal is whether the child should be forced to return immediately or through a more graduated procedure, perhaps after a period at a specialised off-site education unit. Clearly, prolonged absence from school increases the difficulty of reintegration:

> With each day out of school more lessons are missed, difficulties in keeping up with other children mount, work accumulates, the embarrassment in finding suitable excuses for teacher and children increases, and the advantages of 'staying away from it all' become greater every day. Return to school becomes progressively more difficult. These secondary factors . . . very often overshadow the (original) cause and make it difficult to isolate the precipitating events. They may form a barrier to effective treatment.
>
> (Glaser 1959: 219)

Kennedy (1965) argues that forced procedures (technically known as *in vivo* flooding) are appropriate for school refusal, particularly for acute cases where onset is rapid and there has been no prior history of similar problems. The advantage of such an approach is that return to school can be immediately reinforced, opportunities for the child's non-attendance to be reinforced by being at home are minimised, and the problem is not compounded by the factors noted by Glaser above. Such an approach, however, can prove highly stressful for both child and parents and may be perceived as unethical by some parties. In addition, the programme may require a high level of ongoing supervision from support agencies that proves to be unavailable.

One of the strongest advocates of forced-return approaches is Blagg (1987), who outlines a detailed programme focusing upon each of the steps necessary for establishing a return to school. This outline provides helpful and practical guidance, particularly for those practitioners with limited experience of school refusal. Topics covered include: preparing the child, parents and teachers for return; establishing what changes are necessary at school and at home; establishing an effective system for ensuring the child arrives at school each day (initially, with one or more escorts); and establishing monitoring and follow-up procedures. Although forced-return approaches require that the child remain in school all day, it is accepted that the child's placement on the normal school timetable may be introduced in a step-by-step fashion.

In contrast, gradual-exposure approaches involve returning the child to school initially for those situations that cause minimal anxiety. Gradually the period in school is increased until full attendance is achieved. Often an emphasis is put upon attending for the last part of the day in order that the natural reinforcer of going home at the end of the school day is operative. This approach is generally less stressful than full forced return for the child and family, although the risks of the child's non-attendance being reinforced by spending more time at home are greater. Blagg and Yule (1984) compared the relative efficacy of differing intervention techniques for a sample of 66 children who were refusing school. Thirty children received behaviour therapy consisting of contingency contracting and enforced return to school (*in vivo* flooding), twenty received home tuition for two hours a day and psychotherapy on a fortnightly basis at a child guidance clinic. The remaining sixteen were hospitalised, received regular therapy inputs and tranquillisers as appropriate. At a one-year follow-up, the return to school group demonstrated significantly improved attendance with 93% of the sample having been judged as successfully returning to school, while the hospitalised and home tuition groups had made very little progress (38% and 10% success rates respectively). In examining attendance rates at follow-up, it was discovered that 83% of the forced-return group were attending school more than 80% of the time, while only 31% of the hospitalised group and none of the home-tuition group reached this level.

What form of intervention is the most effective?

Despite the relatively detailed literature on intervention with school refusers, it is widely noted that the vast majority of publications refer to individual or multiple case studies that, while potentially informative to clinicians have not been subject to experimental control (Pina *et al.* 2009). Often, the nature of the children's difficulties is inadequately discussed so that it is unclear to what extent problems are related to separation anxiety rather than to school-based factors. There is also no indication of the extent to which there is evidence of severe emotional difficulties, such as clinical depression. Where the outcomes of interventions have been examined (e.g. Blagg and Yule 1984), it has been assumed that school refusers are essentially alike, a proposition that does not appear to be justifiable. As Pina *et al.* (2009) note, it may be the case, for example, that a child who has difficulty making friends may respond to particular types of intervention in ways that are different to other refusers with superior social skills. A further difficulty in judging the efficacy of treatment results from the use of a number of techniques in combination (e.g. systematic desensitisation, contingency management and drug therapy). As a result, it is not easy to ascertain the unique contribution of each.

Provision for school refusers

The role of support services

In most school systems, the first point of contact with non-education professionals will typically be with either social work or medical services. In the UK or US, education social workers will often take up the child case at the outset and coordinate multi-professional involvement (Kearney and Bates 2005), often with important input from the educational (school) psychologist (Miller and Jome 2008). Depending upon local circumstances, children whose absence appears to stem from high levels of fearfulness, anxiety or depression may be referred to mental health services.

Child psychiatry services typically incorporate a range of different professionals, such as psychiatrists, psychologists, social workers, occupational therapists, nurses and child therapists. Most of the techniques outlined in this chapter may be undertaken by any of these professionals, although emphases will differ. It is likely, for example, that the educational (school) psychologist would have a greater role in addressing important school-based factors (e.g. exploring how the child may be assisted with academic difficulties) whereas the child psychiatrist would be more likely to be closely involved in working with medical colleagues and in prescribing medication. Given the differing perspectives that can be held by professionals involved in tackling school refusal, it is essential that close liaison exists and opportunities for the provision of conflicting advice are minimised. As Blagg (1987) notes, a failure to achieve such liaison can result in the anxious parent becoming even more confused and unsure how to proceed. Furthermore, it may help the resistant parent to ignore any recommendations for action. Blagg recommends that educational psychologists, by virtue of their educational and clinical expertise, are best placed to coordinate multi-professional involvement, although changes in UK educational psychologists' work patterns have made this more problematic. Particular stresses result from the pressure upon educational psychology services to undertake increasing numbers of statutory assessments of children with special educational needs and the widespread use of time-contracting, by which educational psychologist time is allocated to each school on a pro rata basis. These factors often reduce the educational psychologist's availability and flexibility in responding to individual cases. There may be little time for intensive, ongoing casework and this may preclude the psychologist from monitoring the child's progress and intervening where necessary on a sufficiently intensive basis.

Provision alternative to school

Home tuition

In some countries, local authorities will provide home tuition for school refusers. This may involve a visit to the home by a peripatetic support teacher for one or two sessions per week with periodic review by an education social worker or educational psychologist. Given that Blagg and Yule's (1984) study found home tuition with psychotherapy to be a highly unsuccessful technique (to such an extent that the authors queried whether this might have even inhibited spontaneous remission), there must be serious doubts as to the efficacy of such an approach. Where such provision is complemented by local authority support services working actively to ensure a return to school, the prognosis may be more favourable (see, for example, Tansey 1995).

Hospitalisation

Inpatient treatment for school refusal is exceedingly rare in the United Kingdom although part-time placement in child psychiatry department day units is more widely employed. Usually, such treatment is associated with more severe symptoms, particularly depression, and greater incidence of family disruption and dysfunction (Borchardt et al. 1994).

Berg (1991) states that while it may be difficult to get the child to accept admission to hospital, once achieved, emotional upset usually improves and a graduated return to school can be planned. The relatively generous availability of psychiatric staff permits support in escorting the child to school and in the provision of a range of appropriate therapies. Murphy and Wolkind (1996) support the use of hospitalisation where other approaches have failed, the child is becoming increasingly anxious or depressed and/or parents have effectively lost control of their child. They add, however, that potential dangers of this procedure are that hospitalisation can increase the likelihood that the child becomes scapegoated for all the family's problems and is emotionally or physically excluded. In return, the hospitalised child may feel rejected by the family and hostile to its members.

Outcomes

As noted above, the likelihood of a positive outcome appears to be related to the severity of the disorder, the age of onset, and the immediacy of treatment intervention. In addition, susceptibility to treatment is greatly reduced where the refusal has persisted for two or more years (Kearney and Tillotson 1998). Studies of adults suffering from neurotic disorders (particularly agoraphobia) indicate that a significant number were school refusers as adolescents (e.g. Berg *et al.* 1974). A number of studies have followed up school refusers in adulthood (e.g. Berg and Jackson 1985; Flakierska *et al.* 1988, 1997). McShane *et al.* (2001, 2004) followed up 117 school refusers six months and three years after treatment. Their findings (see also McCune and Hynes 2005; Kearney 2001) reflect a general picture which suggests that approximately one-third of cases continues to experience severe emotional disorders and/or problematic social relationships into adulthood, although it should be noted that samples often contain children who were hospitalised – usually the most severe cases.

References

Atkinson, L., Quarrington, B. and Cyr, J.J. (1985). School refusal: the heterogeneity of a concept. *American Journal of Orthopsychiatry* 55: 83–101.

Barmish, A.J., and Kendall, P.C. (2005). Should parents be co-clients in cognitive-behavioural therapy for anxious youth? *Journal of Clinical Child and Adolescent Psychology* 34: 569–81.

Beck, A.T. (1976). *Cognitive Therapy and the Emotional Disorders*. New York: International Universities Press.

Beidel, D.C., Turner, S.M., Sallee, F.R. *et al.* (2007). SET-C versus fluoxetine in the treatment of childhood social phobia. *Journal of the American Academy of Child and Adolescent Psychiatry* 46: 1622–32.

Berg, I. (1970). A follow-up study of school phobic adolescents admitted to an inpatient unit. *Journal of Child Psychology and Psychiatry* 11: 37–47.

Berg, I. (1991). School avoidance, school phobia and truancy. In M. Lewis (ed.) *Child and Adolescent Psychiatry: A Comprehensive Textbook*. London: Williams & Wilkins.

Berg, I. and Jackson, A. (1985). Teenage school refusers grow up: A follow-up study of 168 subjects, ten years on average after inpatient treatment. *British Journal of Psychiatry* 119: 167–8.

Berg, I., Nichols, K. and Pritchard, C. (1969). School phobia: Its classification and relationship to dependency. *Journal of Child Psychology and Psychiatry* 10: 123–41.

Berg, I., Marks, I., McGuire, R. *et al.* (1974). School phobia and agoraphobia. *Psychological Medicine* 4: 428–34.

Blagg, N. (1987). *School Phobia and its Treatment*. London: Croom Helm.

Blagg, N. and Yule, W. (1984). The behavioural treatment of school refusal: A comparative study. *Behaviour Research and Therapy* 22: 119–27.

Bools, C., Foster, J., Brown, I. *et al.* (1990). The identification of psychiatric disorders in children who fail to attend school: A cluster analysis of a non-clinical population. *Psychological Medicine* 20: 171–81.

Borchardt, C.M., Giesler, J., Bernstein, G.A. *et al.* (1994). A comparison of inpatient and outpatient school refusers. *Child Psychiatry and Human Development* 24(4): 255–64.

Bouchard, S. (2011). Could virtual reality be effective in treating children with phobias? *Expert Review of Neurotherapeutics* 11(2): 207–13.

Broadwin, I.T. (1932). A contribution to the study of truancy. *American Journal of Orthopsychiatry* 2: 253–9.

Doobay, A.F. (2008). School refusal behavior associated with separation anxiety disorder: A cognitive-behavioral approach to treatment. *Psychology in the Schools* 45(4): 261–72.

Elliott, J.G. (1999). Practitioner review: School refusal: Issues of conceptualisation, assessment and treatment. *Journal of Child Psychology and Psychiatry* 40: 1001–12.

Ellis, A. (1984). *Rational-emotive Therapy and Cognitive Behaviour Therapy*. New York: Springer.

Evans, L.D. (2000). Functional school refusal subtypes: Anxiety, avoidance and malingering. *Psychology in the Schools* 37: 183–91.

Flakierska, N., Linstrom, M. and Gillberg, C. (1988). School refusal: A 15–20-year follow-up study of 35 Swedish urban children. *British Journal of Psychiatry* 152: 834–7.

Flakierska, N., Linstrom, M. and Gillberg, C. (1997). School phobia with separation anxiety disorder: A comparative 20–29-year follow-up study of 35 school refusers. *Comprehensive Psychiatry* 38: 17–22.

Fremont, W.P. (2003). School refusal in children and adolescents. *American Family Physician* 68: 1555–60.

Galloway, D. (1983). Truants and other absentees. *Journal of Child Psychology and Psychiatry* 24(4): 607–11.

Glaser, K. (1959). Problems in school attendance: School phobia and related conditions. *Pediatrics* 23: 371–83.

Gutiérrez-Maldonado, J., Magallón-Neri, E., Rus-Calafell, M. *et al.* (2009). Virtual reality exposure therapy for school phobia. *Anuario de Psicología* 40(2): 223–36.

Hersov, L. (1977). School refusal. In M. Rutter and L. Hersov (eds) *Child Psychiatry. Modern Approaches*. Oxford: Blackwell.

Hersov, L. (1985). School refusal. In M. Rutter and L. Hersov (eds) *Child and Adolescent Psychiatry: Modern Approaches*, Second edition. Oxford: Blackwell.

Johnson, A.M. (1957). School phobia. *American Journal of Orthopsychiatry* 27: 307–9.

Johnson, A.M., Falstein, E.I., Szurek, S.A. *et al.* (1941). School phobia. *American Journal of Orthopsychiatry* 11: 702–11.

Kearney, C.A. (2001). *School Refusal Behavior in Youth: A Functional Approach to Assessment and Treatment*. Washington, DC: American Psychological Association.

Kearney, C.A. (2002). Identifying the function of school refusal behavior: A revision of the School Refusal Assessment Scale. *Journal of Psychopathology and Behavioral Assessment* 24: 235–45.

Kearney, C.A. (2007a). Forms and functions of school refusal behavior in youth: An empirical analysis of absenteeism severity. *Journal of Child Psychology and Psychiatry* 48(1): 53–61.

Kearney, C.A. (2007b). *Getting Your Child to Say 'Yes' to School: A Guide for Parents of Youth with School Refusal Behavior*. New York: Oxford University Press.

Kearney, C.A. (2008). School absenteeism and school refusal behavior in youth: A contemporary review, *Clinical Psychology Review* 28(3), 451–71.

Kearney, C.A. and Albano, A.M. (2007a). *When Children Refuse School: A Cognitive-Behavioral Therapy Approach Parent's Workbook*, Second edition. New York: Oxford University Press.

Kearney, C.A. and Albano, A.M. (2007b). *When Children Refuse School: A Cognitive-Behavioral Therapy Approach Therapist's Guide*, Second edition. New York: Oxford University Press.

Kearney, C.A. and Bates, M. (2005). Addressing school refusal behavior. Suggestions for frontline professionals. *Children and Schools* 27: 207–16.

Kearney, C.A. and Beasley, J.F. (1994). The clinical treatment of school refusal behavior: A survey of referral and practice characteristics. *Psychology in the Schools* 31: 128–32.

Kearney, C.A. and Silverman, W.K. (1993). Measuring the function of school refusal behaviour: The School Refusal Assessment Scale. *Journal of Clinical Child Psychology* 22: 85–96.

Kearney, C.A. and Silverman, W.K. (1995). Family environment of youngsters with school refusal behavior. *American Journal of Family Therapy* 23(1): 59–72.

Kearney, C.A. and Silverman, W.K. (1999). Functionally based prescriptive and nonprescriptive treatment for children and adolescents with school refusal behavior. *Behaviour Therapy* 30: 673–93.

Kearney, C.A. and Tillotson, C.A. (1998). School attendance. In D. Watson and M. Gresham (eds) *Handbook of Child Behavior Therapy* (pp. 143–61). New York: Plenum Press.

Kearney, C.A., Lemos, A. and Silverman, W.K. (2006). School refusal behavior. In R.B. Mennuti, A. Freeman and R.W. Christner (eds), *Cognitive-Behavioral Interventions in Educational Settings: A Handbook for Practice* (pp. 89–105). New York: Brunner-Routledge.

Keeton, C.P. and Ginsburg, G.S. (2008). Combining and sequencing medication and cognitive-behaviour therapy for childhood anxiety disorders. *International Review of Psychiatry* 20: 159–64.

Kennedy, W.A. (1965). School phobia: Rapid treatment of fifty cases. *Journal of Abnormal Psychology* 70: 285–9.

King, N., Ollendick, T.H. and Tonge, B.J. (1995). *School Refusal: Assessment and Treatment*. Boston: Allyn & Bacon.

King, N., Ollendick, T.H., Murphy, G.C. and Molloy, G.N. (1998). Relaxation training with children. *British Journal of Educational Psychology* 68: 53–66.

Knollman, M., Knoll, S., Reissner, V. *et al.* (2010). School avoidance from the point of view of child and adolescent psychiatry. *Deutsches Ärzteblatt International* 107(4): 43–9.

Kovacs, M. and Beck, A.T. (1977). An empirical-clinical approach toward a definition of childhood depression. In J.G. Schulterbrandt and A. Raskin (eds) *Depression in Childhood: Diagnosis, Treatment, and Conceptual Models*. New York: Raven Press.

Kratochwill, T.R. and Morris, R.J. (eds) (1991). *The Practice of Child Therapy*. New York: Pergamon Press.

La Greca, A.M. and Stone, W.L. (1993). Social anxiety scale for children – revised: Factor structure and concurrent validity. *Journal of Clinical Child Psychology* 22: 17–27.

Last, C.G. and Francis, G. (1988). School phobia. In B.B. Lahey and A.E. Kazdin (eds) *Advances in Clinical Child Psychology*, vol. II. New York: Plenum.

Last, C.G., Hansen, M.S. and Franco, N. (1998). Cognitive-behavioral treatment of school phobia. *Journal of the American Academy of Child and Adolescent Psychiatry* 37: 404–11.

Last, C.G., Francis, G., Hersen, M. *et al.* (1987). Separation anxiety and school phobia: A comparison using DSM-III criteria. *American Journal of Psychiatry* 144: 653–7.

Layne, A.E., Bernstein, G.A., Egan, E.A. *et al.* (2003). Predictors of treatment response in anxious-depressed adolescents with school refusal. *Journal of the American Academy of Child and Adolescent Psychiatry* 42(3): 319–26.

Lazarus, A.A. and Abramovitz, A. (1962). The use of 'emotive imagery' in the treatment of children's phobias. *Journal of Mental Science* 108: 191–5.

Lyon, A.R. and Cotler, S. (2007). Toward reduced bias and increased utility in the assessment of school refusal behavior: The case for diverse samples and evaluations of context. *Psychology in the Schools* 44(6): 551–65.

McCune, N. and Hynes, J. (2005). Ten year follow-up of children with school refusal. *Irish Journal of Psychological Medicine* 22: 56–8.

McShane, G., Walter, G. and Rey, J.M. (2001). Characteristics of adolescents with school refusal. *Australian and New Zealand Journal of Psychiatry* 35: 822–6.

McShane, G., Walter, G. and Rey, J.M. (2004). Functional outcomes of adolescents with 'school refusal'. *Clinical Child Psychology and Psychiatry* 9: 53–60.

Meichenbaum, D.H. and Goodman, J. (1971). Training impulsive children to talk to themselves: A means of developing self-control. *Journal of Abnormal Psychology* 77: 115–26.

Miller, D.N. and Jome, L.M. (2008). School psychologists and the assessment of childhood internalizing disorders. *School Psychology International* 29(4): 500–10.

Murphy, M. and Wolkind, S. (1996). The role of the child and adolescent psychiatrist. In I. Berg and J. Nursten (eds) *Unwillingly to School*, Fourth edition. London: Gaskell.

Ollendick, T.H. (1983). Reliability and validity of the Revised Fear Survey Schedule for Children (FSSC-R). *Behaviour Research and Therapy* 21, 685–92.

Ollendick, T.H. and Mayer, J.A. (1984). School phobia. In S.M. Turner (ed.) *Behavioral Theories and Treatment of Anxiety*. New York: Plenum.

Pilkington, C. and Piersel, W.C. (1991). School phobia: a critical analysis of the separation anxiety theory and an alternative conceptualization. *Psychology in the Schools* 28: 290–303.

Pina, A.A., Zerr, A.A., Gonzales, N.A. and Ortiz, C.D. (2009). Psychosocial interventions for school refusal behavior in children and adolescents. *Child Development Perspectives* 3(1): 11–20.

Reynolds, C.R. and Paget, K.D. (1983). National normative and reliability data for the Revised Children's Manifest Anxiety Scale. *School Psychology Review* 12: 324–36.

Silverman, W.K., Pina, A.A. and Viswesvaran, C. (2008). Evidence-based psychosocial treatments for phobic and anxiety disorders in children and adolescents. *Journal of Clinical Child and Adolescent Psychology* 37: 105–30.

Smith, S.L. (1970). School refusal with anxiety: A review of sixty-three cases. *Canadian Psychiatry Association Journal* 15: 257–64.

Spence, S.H., Donovan, C. and Brechman-Toussaint, M. (2000). The treatment of childhood social phobia: The effectiveness of a social skills training-based, cognitive behavioural intervention, with and without parental involvement. *Journal of Child Psychology and Psychiatry* 41: 713–26.

Steinhausen, H., Müller, N. and Metzke, C.W. (2008). Frequency, stability and differentiation of self-reported school fear and truancy in a community sample. *Child and Adolescent Psychiatry and Mental Health* 2(17): DOI: 10.1186/1753-2000-2-17.

Tansey, K. (1995). This can't be my responsibility: It must be yours! An analysis of a reintegration programme for a school refuser. *British Journal of Special Education* 22(1): 12–15.

Trueman, D. (1984). What are the characteristics of school phobic children? *Psychological Reports* 54: 191–202.

Tyrrell, M. (2005). School phobia. *Journal of School Nursing* 21: 147–51.

Weissman, A.S., Antinoro, D. and Chu, B.C. (2009). Cognitive behavioral therapy for anxious youth in school settings. In M. Mayer, R. Van Acker, J.E. Lochman and F.M. Gresham (eds), *Cognitive-Behavioral Interventions for Emotional and Behavior Disorders* (pp. 173–203). New York: Guilford Press.

Wiederhold, B.K. and Wiederhold, M. (2005). *Virtual Reality Therapy for Anxiety Disorders: Advances in Evaluation and Treatment*. Washington, DC: American Psychological Association.

Wood, J.J., and McLeod, B.D. (2008). *Child Anxiety Disorders: A Family-based Treatment Manual for Practitioners*. Norton: New York.

Wood, J.J., McLeod, B.D., Piacentini, J.C. *et al.* (2009). One year follow-up of family versus child CBT for anxiety disorders: Exploring the roles of child age and parental intrusiveness. *Child Psychiatry and Human Development* 40: 301–16.

Wood, J.J., Piacentini, J.C., Southam-Gerow, M. *et al.* (2006). Family cognitive behavioral therapy for child anxiety disorders. *Journal of the American Academy for Child and Adolescent Psychiatry* 45: 314–21.

Chapter 4

Oppositional defiance, conduct and attachment disorders

Attachment and its impact upon child development

An area that is now recognised to be of great influence upon a person's long-term functioning is their capacity to form meaningful attachments. Attachment is defined as a 'lasting psychological connectedness between human beings' (Bowlby 1969). It fosters a sense of security by maintaining proximity – giving a firm base from which to learn about wider environments. It gives a sense of 'felt' security and provides the internal representation upon which to model all future relationships. Having a sense of secure attachment allows the child to correctly recognise emotions, show empathy and behave morally. It also makes a significant contribution towards helping the child develop feelings of self-worth and develop a positive view about life. Indeed it is one of the most important building blocks for human development, because it establishes the internal working models of emotional experiences and significant relationships (Bowlby 1980).

Of all bonds that contribute to the sense of attachment, the mother-infant bond is the most crucial. A mother's sensitivity to her infant's needs is a critical factor for the establishment of a secure attachment (De Wolff and van Ijzendoorn 1997), but the development of attachment is not a passive process. The parental reactions shape the infant's behaviour, but it is also the positive responses from the infant that in turn shape the parent's responding behaviour. Mutual satisfaction and enjoyment must exist between mother and infant if a positive and strong attachment capacity is to be established. It is also worthy of note that father-child attachments have the same impact as mother-child attachments (Brumariu and Kerns 2010).

From the age of about 3 months the infant becomes increasingly aware of this subtle communication. As the parent responds to the child's needs, the child detects warmth and affection from the parent, and begins to develop trust in their carer, an essential foundation upon which all subsequent development hinges. Specific interactions necessary in the development of the parent-child bond include eye contact, skin-to-skin contact, rocking and vocalisations.

The structure provided by Erikson (1969) that was described in Chapter 1 illustrates the importance of parenting in the early stages of this process. The attachment stages can be viewed in three phases, the first of which is the pre-attachment phase of the newborn. From 6 weeks to 6 months the infant shows a growing sense of recognition of their main caregiver but, there is no separation anxiety, suggesting that attachment capacity formation is yet to truly commence. Between 6 months and 2 years the capacity for attachment is being developed and separation anxiety is evident when the principle caregiver is absent. The situation is consolidating over the next year, and from the age of 3 years the capacity for attachment formation is established and utilised. The potential for varying the timing of these stages is probably quite limited (Upton and Sullivan 2010), making any disruption to the process quite critical.

Positive attachment in mothers can be demonstrated by seeing specific brain activation when they are shown their own children's pictures being settled or crying. Also, early maternal separation produces enduring changes to various brain structures, some of which may not become evident until adulthood (Andersen and Teicher 2004).

Impact of attachment failings

As the knowledge about this crucial developmental stage has increased the impact of disruption has gradually been recognised. Children whose parenting has been abusive or rejecting show avoidant attachment – their behaviour is confusing and contradictory. A burst of anger may be followed by a sudden frozen watchfulness, and they will, without fear, ask to be taken home by a stranger. These children are unable to regulate emotions and are prone to impulsive, often violent behaviour, and respond poorly to environmental stress and challenges (Oosterman et al. 2010). They also show features of disorders such as anxiety and depression (Brumariu and Kerns 2010).

As they get older, children with damaged attachment capacity show an increasing inability to form normal relationships with others, with a pattern of behaviours that can include:

- superficially engaging and charming;
- indiscriminately affectionate with strangers;
- destructive of self, others, things;
- developmental lags;
- avoids direct eye contact;
- not cuddly with parents;
- cruel to animals, siblings;
- poor peer relations;
- inappropriately demanding or clingy;
- stealing, lying;
- lack of conscience about misbehaviour;
- persistent nonsense questions or incessant chatter;
- poor impulse control;
- abnormal speech patterns;
- fights for control over everything;
- hoardes or gorges on food;
- preoccupation with fire, blood or gore.

Often the pace of emergence of these difficulties accelerates in adolescence, and the difficulties that stem from it tend to recur throughout their lives. When they are teenagers and young adults they are likely to have romantic relationships which are punctuated by violent and abusive episodes (Riggs *et al.* 1990). They are particularly prone to depression, and various forms of mental health problems later in life (Belsky *et al.* 2007), as well as commonly having aggressive outbursts (Frazzetto *et al.* 2007). When they themselves become parents they often have poorer parenting practices, and find it difficult to develop emotional attachments with their own children (Broussard and Cassidy 2010).

The impact of life stresses upon this process increases with their severity (Rutter *et al.* 2006), but if toddlerhood is without major incident, and the negative experiences begin later in life then the risk of disturbing attachment markedly decreases (Lynch and Cicchetti 1991). These observations add weight to the importance that early environmental experiences have on the attachment formation process, and upon the developing brain (see Chapter 1).

Family and environmental issues

The fundamental influence upon attachment capacity formation is the family, and in particular the main caregiving parent. Children who have significant upheavals of parenting in the first three years of life experience disruption to this process. If the maltreatment is associated with socioeconomic risks such as poverty, then the risk of damaged attachment increases (Cyr *et al.* 2010). The intensity of these difficulties is positively associated with the duration of the child's exposure to severe deprivation, although not all children who suffer severe deprivation develop an attachment disorder (O'Connor *et al.* 2000).

As described above, attachment is an interactive process and requires both parent and infant to positively participate. For instance, research suggests that cocaine-exposed mothers, even when not actively using the drug, may be less able to respond appropriately to their infants' cues, or may find these interactions less intrinsically rewarding. Also cocaine disrupts the brain circuits that normally regulate parenting, because infant cues, such as facial expressions and cries, activate the same brain reward regions as does cocaine (Swain *et al.* 2007).

Hormonal mechanisms that influence attachment

The mechanisms that bring about these changes in attachment capacity formation are gradually being understood through a strand of research described as stress neurobiology. It has been known for some time that emotional stress changes our brain chemistry, the main mechanism of which is the hypothalamic–pituitary–adrenal (HPA) axis. This involves many hormones but one of the most studied is cortisol, which has a major role in helping the body respond to stress (see Chapter 6).

Behavioural difficulties have been shown to be linked to having an unusually low cortisol level in the morning (Luijk *et al.* 2010), and it is now clear that the levels of cortisol in the newborn are influenced by their mother's levels of cortisol (Stenius et al. 2008), especially if the mother has mental health problems (Oberlander et al. 2008), or she herself has been the victim of abuse (Rice and Records 2008).

Dopamine has also been shown to be influential in mediating the impact of early life experiences (Schultz 2006), particularly through its role in giving a sense of reward for carrying out positive actions (McClure et al. 2003). It is a mechanism that is particularly active during attachment capacity formation (Lorberbaum et al. 2002), with positive maternal care increasing dopamine activity in the mother (Champagne et al. 2004). However, repeated maternal separations reduce dopamine levels in both the infant and the mother (Pruessner et al. 2004).

Oxytocin has long been recognised as significant in birth. It is important in forming social and spatial memories, and in emotional regulation (Kirsch et al. 2005). It also increases nurturing behaviour between a mother and her infant (Insel and Young 2001). Suckling and offering positive maternal care increase the mother's levels of oxytocin, and explains the positive link between breastfeeding and a reduced risk of behavioural problems in the child (Heikkilä et al. 2011). It has a significant role in developing a sense of trust (Petrovic et al. 2008), a key element in positive attachment capacity formation.

Given that most of the research has been focused upon maternal responses, what about fathers? The small amount of work that has been done shows that both mothers and fathers show higher concentrations of cortisol in the period just before the birth, and lower post-natal concentrations of sex hormones (Storey et al. 2000). Work with fathers has shown that these lowered levels of testosterone increase the father's need to respond to infants when they cry (Fleming et al. 2002).

Genetic issues that influence attachment

A further element of this complex story comes from work which is trying to understand mechanisms by which genetic predisposition and environmental factors interact to influence nurturing parental behaviour. Of interest in the area of child neglect and abuse is the work of Caspi and his colleagues (Caspi et al. 2002), which looked at the genetic mechanism that controls monoamine oxidase A (MAOA), an enzyme that destroys amines, and is significant in regulating emotion. Low MAOA activity in children who are maltreated significantly increases the likelihood of antisocial behaviour, whereas in children who are not abused, the low MAOA has little effect on behaviour (Kim-Cohen et al. 2006). The timing of the abuse may also be important (Andersen and Teicher 2004).

Similar interest has been focused upon another genetic marker, the DRD4 7-repeat polymorphism. This appears to make infants vulnerable to difficulties if they receive poor parenting (van Ijzendoorn and Bakermans-Kranenburg 2006), and is also a marker for the quality of attachment that adults themselves received (Reiner and Spangler 2010).

Studies have also looked at subtle changes on the gene itself – known as polymorphisms – and the way the environment influences gene expression (epigenetics) is of growing importance as the mechanism by which poor care in one generation is transmitted to the next by changing the infant's response to stressful situations (Weaver *et al.* 2004) (see Chapter 1).

Interventions

A child with attachment difficulties is persistently frustrating, and emotionally demanding, and parents can quickly become exhausted in trying to maintain appropriate limits and boundaries. Carers need to demonstrate patience, and make a concerted effort to provide a calm, yet firm approach to managing the child. The adults must:

- have realistic expectations of the child's behaviour;
- have patience;
- have the ability to stay positive and hopeful;
- set consistent limits and boundaries;
- remain calm when the child is upset or misbehaving;
- be able to immediately emotionally reconnect with the child following a conflict;
- maintain predictable routines and schedules;
- demonstrate emotional care;
- respond to the child's emotional age;
- help the child identify emotions and express his or her needs appropriately.

These requirements, while features of good parenting, are essential for children with attachment problems, and are very difficult to maintain against the persistent background of challenge, and threat that such children present.

As they grow up, these children and young people have a myriad problems to deal with, but it appears that living in a stable placement helps them function much better as an adult. In view of this need for persistent and intensive positive parenting there has been growing interest in the potential benefit of alternative family care, either through foster care or adoption. Given the process and timing for attachment capacity formation, it is perhaps not surprising that children placed before 12 months are more likely to eventually have more secure attachments than children placed later in life (van Ijzendoorn and Juffer 2006).

Whatever the type of placement, alternative carers benefit from training and advice about positive management of children with attachment difficulties. These children bring to their new placements the strategies that have helped them cope with and, to an extent, survive their abusive and neglectful family life (Allen and Vostanis 2005). It is also important to recognise that the attitude to the child of the new parental figures can be hugely influential on the success of the placement.

It is the nature of attachment difficulties that they are relatively resistant to therapeutic work. An attachment-based intervention which focuses upon improving parent sensitivity, and promoting the sense of secure attachment, can lead to improved functioning. However the evidence is that an exclusive focus on improving parent sensitivity is not sufficient to reduce the main behavioural difficulties (Bakermans-Kranenburg *et al.* 2003); rather it is also management of the day-to-day living experience that helps such children achieve a better pattern of functioning.

Recognising that these children have significant difficulties with managing emotion and with eliciting care and attention in an appropriate and positive way, there have been several specific therapies developed to help children and their new families improve their emotional regulation. These usually involve correcting unacceptable behaviour, and advising about alternative responses within the context of a safe relationship (Redl and Wineman 1952). This type of intervention needs to be delivered carefully, for it is the non-verbal messages that the child will register rather than the explicit ones, because children who have been maltreated tend to process actions not words (Schore 2001).

These interventions also have a behavioural component which offer effective interventions for unacceptable behaviours. For instance, they demonstrate how to deal with rather paradoxical responses, such as when a child becomes angry even though the carer's aim is to offer comfort and solace. Such interventions are on a continuum which, at its most extreme, takes the form of 'holding therapy'. Here the child is held for periods in an effort to erode their belief that parents will not persist in being caring. This approach has been heavily criticised (e.g. O'Connor and Zeanah 2003) and is not generally considered mainstream practice.

More appropriate is the approach based around positive parenting. This develops a persistent, sensitive response to emotional needs while demonstrating great consistency of management. It is generally combined with elements such as providing the child with multisensory and stimulating experiences, or play activities which focus around the child's developmental age rather than their chronological one (Howe and Fearnley 2003). Experience with children who have been adopted from institutions has found that difficulties may be reduced by initially offering care that mimics early life experiences, such as offering close physical contact, reducing exposure to stressful situations and, in the early stages of placement, co-sleeping and regressed feeding patterns (Gribble 2007).

Alongside such positive life experiences the child usually requires specific and focused therapeutic work. This is often quite lengthy, with the progress being marked by quite small, but significant improvements.

As well as psychological interventions there may be benefit in medication programmes, especially if there are other conditions that are exacerbating the attachment difficulties. If impulsive behaviour becomes too troublesome, stimulant medication can reduce its expression, and if violent episodes become a major issue then there are medications that can be considered (Findling 2008).

Jay was adopted at the age of 11, having spent his early years with his parents who made several moves of home and area throughout that time. Both had significant mental health problems, and in addition Jay's father was a heavy user of drugs, and there were several episodes where he was imprisoned because of violent outbursts. Jay's mother drank heavily, and although Jay had several brief periods in foster care, by regularly moving area, definitive intervention to remove Jay was not achieved until he was 5 years of age. His foster placement quickly broke down because he was violent and aggressive whenever the carers attempted to limit or correct his actions, and his school quickly adopted a regime which had Jay spending the day in the headmaster's office.

The next foster placement saw a reduction in his outbursts, but found his persistent negative attitude quite emotionally draining, and after two years he moved to another foster carer, which also necessitated a change of school. This school had little difficulty with his behaviour, and within his foster placement he showed more response to adult wishes, though he could become very angry and destructive over very trivial issues. Because there was an association between such episodes and contact with his mother it was decided this should cease, and the episodes did show a reduction after this was achieved.

At the age of 11 Jay was adopted, and for the first year his behaviour both at home and at school was positive and settled. There then began to emerge explosive outbursts of temper which could last for up to two hours and during which Jay smashed furniture, kicked doors, and resisted any efforts at being offered comfort. Afterwards he would sob and permit his adoptive parents to hold him and would then usually fall asleep.

Jay commenced an individual sequence of psychotherapy, which focused on his understanding of emotion, and how this was expressed. Over time, issues around his early life experiences, his sense of abandonment by his parents, his confusion that he was angry with adults for whom he should care, and his bewilderment at how to respond to parents who care were all explored. After three years his behaviour could still show episodes of destructive anger, but these were brief and occurring only sporadically.

Jay's difficulties were eased by the therapeutic process, and his positive success within the school environment offered an element of resilience and a source of positive self-image. However his functioning was still emotionally troubled at times, and he had only a limited understanding of relationships.

Outcome

Children whose early life experiences have been so poor that their attachment capacity has been significantly damaged usually spend a significant period of their childhood in alternative care settings. If very young they tend to be placed with permanent families and many go on to have very settled and positive developmental experiences (Triseliotis 2002), with children placed for adoption before 12 months of age showing better physical and emotional adjustment than children placed at an older age (van Ijzendoorn and Juffer 2006).

The results from psychotherapy with such children show that they gradually do develop a degree of secure attachment, and achieve a more appropriate understanding of families and parents (Steele et al. 2010). However this improvement is not complete, and children with attachment difficulties tend to be very vulnerable to mood disorders and substance abuse as they get older, and these are intrinsic difficulties, not merely problems prompted by the memory of abuse (Scott et al. 2010).

As adults such experiences can also exert long-term difficulties, with a third of adults with depression attributing their illness to adverse childhood experiences (Danese *et al.* 2009), and many having long-term physical health difficulties (Irish *et al.* 2010).

Oppositional defiance and conduct disorder

Oppositional or noncompliant behaviour is common in childhood, but if severe can become problematic. The child watching the television who does not 'hear' the call for bed, or the child who won't turn down the volume on the radio, are failing to comply with adult instructions or requests.

Simon was an 8-year-old boy who, although highly intelligent and generally friendly with visitors, frequently found himself in conflict with parents and teachers. At home he repeatedly engaged in a variety of attention-seeking behaviours such as waving household materials in front of an open fire, switching television channels with the remote control and jumping on the furniture. When admonished by his mother he immediately sought to engage her in an argument and clearly delighted in her subsequent inability to manage him.

Part of understanding whether such behaviour should require professional intervention is assessing where it fits with the developmental processes that a child undergoes. The infant years are marked by a growing sense of individuation and autonomy and, as such, the emergence of oppositional behaviour in the toddler is age-appropriate, and largely desirable. Stable individual differences in anger expression emerge towards the end of the first year, and in the second year conflict, anger, and aggression increase in frequency and intensity. For most infants, physical aggression decreases between 2 and 4 years of age, while non-compliance increases as an age-appropriate expression of emerging independence. Subsequently, direct defiance decreases as the young child acquires more mature forms of self-assertion, a development which coincides with the growth in language ability. These patterns of behaviour remain relatively stable until adolescence, with about 25% of children showing persistent features of non-compliance (Johnson *et al.* 1973). However even with this developmentally appropriate pattern of physical aggression, less than 10% of toddlers are reported by their parents to 'often' hit others (Wakschlag *et al.* 2010).

There are relatively few sex differences in this behaviour in infancy, but from 4 years of age girls show increasingly less physical aggression, with social aggression becoming the typical behavioural concern (Crick and Zahn-Waxler 2003). The phase of social consolidation that follows is dependent upon having positive social interaction, and learning how to achieve goals through non-aggressive means. Success with these developing social skills reinforces the potential value of delaying gratification, and also contributes to the development of managing emotional situations appropriately, elements of the child's emerging executive function (Schultz *et al.* 2004).

It is those children whose oppositional behaviour appears particularly intense or long-lasting who become the subject of parental and professional concern. These children also cause a wider degree of difficulty within their community. Their actions and behaviour within school significantly decrease their peers' academic focus, and their presence is associated with increased misbehaviour generally within the classroom (Carrell and Hoekstra 2009). However the principal concerns have to be for the index child because the early emergence of behavioural problems has been shown to be the most important predictor of future delinquency, violence and substance abuse (Snyder 2001). Given this scenario, the importance of intervening at an early stage is clear.

Reaching a diagnosis

Disruptive behaviour can stem from a variety of sources. Oppositional defiance disorder (ODD), conduct disorder (CD) and attention deficit hyperactivity disorder (ADHD) can all present with disruptive behaviour. Delinquency is a term used for conduct difficulties that have come to the notice of the legal authorities. ODD is 'a recurrent pattern of negativistic, defiant, disobedient and hostile behaviour toward authority figures that persists for at least six months' (American Psychiatric Association 1994). These behaviours must occur more frequently than is typically observed in individuals of comparable age, and at a similar developmental level. Furthermore, they must lead to significant impairment in social, academic or occupational functioning. If, in addition, there is aggression towards others, the destruction of property, theft or deceit, then the child is considered to be showing a conduct disorder.

ODD and CD are increasingly being viewed as a continuum. Young people with severe conduct traits often have difficulty understanding and processing emotional information, and struggle to correctly recognise facial expressions. However it is interesting to note that the one facial expression they can accurately recognise is that of fear (Woodworth and Waschbusch 2008).

Prevalence

Estimates as to the prevalence of major behavioural difficulties depend upon the community and culture. In Western society, CD and ODD affects 8.1% of boys and 2.8% of girls aged between 11 and 16 (Green et al. 2005). The nature of these difficulties also changes with the child's age. The frequency of physical aggression decreases substantially from the preschool years to the end of adolescence, while the frequency of theft increases from 10 onwards (Tremblay 2010).

Impact of the disorder

There is evidence that conduct problems commencing before the age of 10 differ from those that commence in adolescence. It has been suggested this early onset indicates specific neuropsychological deficits (Moffitt et al. 1993), although young people who begin having their conduct difficulties in adolescence still show some neurophysiological abnormalities (Passamonti *et al.* 2010). However, individuals with early onset disorder are more likely to display aggressive symptoms, and to develop antisocial personality disorder in adulthood (Moffitt *et al.* 2007).

Antisocial behaviour has been associated with deficiencies in the brain's executive functions, which include operations such as sustaining attention and concentration, and there is the frequent presence of ADHD (see Chapter 7). There are also links to wider emotional difficulties, but in general these are reactions to the difficulties the child is experiencing rather than having any role in prompting the conduct difficulties.

Causes of disruptive behaviour

Parental and family factors

General behavioural difficulties in young children have been found to be associated with parental conflict, and it is this conflict rather than legal actions such as divorce which is the most important causative element (O'Leary and Emery 1982).

It has been well recognised for some time that parents of young children with behavioural difficulties tend to encounter a greater incidence of major stressors (e.g. unemployment, divorce, poverty), and tend to adopt a coercive approach to family relations (Robinson *et al.* 2008). There is also a strong association with mothers who have shown antisocial behaviour during their adolescence, given birth before 21 years of age, and have not completed their school career (Tremblay *et al.* 2004).

Most practitioners will recognise the behaviours frequently exhibited by parents with oppositional children. Commands are given in an anxious or irritable voice, and spoken rapidly. Alternatively, the parent may deliberately avoid following up a request as noncompliance is expected and, as such, an effort is made to avoid conflict.

In their effort to establish control, parents can resort to physical punishment, and there is a clear correlation between physical punishment and child aggressive behaviour (Gershoff 2002), with harsh discipline at age 8 being an important predictor of the early onset of delinquency (Farrington and Hawkins 1991). This correlation is moderated by other factors such as the quality of the parent–child relationship, and the degree of parent–child warmth. However it is only a short step from physical chastisement to abusive parenting, with the experience of physical abuse being one of the most important factors in prompting the emergence of antisocial behaviour (Jaffee *et al.* 2004).

Other factors have also been considered as influencing the emergence of such difficulties. Smoking during pregnancy is associated with later oppositional defiance through a mechanism which is thought to involve disruption to the development of the foetal brain (Jacobsen *et al.* 2007). As discussed below, the quality of life which the mother experienced during her pregnancy is increasingly seen as a major influence on the child's functioning and development.

Within-child factors

All parents know that some children seem to find it harder to socialise than others, and differences between children within the same family cannot be sufficiently explained solely by environmental factors. Temperamental factors are likely to play an important mediating role between the child's genetic make-up, environmental experiences and behaviour. Research suggests that negative temperamental characteristics in infants (e.g. struggles to adapt, prone to negative emotions and feelings) are associated with later behavioural difficulties, although this relationship is substantially weaker than parental and family factors (Bates *et al.* 1991).

Children with CD are less able to recognise and understand social cues, and have difficulty understanding emotion and facial expressions, factors which make them prone to misunderstanding situations and approaches (Woodworth and Waschbusch 2008). These difficulties limit their ability to develop beyond the infant phases of demand and aggression, leaving them with a tendency to continue to use these immature mechanisms (Bongers *et al.* 2004).

Peer and social issues

It has been shown that the more peers who are aggressive in a child's classroom the greater the tendency for the child to become aggressive and to value aggression as a method of coping with challenging situations (Stormshak *et al.* 1999). However peer groups are not instrumental in causing conduct problems, because disruptive individuals tend to seek out friends who share similar interests and have similar behavioural tendencies (Galbaud du Fort *et al.* 2002).

After puberty, peers exert a much stronger influence than in childhood, and while younger children would tend to reject and exclude disruptive or aggressive children, at this time of development such rebellion can appear attractive (Cillessen and Mayeux 2004). Allegiance to the peer group, and its minor rebellions against adult-imposed norms, helps develop peer interaction skills, and strengthen the social network (Engels and Bogt 2001). However this allegiance can prompt the adolescent to try to comply with the group's expectations, which may be changing to a pattern of more challenging behaviour (Berndt 2002).

Although generally peer group membership does not initiate conduct problems, the exception is communities where gang culture is prevalent. In such neighbourhoods, being in the gang is sometimes a means of survival, and membership demands committing violent and criminal acts. Work in some US city schools has found that 8.8% of students report gang membership, with these young people often drinking alcohol and using drugs from a young age, as well as being involved in other delinquent activity (Swahn *et al.* 2010). This pattern of behaviour often becomes quite entrenched as the need to remain part of the gang dominates the young person's decisions and actions.

The effects of media violence

It has been estimated that currently children and adolescents spend up to 7 hours a day watching television, or using modern media (Strasburger et al. 2010). For some time this degree of exposure has prompted concern because children learn by observing and imitating what they see around them, and are particularly keen to imitate behaviour they have seen on the screen if it seems realistic, or the programme shows the actions carry significant reward (Worth et al. 2008). The influence of violence on television is of particular concern because of its impact upon children's own aggressive behaviour (Huesmann et al. 2003). Repeated exposure to media violence can lead to an acceptance of violence as an appropriate means of solving conflict, with evidence that it also reduces a child's ability to recognise friendly overtures, and even signs of distress in others (Mueller and Silverman 1989). It also makes the child more willing to use violence themselves (Boxer et al. 2009).

Today there is perhaps no greater source of active participation in violence than through video games, and it has been shown that such participation has a significant association with subsequent aggressive behaviour (Anderson 2004). Also, the easy access to interactive media gives young people the opportunity to behave aggressively through Internet bullying and harassment (Ybarra and Mitchell 2007), a medium which can quickly engage others into like-minded behaviour, resulting in significant distress to victims (Patchin and Hinduja 2006).

Mechanisms mediating disruptive behaviour

The growing recognition that persistent behaviour requires changes to brain functioning at a cellular level has prompted significant effort in trying to understand the mechanisms involved. Whether children with conduct difficulties show specific genetic patterns has been the focus of considerable research. This shows that the variations to genetic make-up are significant with, for instance, boys who show persistently aggressive behaviours having different patterns of gene expression to those who do not (Broidy et al. 2003). However it is increasingly clear that these gene variations (known as polymorphisms) require other factors and events to occur for the disruptive behaviour to emerge (see Chapter 1).

As discussed above, studies have persistently found a significant interaction between childhood maltreatment and MAO-A genotype, with 85% of the males with the low-activity allele and a history of childhood maltreatment showing some form of antisocial behaviour (van der Vegt et al. 2009). These young people also show a tendency to be persistently aggressive (Beitchman et al. 2004).

Many other gene patterns have been studied. For instance, the 7-repeat allele of the dopamine D4 receptor gene has been found to be associated with impulsivity and poor executive function (see Chapter 7). It also has a moderate association with disruptive behaviour and cognitive ability (Forbes et al. 2009), as does the DAT1 genetic polymorphism, which may make a young person more prone to seek out delinquent peer networks (Beaver et al. 2008). However, the difficulty with all such studies is that the links are statistical rather than direct, and overall these gene x environment interactions appear to be dependent on age, severity of maltreatment, situational factors, and the presence of other behaviour problems to express themselves (Weder *et al.* 2009).

A more immediate pattern of expression that is generating considerable interest is epigenetics (see Chapter 1). The mechanism of action for these genetic influences is through the body's attempt to manage stressful events, and particularly cortisol (Alink *et al.* 2008). However its association with conduct problems is rather complex because the pattern is not easily predictable between different groups of children (Dadds and Rhodes 2008), but generally low cortisol reactivity is linked to aggression and disruptive behaviour (van Goozen *et al.* 2007).

Associations with other disorders

Difficult behaviour has strong associations with various disorders. For instance 80% of children with ADHD show ODD (Hartman *et al.* 2003), and up to 40% of long-term inmates in prison have ADHD (Ginsberg *et al.* 2010). There is also a significant link between conduct difficulties and drug misuse, with the conduct problems usually starting before the misuse of drugs (Hser *et al.* 2003). Depression occurs in about a third of young people who have conduct problems (Kovacs *et al.* 1988). When faced with quite challenging young people it can be quite difficult to be alert to such problems, but recognising their presence, and addressing them appropriately, can significantly reduce the overall level of difficulty as well as making reduction in the disruptive behaviour more probable.

Intervention

Parent training programmes

Behavioural approaches to non-compliance are the most effective means of altering function in this group, with parent management programmes being the most intensively evaluated. These programmes use various means of offering advice and guidance, including the provision of written materials, telephone contact and audio and videotaped sequences. They are more successful if emphasis is upon the discussion of difficulties, modelling responses and practising skills rather than simply teaching behavioural principles (Behan and Carr 2000).

There is a range of other programmes which have a different focus for their therapeutic intervention. For instance the Parenting with Love and Limits (PLL) is a group parent training programme for parents of teenagers with challenging behaviour. It emphasises appropriate management while focusing on the emotional interaction within the family, and has proved helpful in reducing both emotional and behavioural problems (Baruch *et al.* 2011). Similarly Parent Management Training (PMT) seeks to alter the pattern of exchanges between parent and child. It has been intensively studied and shown to improve family interaction (Hinshaw *et al.* 2000).

Individual family interventions

Research has consistently found that family-based treatments for adolescent conduct disorder are more effective than routine treatment (Woolfenden *et al.* 2002), and systemic family therapy is effective for those cases where dynamic issues within the family are making a significant contribution to the difficulties (Carr 2009).

One of the most intensive forms of intervention for young people with significant conduct difficulties is Multisystemic Therapy (MST) (Henggeler *et al.* 1998). This approach to the treatment of adolescent conduct disorder combines intensive family therapy with individual skills training for the adolescent, and intervention in the wider school and interagency network. It has consistently been found to reduce antisocial behaviour, with positive effects being maintained up to four years after treatment (Borduin *et al.* 2004). By its very nature it is an intensive approach, and hence an expensive form of intervention. However it has been calculated from studies done in the United States that every dollar spent on MST provides $9.51 to $23.59 in savings to taxpayers and to crime victims in the years ahead (Klietz *et al.* 2010).

Individual behavioural programmes

Many interventions involve both an individual behavioural programme and an element of parent training (although the training element may often be rather less structured and overt than that described above). In such cases, the focus may be upon what the child gains from the disruptive behaviour and how this may be changed. In this approach parental handling and management of the child is important, with key elements including the reduction of the child's capacity for negotiation, ensuring that instructions are complied with, and taking care that rewards and sanctions are clearly signalled and operate contingently.

Adam, aged 8, was referred to the educational psychologist by his school at parental request. He was perceived by his teachers as being rather idiosyncratic – he would occasionally make funny noises in class, demonstrated some rather unappealing personal habits, was something of a loner and, in his interests and sense of humour, appeared to function as a somewhat younger child. Although he had some learning difficulties – for example, he was only a beginning reader and required additional help from a support teacher – he was generally well behaved in class and responsive to his teachers. On occasions he had been brought to the headteacher for his involvement in minor misdemeanours (e.g. writing on the walls, teasing younger children).

At home, his behaviour was radically different. Here he was often argumentative, irritating, destructive and refused to respond to his parents' direction. Many of the arguments centred upon requests for sweets, toys and television, or refusal to undertake self-help tasks such as washing himself. Adam's father worked long hours and was often away from home. When his father was at home, Adam's behaviour was markedly better and this resulted in his father becoming frustrated at his wife's inability to cope at other times. His mother, a caring, concerned parent, was frequently overwhelmed by the demands of her son, particularly in public settings where his noisy and over-bearing manner frequently brought anxious glances from members of the public. Adam's maternal grandparents, while indulging the boy, were exasperated by his behaviour and often fuelled the tension within the family. For them Adam was a lost cause who was regularly compared unflatteringly with his younger sister (Sasha, aged five) who could 'do no wrong'.

Baseline measures of Adam's non-compliant behaviour, completed by his mother, indicated that bickering and non-compliance were almost continuous occurrences. As a result, it was agreed to set up a behavioural programme which would monitor sequences of thirty minutes – a highly intrusive and demanding schedule. Capitalising upon Adam's love of the *Power Rangers* television characters, Adam and his mother designed a Monopoly-style Power Rangers game board on a large piece of card. Each segment of the pathway represented a thirty-minute time period. The number of boxes totalled approximately one hundred.

At the end of each thirty-minute period an entry was made. If the target behaviours were achieved (no arguing with parents, compliance with instructions), Adam drew or coloured in the square. If these were not achieved, a large cross was drawn in the square with a felt pen. Rewards, in the form of pocket money, sweets and television programmes, were tied in tightly and explicitly to daily and weekly targets. It was made clear to Adam that there would be no negotiation or debate about parental judgements or the operation of reinforcement. Adam was required to take the chart to school at the end of each week to show his class teacher and headteacher.

Although somewhat daunted by the schedule, Adam's parents agreed to establish the programme and to adhere to the measures agreed. His grandparents, however, thought that the scheme was 'daft' and was unlikely to be any more effective than earlier attempts to tackle Adam's misbehaviour, but reluctantly agreed to 'give it a try'. Discussion focused upon the ways to give instructions, to pause afterwards to permit time for compliance, and to ensure that all verbal and non-verbal messages signalled an air of authority.

This case demonstrates the complex interaction between a simple behavioural model, the nature and quality of child–adult communication and the wider family and school contexts within which these operate. Many behavioural interventions fail because they focus too much upon the behavioural mechanics, and don't appreciate the contribution being made by interpersonal/parenting skills and wider family dynamics.

Commonly there is an assumption that helping the young person manage anger issues will make a very positive contribution, but so-called anger management rarely works in isolation, and is only really successful when part of a wider intervention which improves emotion awareness and problem solving for social situations (Lochman *et al.* 2011).

It is not uncommon for young people with significant conduct difficulties to also show other emotional problems, and the evidence suggests that in depressed young people cognitive behaviour therapy has a positive effect upon the mood, but not conduct difficulties (Rohde *et al.* 2004). Similar results have been found with solution-focused interventions (Corcoran 2006).

School-based approaches

Difficulties with disruptive behaviour within schools are discussed in Chapter 8, but there is a clear overlap between these children and those who are disruptive, and perhaps delinquent, in other settings. Children spend a considerable part of their lives in school, and it is an environment that does not have the emotional elements that are associated with family life. It has therefore frequently been used as a dependable setting in which to deliver interventions, but it is increasingly clear that school-only programmes are only effective in younger children (Petras *et al.* 2011).

However such programmes still have value in older children. The changes they bring can often make the child more popular with peers, and also help staff to recognise which youngsters need more focused and intensive help (Hall *et al.* 2009). These interventions often have behavioural and emotional components, with the behavioural elements showing the most immediate effects (Kolvin *et al.* 1981), while the benefits of interventions such as psychodynamic group work can take some time to emerge (Kolvin *et al.* 1988). However it is worth noting that the methods chosen to manage difficult behaviour within school can have repercussions in the wider community, with evidence that, for instance, school suspensions as a method of behavioural control appear to increase the likelihood of future conduct problems (Hemphill *et al.* 2006).

Medication

Conduct disorder is generally not responsive to medication alone, but if there are associated difficulties, such as ADHD and mood disorders, then the treatment of these may well reduce the overall degree of difficulty the young person is experiencing. There has been considerable interest in medication that is capable of reducing aggression, with a wide range of preparations being studied. The most recent interest has focused upon the atypical antipsychotics, such as risperidone, which have been shown to have a moderate to large effect upon reducing aggression (Pappadopulos *et al.* 2006). Medications such as clonidine, and occasionally lithium, may also be used to curb aggressive behaviour, but no medication appears to alter behaviour that is premeditated or planned.

Community treatment

The research on how the influence of peers can change behaviour in adolescence has shown that to place conduct-disordered young people with peers who show the same behaviour is likely to entrench rather than reduce such difficulties because within such settings criminal behaviour may actually be valued, and increase a youth's status (Dishion *et al.* 1999). Such concerns have prompted other forms of intervention to be considered, and one of the most promising is Multi-dimensional Treatment Foster Care, which has been used successfully with offenders in Oregon for some time (Chamberlain and Reid 1998). The young person is placed for up to a year in a foster family where the foster parents have been trained in behavioural interventions. The model is based on a system of points and levels which reward appropriate behaviour. It has a core aim of holding the young person to account for their crimes, while ensuring they get the support they need within their community to address factors which may have contributed to their offending behaviour. As well as reducing the rate of violent offending (Eddy *et al.* 2004), and offending generally, it also has been shown to help the young person back into education and community activities (Youth Justice Board 2010).

Outcome

Children who are disruptive and oppositional often become anxious as adults, while those who also have issues around truancy and drug misuse tend to continue to show such difficulties into adulthood (Reef *et al.* 2010). The developmental courses of the two types of CD are somewhat predictable. Without appropriate intervention, children with childhood-onset CD develop high rates of substance abuse, risky sexual behaviour, and self-harm behaviour as they move toward adulthood (Broidy *et al.* 2003). They commit more serious and violent acts than young people without an early history of conduct problems (Farrington *et al.* 2003), and graduate into adult criminality, with a continuing tendency to violent behaviour (Tremblay 2006). They also tend to have poor mental health, be less successful in their family lives, and have poorer social and economic prospects in adulthood (Colman *et al.* 2009). Thus, left untreated, conduct disorders are costly to both the individual and society.

Interventions which focus upon behavioural parent training have been shown to be effective in reducing childhood behaviour problems, with about two-thirds showing an improvement which lasted at least a year. Programmes which include sessions on parental support and stress management are more effective than standard management-focused programmes. No matter what the specific form of parent training programme, there appears to be benefit to the young person's functioning, and such programmes have been shown to be cost effective (Charles *et al.* 2011). The gains can be best sustained if periodic follow-up sessions are offered, but parents with limited social support, high levels of poverty-related stress, and mental health problems appear to derive least benefit from them (Reyno and McGrath 2006).

Preventative strategies

Conduct and behavioural difficulties have a tendency to bring enduring disruption to the child and family, and there have been major efforts to develop interventions which have the potential to prevent such difficulties emerging. Most of these programmes focus on children or families where the risk is considered high, with many of them echoing the parent training programmes described above. Perhaps the best known of these is the Incredible Years Programme (Webster-Stratton 1998), which has been used in many settings and has demonstrated that it can reduce the incidence of disruptive behaviour that children show when they reach adolescence (Webster-Stratton *et al.* 2011). It has also been shown to help children function better in school (Webster-Stratton *et al.* 2008). In view of the role that cortisol plays in the manifestation of aggressive behaviour it is interesting to note that children who responded to this approach, and showed an improvement in their behaviour, did show a normalisation of their cortisol responses (O'Neal *et al.* 2010).

The work with epigenetics suggests that prevention programmes may achieve most by markedly improving the family environment during the period of the pregnancy and in the infant's early weeks of life (Gluckman *et al.* 2008). However, most preventative strategies have focused upon children of school age (Wilson and Lipsey 2007). In those programmes that are offered to younger children, an intensive intervention with preschool children brings improvements in the child's behaviour, with the parents having lower rates of depression and reporting less stress (Bywater *et al.* 2009). In the longer term there is an improvement in the child's overall school performance, and there is a reduced risk of adulthood criminality (Barker *et al.* 2010).

Conclusion

Disruptive behaviour disorders and conduct difficulties can be enduring sources of disturbance and distress both to the young people themselves, and their communities. Once criminal activity is established it is very difficult to make meaningful change, and the evidence is that if intervention is focused in childhood, not only are the behaviours moderated at the time, but the future risk is significantly reduced. Genetic science points to even earlier intervention having potentially much greater impact, and as the research into this area continues the hope must be that future generations of children who appear at a high risk of conduct difficulties will be able to avoid becoming delinquent adolescents, and having criminal careers as adults.

Sources of further help

www.baaf.org.uk/webfm_send/2066
www.nlm.nih.gov/medlineplus/ency/article/001547.htm
www.mayoclinic.com/health/reactive-attachment-disorder/DS00988
www.incredibleyears.com
www.nlm.nih.gov/medlineplus/childbehaviordisorders.html
www.aacap.org/galleries/eAACAP.ResourceCenters/ODD_guide.pdf

www.bullying.co.uk/
www.antisocialbehaviour.org.uk/

References

Allen, J. and Vostanis, P. (2005). The impact of abuse and trauma on the developing child: An evaluation of a training programme for foster carers and supervising social workers. *Adoption and Fostering* 29: 68–81.

Alink, L., Van Ijzendoorn, M.H., Bakermans-Kranenburg, M.J. *et al.* (2008). Cortisol and externalizing behavior in children and adolescents: Mixed meta-analytic evidence for the inverse relation of basal cortisol and cortisol reactivity with externalizing behavior. *Developmental Psychobiology* 50: 427–50.

American Psychiatric Association (APA) (1994). *Diagnostic and Statistical Manual of Mental Disorders*, Fourth edition. Washington, DC: American Psychiatric Association.

Anderson, C.A. (2004). An update on the effects of violent video games. *Journal of Adolescence* 27: 113–22.

Andersen, S.L. and Teicher, M.H. (2004). Delayed effects of early stress on hippocampal development. *Neuropsychopharmacology* 29: 1988–93.

Bakermans-Kranenburg, M.J., van Ijzendoorn, M.H. and Juffer, F. (2003). Less is more: Meta-analysis of sensitivity and attachment interventions in early childhood. *Psychological Bulletin* 129: 195–215.

Barker, E.D., Vitaro, F., Lacourse, E. *et al.* (2010). Testing the developmental distinctiveness of male proactive and reactive aggression with a nested longitudinal experimental intervention. *Aggressive Behavior* 36: 127–40.

Baruch, G., Vrouva, I. and Wells, C. (2011). Outcome findings from a parent training programme for young people with conduct problems. *Child and Adolescent Mental Health* 16: 47–54.

Beaver, K.M., Wright, J.P. and De Lisi, M. (2008). Delinquent peer group formation: Evidence of a gene x environment correlation. *The Journal of Genetic Psychology* 169: 227–44.

Behan, J. and Carr, A. (2000). Oppositional defiant disorder. In A. Carr (ed.) *What Works with Children and Adolescents*. London: Routledge.

Beitchman, J.H., Mik, H.M., Ehtesham, S. *et al.* (2004). MAOA and persistent, pervasive childhood aggression. *Molecular Psychiatry* 9: 546–7.

Belsky, J., Bakermans-Kranenburg, M.J. and van IJzendoorn, M.H. (2007). For better and for worse: Differential susceptibility to environmental influences. *Current Directions in Psychological Science* 16: 300–4.

Berndt, T.J. (2002). Friendship quality and social development. *Current Directions in Psychological Sciences* 11: 7–10.

Bongers, I.L., Koot, H.M., Van Der Ende, J. *et al.* (2004). Developmental trajectories of externalizing behaviors in childhood and adolescence. *Child Development* 75: 1523–37.

Borduin, C., Curtis, N. and Ronan, K. (2004). Multisystemic treatment: A meta-analysis of outcome studies. *Journal of Family Psychology* 18: 411–19.

Bowlby, J. (1969). *Attachment and Loss (Vol. I)*. New York: Basic Books.

Bowlby J. (1980). *Attachment and Loss (Vol. 3): Loss: Sadness and Depression*. London: Hogarth Press.

Boxer, P., Huesmann, L.R., Bushman, B.J. *et al.* (2009). The role of violent media preference in cumulative developmental risk for violence and general aggression. *Journal of Youth and Adolescence* 38: 417–28.

Broidy, L.M., Nagin, D.S., Tremblay, R.E. *et al.* (2003) Developmental trajectories of childhood disruptive behaviors and adolescent delinquency: A six site, cross national study. *Developmental Psychology* 39: 222–45.

Broussard, E.R. and Cassidy, J. (2010). Maternal perception of newborns predicts attachment organization in middle adulthood. *Attachment and Human Development* 12: 159–72.

Brumariu, L.E. and Kerns, K.A. (2010). Parent–child attachment and internalizing symptoms in childhood and adolescence: A review of empirical findings and future directions. *Development and Psychopathology* 22: 177–203.

Bywater, T., Hutchings, J., Daley, D. *et al.* (2009). Long-term effectiveness of a parenting intervention for children at risk of developing conduct disorder. *British Journal of Psychiatry* 195: 318–24.

Carr, A. (2009). The effectiveness of family therapy and systemic interventions for child-focused problems. *Journal of Family Therapy* 31: 3–45.

Carrell, S.E. and Hoekstra, M.L. (2009). Domino effect: Domestic violence harms everyone's kids. *Education Next* 9: 3.

Caspi, A., McClay, J., Moffitt, T.E. *et al.* (2002). Role of genotype in the cycle of violence in maltreated children. *Science* 297: 851–5.

Caspi, A., Moffitt, T.E., Harrington, H. *et al.* (2009). Adverse childhood experiences and adult risk factors for age-related disease: Depression, inflammation, and clustering of metabolic risk markers. *Archives of Pediatric and Adolescent Medicine* 163: 1135–43.

Chamberlain, P. and Reid, J. (1998). Comparison of two community alternatives to incarceration for chronic juvenile offenders. *Journal of Consulting and Clinical Psychology* 66: 624–33.

Champagne, F., Chretien, P., Stevenson, C.W. *et al.* (2004). Variations in nucleus accumbens dopamine associated with individual differences in maternal behavior in the rat. *Journal of Neuroscience* 24: 4113–23.

Charles, J.M., Bywater, T. and Edwards, R.T. (2011). Parenting interventions: A systematic review of the economic evidence. *Child: Care, Health and Development* 37: 462–74.

Cillessen, A.H.N. and Mayeux, L. (2004). From censure to reinforcement: Developmental changes in the association between aggression and social status. *Child Development* 75: 147–63.

Colman, I., Murray, J., Abbott, R. *et al.* (2009). Outcomes of conduct problems in adolescence: 40 year follow-up of national cohort. *British Medical Journal* 338: a2981.

Corcoran, J. (2006). A comparison group study of solution-focused therapy versus 'treatment-as-usual' for behavior problems in children. *Journal of Social Service Research* 33: 69–81.

Crick, N.R. and Zahn-Waxler, C. (2003). The development of psychopathology in females and males: Current progress and future challenges. *Development and Psychopathology* 15: 719–42.

Cyr, C., Euser, E.M., Bakermans-Kranenburg, M.J. *et al.* (2010). Attachment security and disorganization in maltreating and high-risk families: A series of meta-analyses. *Development and Psychopathology* 22: 87–108.

Dadds, M.R. and Rhodes, R. (2008). Aggression in young children with concurrent callous-unemotional traits: Can the neurosciences inform progress and innovation in treatment approaches? *Philosophical Transactions of the Royal Society B: Biological Sciences* 363: 2567–76.

De Wolff, M.S. and van Ijzendoorn, M.H. (1997) Sensitivity and attachment: A meta-analysis on parental antecedents of infant attachment. *Child Development* 68: 571–91.

Dishion, T.J., McCord, J. and Poulin, F. (1999). When interventions harm: Peer groups and problem behavior. *American Psychologist* 54: 1–10.

Eddy, J.M., Whaley, R.B. and Chamberlain, P. (2004). The prevention of violent behavior by chronic and serious male juvenile offenders: A 2-year follow-up of a randomized clinical trial. *Journal of Emotional and Behavioral Disorders* 12: 2–8.

Engels, R.C.M.E. and ter Bogt, T.F.M. (2001). Influences of risk behaviors on the quality of peer relations in adolescence. *Journal of Youth and Adolescence.* 30: 675–95.

Erikson, E. (1969*). Identity, Youth and Crisis.* London: Faber & Faber.

Farrington, D.P. and Hawkins, J.D. (1991). Predicting participation, early onset and later persistence in officially recorded offending. *Criminal Behavior and Mental Health* 1: 1–33.

Farrington, D.P., Joliffe, D., Hawkins, J.D. *et al.* (2003). Comparing delinquency careers in court records and self-reports. *Criminology* 41: 933–58.

Findling, R.L. (2008). Atypical antipsychotic treatment of disruptive behavior disorders in children and adolescents. *Journal of Clinical Psychiatry* 68: 9–14.

Fleming, A.S., Corter, C., Stallings, J. *et al.* (2002) Testosterone and prolactin are associated with emotional responses to infant cries in new fathers. *Hormones and Behavior* 42: 399–413.

Forbes, E.E., Brown, S.M., Kimak, M. *et al.* (2009). Genetic variation in components of dopamine neurotransmission impacts ventral striatal reactivity associated with impulsivity. *Molecular Psychiatry* 14: 60–70.

Frazzetto, G., Di Lorenzo, G., Carola, V. *et al.* (2007). Early trauma and increased risk for physical aggression during adulthood: The moderating role of MAOA genotype. *PLoS ONE 2*: e486.

Galbaud du Fort, G.L., Boothroyd, J., Bland, R.C. *et al.* (2002). Spouse similarity for antisocial behavior in the general population. *Psychological Medicine* 32: 1407–16.

Gershoff, E.T. (2002). Parental corporal punishment and associated child behaviors and experiences: A meta-analytic and theoretical review. *Psychological Bulletin* 128: 539–79.

Ginsberg, Y., Hirvikoski, T. and Lindefors, N. (2010). Attention deficit hyperactivity disorder (ADHD) among longer-term prison inmates is a prevalent, persistent and disabling disorder. *BMC Psychiatry* 10(1): 1–13.

Gluckman, P.D., Hanson, M.A., Cooper, C. *et al.* (2008). Effect of in utero and early-life conditions on adult health and disease. *New England Journal of Medicine* 359: 61–73.

Green, H., McGinnity, A., Meltzer, H. *et al.* (2005) *Mental Health of Children and Young People in Great Britain, 2004.* Basingstoke: Palgrave Macmillan.

Gribble, K.D. (2007). A model for caregiving of adopted children after institutionalization. *Journal of Child and Adolescent Psychiatric Nursing* 20: 14–26.

Hall, B., Haddow, S. and Place, M. (2009). VAST – a tool for recognising vulnerable children in the classroom and developing a care pathway of intervention. *International Journal of Education* 1: E10.

Hartman, R.R., Stage, S.A. and Webster-Stratton, C. (2003). A growth curve analysis of parent training outcomes: Examining the influence of child risk factors (inattention, impulsivity and hyperactivity problems), parental and family risk factors. *Journal of Child Psychology and Psychiatry* 44: 388–98.

Heikkilä, K., Sacker, A., Kelly, Y. *et al.* (2001). Breast feeding and child behaviour in the Millennium Cohort Study. *Archives of Diseases in Childhood* doi:10.1136/adc.2010. 201970.

Hemphill, S.A., Toumbourou, J.W., Herrenkohl, T.I. *et al.* (2006) The effect of school suspensions and arrests on subsequent adolescent antisocial behavior in Australia and the United States. *Journal of Adolescent Health* 39: 736–44.

Henggeler, S.W., Schoenwald, S.K., Borduin, C.M. *et al.* (1998). *Multisystemic Treatment of Antisocial Behavior in Children and Adolescents.* New York: Guilford.

Hinshaw, S.P., Owens, E.B., Wells, K.C. *et al.* (2000). Family processes and treatment outcome in the MTA: Negative/ineffective parenting practices in relation to multimodal treatment. *Journal of Abnormal Child Psychology* 28: 555–68.

Howe, D. and Fearnley, S. (2003). Disorder of attachment in adopted and fostered children: Recognition and treatment. *Clinical Child Psychology and Psychiatry* 8: 369–87.

Hser, Y.I., Grella, C.E., Collins, C. *et al.*(2003). Drug-use initiation and conduct disorder among adolescents in drug treatment. *Journal of Adolescence* 26: 331–45.

Huesmann, L.R., Moise-Titus, J., Podolski, C. *et al.* (2003). Longitudinal relations between children's exposure to TV violence and their aggressive and violent behavior in young adulthood, 1977–1992. *Developmental Psychology* 39: 201–21.

Insel, T.R. and Young, L.J. (2001) The neurobiology of attachment. *Nature Reviews in Neuroscience* 2: 129–36.

Irish, L., Kobayashi, I. and Delahanty, D.L. (2010). Long-term physical health consequences of childhood sexual abuse: A meta-analytic review. *Journal of Pediatric Psychology* 35: 450–61.

Jacobsen, L.K., Slotkin, T.A., Mencl, W.E. *et al.* (2007). Gender-specific effects of prenatal and adolescent exposure to tobacco smoke on auditory and visual attention. *Neuropsychopharmacology* 32: 2453–64.

Jaffee, S.R., Moffitt, T.E., Caspi, A. *et al.* (2002). Influence of adult domestic violence on children's internalizing and externalizing problems: An environmentally informative twin study. *Journal of the American Academy of Child and Adolescent Psychiatry* 41: 1095–103.

Johnson, S.M., Wahl, G., Martin, S. *et al.* (1973). How deviant is the normal child? A behavioural analysis of the preschool child and his family. In R.D. Rubin, J.P. Brady and J.D. Henderson (eds) *Advances in Behavior Therapy*, vol. 4. New York: Academic Press.

Kim-Cohen, J., Caspi, A., Taylor, A. *et al.* (2006). MAOA, maltreatment, and gene–environment interaction predicting children's mental health: New evidence and a meta-analysis. *Molecular Psychiatry* 11: 903–13.

Kirsch, P., Esslinger, C., Chen, Q. *et al.* (2005). Oxytocin modulates neural circuitry for social cognition and fear in humans. *Journal of Neuroscience* 25: 11489–93.

Klietz, S.J., Borduin, C.M., Schaeffer, C.M. (2010). Cost-benefit analysis of multisystemic therapy with serious and violent juvenile offenders. *Journal of Family Psychology* 24: 657–66.

Kolvin, I., Garside, R.F., Nicol, A.R. *et al.* (1981). *Help Starts Here: The Maladjusted Child in the Ordinary School.* London: Tavistock.

Kolvin, I., Macmillan, A., Nicol, A.R. *et al.* (1988). Psychotherapy is effective. *Journal of the Royal Society of Medicine* 81: 261–6.

Kovacs, M., Paulaskas, S., Gastoris, C. *et al.* (1988). Depressive disorders in childhood: III. A longitudinal study of comorbidity with and risk for conduct disorder. *Journal of Affective Diseases* 15: 205–17.

Lochman, J.E., Powell, N.P., Boxmeyer, C.L. *et al.*(2011). Cognitive-behavioral therapy for externalizing disorders in children and adolescents. *Child and Adolescent Psychiatric Clinics of North America* 20: 305–18.

Lorberbaum, J.P., Newman, J.D., Horwitz, A.R. *et al.* (2002) A potential role for thalamocingulate circuitry in human maternal behavior. *Biological Psychiatry* 51: 431–45.

Luijk, M.P., Saridjan, N., Tharner, A. *et al.* (2010). Attachment, depression, and cortisol: Deviant patterns in insecure-resistant and disorganized infants. *Developmental Psychobiology* 52: 441–52.

McAuley, R. and McAuley, P. (1977). *Child Behaviour Problems.* London: Macmillan.

McClure, S.M., Daw, N.D. and Montague, P.R. (2003) A computational substrate for incentive salience. *Trends in Neuroscience* 26: 423–8.

Mueller, E. and Silverman, N. (1989). Peer relationships in maltreated children. In D. Cicchetti and V. Carlson (eds) *Child Maltreatment: Theory and Research on the Causes and Consequences of Child Abuse and Neglect.* New York: Cambridge University Press.

Oberlander, T.F., Weinberg, J., Papsdorf, M. *et al.* (2008). Prenatal exposure to maternal depression, neonatal methylation of human glucocorticoid receptor gene (NR3C1) and infant cortisol stress responses. *Epigenetics* 3: 97–106.

O'Connor, T. and Zeanah, C. (2003). Attachment disorders: Assessment strategies and treatment approaches. *Attachment and Human Development* 5: 223–44.

O'Connor, T.G., Rutter, M. and the English and Romanian Adoptees Study Team (2000). Attachment disorder behavior following severe deprivation: Extension and longitudinal follow-up. *Journal of American Academy of Child and Adolescent Psychiatry* 39: 703–12.

O'Leary, K.D. and Emery, R.E. (1982). Marital discord and child behavior problems. In M.D. Levine and P. Satz (eds) *Middle Childhood: Developmental Variation and Dysfunction.* New York: Academic Press.

O'Neal, C.R., Brotman, L.M., Huang, K.-Y. *et al.* (2010). Understanding relations among early family environment, cortisol response, and child aggression via a prevention experiment. *Child Development* 81: 290–305.

Oosterman, M., de Schipper, J.C., Fisher, P. *et al.* (2010). Autonomic reactivity in relation to attachment and early adversity among foster children. *Development and Psychopathology* 22: 109–18.

Pappadopulos, E., Woolston, S., Chait, A. *et al.* (2006) Pharmacotherapy of aggression in children and adolescents: efficacy and effect size. *Journal of the Canadian Academy of Child and Adolescent Psychiatry* 15: 27–39.

Passamonti, L., Fairchild, G., Goodyer, I.M. *et al.* (2010). Neural abnormalities in early-onset and adolescence-onset conduct disorder. *Archives of General Psychiatry* 67: 729–38.

Patchin, J.W. and Hinduja, S. (2006). Bullies move beyond the schoolyard: A preliminary look at cyberbullying. *Youth Violence and Juvenile Justice* 4: 148–69.

Petras, H., Masyn, K. and Ialongo, N. (2011). The developmental impact of two first grade preventive interventions on aggressive/disruptive behavior in childhood and adolescence: An application of latent transition growth mixture modeling. *Prevention Science* 12: 300–13.

Petrovic, P., Kalisch, R., Singer, T. *et al.* (2008). Oxytocin attenuates affective evaluations of conditioned faces and amygdala activity. *Journal of Neuroscience* 28: 6607–15.

Pruessner, J.C., Champagne, F., Meaney, M.J. *et al.* (2004) Dopamine release in response to a psychological stress in humans and its relationship to early life maternal care: A positron emission tomography study using 11C-raclopride. *Journal of Neuroscience* 24: 2825–31.

Redl, F. and Wineman, D. (1952). *Controls From Within: Techniques for the Treatment of the Aggressive Child.* New York: Free Press.

Reef, J., Diamantopoulou, S., van Meurs, I. *et al.* (2010). Developmental trajectories of child to adolescent externalizing behavior and adult DSM-IV disorder: Results of a 24-year longitudinal study. *Social Psychiatry and Psychiatric Epidemiology:* Oct 10. *Early View.*

Reiner, I. and Spangler, G. (2010). Adult attachment and gene polymorphisms of the dopamine D4 receptor and serotonin transporter (5-HTT). *Attachment and Human Development* 12: 209–29.

Reyno, S. and McGrath, P. (2006) Predictors of parent training efficacy for child externalizing behaviour problems: A meta-analytic review. *Journal of Child Psychology and Psychiatry* 47: 99–111.

Rice, M.J. and Records, K. (2008). Comparative analysis of physiological adaptation of neonates of abused and nonabused mothers. *Journal of Forensic Nursing* 4: 80–90.

Riggs, D., O'Leary, K. and Breslin, F. (1990). Multiple correlates of physical aggression in dating couples. *Journal of Interpersonal Violence* 5: 61–73.

Robinson, M., Oddy, W.H., Li, J.H. *et al.* (2008). Pre- and postnatal influences on preschool mental health: A large-scale cohort study. *Journal of Child Psychology and Psychiatry* 49: 1118–28.

Rohde, P., Clarke, G.N., Mace, D.E. *et al.* (2004). An efficacy/effectiveness study of cognitive-behavioral treatment for adolescents with comorbid major depression and conduct disorder. *Journal of the American Academy of Child and Adolescent Psychiatry* 43: 660–8.

Rutter, M., Moffitt, E.R. and Caspi, A. (2006). Gene–environment interplay and psychopathology: Multiple varieties but real effects. *Journal of Child Psychology and Psychiatry* 47: 226–61.

Schore, A.N. (2001). The effects of early relational trauma on right brain development, affect regulation, and infant mental health. *Infant Mental Health Journal* 22: 201–69.

Schultz, W. (2006) Behavioral theories and the neurophysiology of reward. *Annual Review of Psychology* 57: 87–115.

Schultz, D., Izard, C.E. and Bear, G. (2004). Children's emotion processing: Relations to emotionality and aggression. *Development and Psychopathology* 16: 371–87.

Scott, K.M., Smith, D.R. and Ellis, P.M. (2010). Prospectively ascertained child maltreatment and its association with DSM-IV mental disorders in young adults. *Archives of General Psychiatry* 67: 712–19.

Snyder H. (2001). Epidemiology of official offending. In R. Loeber and D.P. Farrington (eds). *Child Delinquents: Development, Intervention and Service Needs.* Thousand Oaks, CA: Sage.

Steele, M., Hodges, J., Kaniuk, J. (2010). Mental representation and change: developing attachment relationships in an adoption context. *Psychoanalytic Inquiry* 30: 25–40.

Stenius, F., Theorell, T., Lilja, G. *et al.* (2008). Comparisons between salivary cortisol levels in six-months-olds and their parents. *Psychoneuroendocrinology* 33: 352–9.

Storey, A.E., Walsh, C.J., Quinton, R.L. *et al.* (2000) Hormonal correlates of paternal responsiveness in new and expectant fathers. *Evolution and Human Behavior* 21: 79–95.

Stormshak, E.A., Bierman, K.L., Bruschi, C. *et al.* (1999). The relation between behavior problems and peer preference in different classroom contexts. *Child Development* 70: 169–82.

Strasburger, V.C., Jordan, A.B. and Donnerstein, E. (2010). Health effects of media on children and adolescents. *Pediatrics* 125: 756–67.

Swahn, M.H., Bossarte, R.M., West, B. *et al.* (2010) Alcohol and drug use among gang members: Experiences of adolescents who attend school. *Journal of School Health* 80: 353–60.

Swain, J.E., Lorberbaum, J.P., Kose, S. *et al.* (2007) Brain basis of early parent–infant interactions: psychology, physiology, and in vivo functional neuroimaging studies. *Journal of Child Psychology and Psychiatry* 48: 262–87.

Tremblay, R.E. (2006). Prevention of youth violence: Why not start at the beginning? *Journal of Abnormal Child Psychology* 34: 481–87.

Tremblay, R.E. (2010). Developmental origins of disruptive behaviour problems: The 'original sin' hypothesis, epigenetics and their consequences for prevention. *Journal of Child Psychology and Psychiatry* 51: 341–67.

Tremblay, R.E, Nagin, D., Séguin, J.R *et al.* (2004). Physical aggression during early childhood: Trajectories and predictors. *Pediatrics* 114: e43–50.

Triseliotis, J. (2002). Long-term foster care or adoption? The evidence examined. *Child and Family Social Work* 7: 23–33.

Upton, K.J. and Sullivan, R.M. (2010). Defining age limits of the sensitive period for attachment learning in rat pups. *Developmental Psychobiology* 52: 453–64.

van der Vegt, E.J.M., Oostra, B.A., Arias-Vasquez, A. *et al.* (2009). High activity of monoamine oxidase A is associated with externalizing behaviour in maltreated and non-maltreated adoptees. *Psychiatric Genetics* 19: 209–11.

van Goozen, S., Fairchild, G., Snoek, H. *et al.* (2007). The evidence for a neurobiological model of childhood antisocial behavior. *Psychological Bulletin* 133: 149–82.

van Ijzendoorn, M.H. and Bakermans-Kranenburg, M.J. (2006). DRD47- repeat polymorphism moderates the association between maternal unresolved loss or trauma and infant disorganization. *Attachment and Human Development* 8: 291–307.

van Ijzendoorn, M.H. and Juffer, F. (2006). Adoption as intervention: Meta-analytic evidence for massive catch-up and plasticity in physical, socio-emotional, and cognitive development. *Journal of Child Psychology and Psychiatry* 47: 1228–45.

Wakschlag, L.S., Tolan, P.H. and Leventhal, B.L. (2010). Research review: 'Ain't misbehavin': Towards a developmentally specified nosology for preschool disruptive behavior. *Journal of Child Psychology and Psychiatry* 51: 3–22.

Walton, A. and Flouri, E. (2010). Contextual risk, maternal parenting and adolescent externalizing behaviour problems: The role of emotion regulation. *Child: Care, Health and Development* 36: 275–84.

Weaver, I.C.G., Cervoni, N., Champagne, F.A. *et al.* (2004). Epigenetic programming by maternal behavior. *Nature Neuroscience* 7: 847–54.

Webster-Stratton, C. (1998) Preventing conduct problems in Head Start children: Strengthening parent competencies. *Journal of Consulting and Clinical Psychology* 66: 715–30.

Webster-Stratton, C, Reid, M.J. and Stoolmiller, M. (2008) Preventing conduct problems and improving school readiness: Evaluation of the Incredible Years teacher and child training programs in high-risk schools. *Journal of Child Psychology and Psychiatry* 49: 471–88.

Webster-Stratton, C., Rinaldi, J. and Reid, J.M. (2011). Long-term outcomes of Incredible Years parenting program: Predictors of adolescent adjustment. *Child and Adolescent Mental Health* 16: 38–46.

Weder, N., Yang, B.Z., Douglas-Palumberi, H. *et al.* (2009). MAOA genotype, maltreatment, and aggressive behavior: The changing impact of genotype at varying levels of trauma. *Biological Psychiatry* 65: 417–24.

Wilson, S.J. and Lipsey, M.W. (2007). School-based interventions for aggressive and disruptive behavior: Update of a meta-analysis. *American Journal of Preventive Medicine* 33: S130–43.

Woodworth, M. and Waschbusch, D. (2008). Emotional processing in children with conduct problems and callous/unemotional traits. *Child: Care, Health and Development* 34: 234–44.

Woolfenden, S., Williams, K. and Peat, J. (2002) Family and parenting interventions for conduct disorder and delinquency: A meta-analysis of randomised controlled trials. *Archives of Diseases in Childhood* 86: 251–6.

Worth, K.A., Chambers, J.G., Naussau, D.H. *et al.* (2008). Exposure of US adolescents to extremely violent movies. *Pediatrics* 122: 306–12.

Ybarra, M. and Mitchell. K. (2007). Prevalence and frequency of internet harassment instigation: Implications for adolescent health. *Journal of Adolescent Health* 41: 189–95.

Youth Justice Board (2010). www.yjb.gov.uk/en-gb/practitioners/Reducingreoffending/IntensiveFostering. Accessed 19 May 2011.

Chapter 5

Eating disorders

Introduction

Eating is, along with breathing, a fundamental necessity to sustain life. If a person does not breathe for some minutes, death occurs very quickly. For someone not eating, although it may take several weeks, death is no less inevitable. Perhaps this is why, throughout the animal kingdom, feeding is such a major part of the daily routine and has become in some species a part of ritual. In primates in particular, feeding routines have assumed particular importance, and are regularly used to placate aggressors. In humans, mutual feeding has also evolved as a major mechanism for showing affection or sexual interest (Morris 1967).

This may go some way to explain why children's problems with eating can so quickly become emotionally charged, and can so often become an area of persisting conflict and difficulty. The high level of concern which feeding problems can provoke provides an excellent mechanism for children to manipulate adult views and achieve their own desires over the expressed wishes of their parents. It can also be a mechanism by which a young person manages emotional difficulties or stressful life events. This can result in a young person either seeking to significantly restrict food intake, eat a poor diet, or eat to excess.

Food refusal

The newborn infant has no capacity to feed itself, and can only respond to danger or discomfort by crying. The main caregiver, usually the mother, has to respond to these signals if the baby is to be reassured. Feeding is an integral part of this process, and so if it becomes disrupted in any way, the impact for both mother and child can be quite profound.

In the first two months of life the baby is learning the mechanics of feeding, and so it is most likely that feeding problems at this very young age are physical ones. They may be mechanical in that the baby cannot coordinate the movements necessary for effective feeding, or they may be medical – for instance, colic or respiratory problems that make sucking a problem. The main focus then for a young infant with difficulties in feeding is the mechanics of the process, and the nature of the difficulties can usually be determined by means of a careful medical review.

Between two and six months the infant begins the crucial process of developing a specific emotional attachment to the primary caregiver. Therefore, problems arising in this age group usually reflect problems in this developing relationship. The commonest cause is for the mother to be depressed, or simply worn out with the childcare routine. The responses to the young person are then poorer, and the child becomes fretful and upset. If this continues, the baby may start to reduce its demands and become remote and self-stimulating, but usually the response is to demand attention by escalating resistance, and so force the mother to interact, albeit in an irritated and perhaps punitive way. These sorts of interaction are very commonly seen in children who present as being very small, and apparently undernourished – the non-organic failure to thrive syndrome (NOFTS). When in a different environment these children usually have insatiable appetites, and characteristically put on significant weight and growth spurts. If the resistance becomes extreme then the conflict between parent and child can become very marked.

About 25% of children will experience some type of feeding difficulties during infancy or early childhood, and this rate can be even higher in children with developmental disabilities. The issues can range from 'picky' eating, and strong food preferences, to behaviours that are designed to end the meal prematurely. For children who are simply very selective in their choice of food, as long as the child is choosing nutritious foods, they can be allowed to choose what to eat. Sometimes they may want to eat a particular food again and again for a while, and then not want to eat it at all. The approach to such difficulties is to encourage the child to explore new foods without insistence; to be aware of how foods look, and try to offer only small amounts; not to insist on a clean plate; and avoid bribes, threats or punishments. Most children will respond to these straightforward strategies, and do not require more vigorous intervention (Farrow and Blissett 2008).

Between 3% and 5% of children will go on to have persistent feeding issues, and of these a proportion have significant medical issues, especially gastrointestinal problems. If a child is refusing to eat on a regular basis it is important not to fight this. Many parents become very concerned when their toddler refuses to eat, but it is important to accept the refusal, and not to show upset. If the child is seeking attention, disapproval fills that need, and makes it more likely that the defiance will continue. The approach here involves ensuring meals occur at predictable times, and that they are a pleasant experience. This does not mean allowing the child to watch TV or playing with toys at the table – it needs to be clear that the mealtime is for eating. It is often helpful if the family sit together to eat, and use the same seats at the table. This type of family gathering gives good role models to the child of how to behave at mealtimes. If the child's resistance to food is very marked, then specific and focused behavioural programmes may need to be adopted. Often in these situations patterns of behaviour have been established in which the parents are attempting to coax or threaten the child. The child may be avoiding eating by leaving the table or keeping their mouth firmly closed. Spitting out the food can be managed by replacing the food that has been expelled. Changing the amount on the spoon, the texture of the food, and blending new items with preferred foods in increasing quantities can all help to improve the child's eating pattern (Williams et al. 2010).

If the purpose of a child's inappropriate mealtime behaviour is to gain attention, then ignoring the demanding behaviour can sometimes be sufficient to eliminate it. However if the food refusal has persisted for some time the child will have developed robust tantrum-type behaviours, and it is important to recognise that the programme must continue despite these, but they will eventually fade.

Childhood obesity

Over recent years there has been a growing concern about the degree of childhood obesity. This has shown a significant increase, with as many as 30% of children being clinically obese, though the rate may have peaked (McPherson et al. 2009). This increase has been attributed to a number of factors from infant feeding practices to a growing preference for fast foods amongst the young. Although it is not surprising that there is a clear link between children who are overweight and parental obesity, what is perhaps slightly more surprising is the link that has recently been found with maternal employment (de Moira et al. 2010).

Perhaps of equal significance are parental responses to infant temperament, because pacifying a fractious child with food can lead to significant weight gain (Darlington and Wright 2006). There has also been interest in how mothers' perception of their infant's growth and appetite might influence the amount of feeding (Baughcum et al. 2001).

A very different strand of research has explored whether leptin, a hormone involved in fat metabolism, influences the brain's ability to sense and control energy balance (Montague and Farooqi 1997). Changes in this hormone can make the child feel greater hunger, and not feel full after a meal. This suggests that childhood obesity may also be linked to a number of genetic and environmental factors, and opens the possibility for treatments beyond diet and exercise programmes.

Preschool-aged children who are obese are likely to continue to be obese as adolescents and adults, and they are at increased risk for poor health problems such as asthma, diabetes and cardiovascular diseases (Fagot-Campagna 2000). Indeed in one study it was found that the carotid arteries of children who were obese had prematurely aged by as much as thirty years (Raghuveer 2010).

If a child is obese then there is a reduction in physical activity which in itself increases health risks, but perhaps a more immediate impact for the child is the effect upon peer acceptance and general mental health. Depression and anxiety tend to be far more common in obese children (Rofey et al. 2009), and this can be persistent into adulthood. Being obese also increases the potential to be bullied by peers (Janssen et al. 2004), which in turn often causes low self-esteem (Ali et al. 2010).

Anorexia nervosa

Anorexia nervosa is a condition which has been known for some time, but was first formally identified by Gull in 1873. It has, however, become far better known in recent years as the image of being thin dominates our lives. This idealised image is experienced by the young at a time when they are searching for a personal identity, and trying to navigate the difficult route from childhood to becoming an adult. As has been mentioned in Chapter 1, one way that adolescents cope with these pressures is to seek conformity with stereotypes, and peer-group expectations. It is perhaps not surprising then that becoming totally focused on body image is a mechanism that some young people use to cope with these difficult pressures. In one survey, 40% of teenage girls and 10% of teenage boys were dieting significantly, and for 7% of the girls (and 1% of the boys) this was extreme (Patton *et al.* 1997).

Anorexia nervosa rarely emerges before puberty, and if a younger child is showing problems with weight loss and a reluctance to eat, it is very important that all physical illnesses are carefully excluded. In these younger children it is easy for bowel problems to masquerade as anorexia, and caution is therefore very important. The key factor for diagnosis in this age group, as in all others, is the presence of distortion in how the young person sees his or her body.

Early assessments found that anorexia nervosa affected 0.1–0.2% of the adolescent population (Whitaker *et al.* 1990), and occurred in girls ten times more commonly than in boys (Lucas *et al.* 1991). More recent studies have found the lifetime prevalence estimates of anorexia nervosa in women to be 0.9%, and for men 0.3% (Hudson *et al.* 2007), and that it is tending to emerge at a younger age.

Anna, at 15 years of age, was a girl who greatly enjoyed tennis. In the winter her relative inactivity caused her to put on weight, and several people within school began calling her 'Pug'. This made her quite distressed, and she determined to lose the extra weight. Over the next few weeks she embarked upon a severe diet which involved eating low-fat yoghurt for breakfast and lunch and a salad for tea. On occasions Anna would 'cheat' by eating biscuits or chocolate, and afterwards she felt so guilty that she would sometimes not eat for two days to remove this 'weight'.

After three months her periods had stopped and she was 15% below the weight that was typical for her height and age. When seen in individual sessions Anna could not accept that she was thin and was worried that if she began eating again she would rapidly become overweight. Family reassurance did not seem to help ease this anxiety for her. The problems presented by Anna are relatively clear, although for many young people with anorexia there are underlying problems of which the unwillingness to eat is merely an external manifestation.

This case illustrates the importance of recognising the key elements which lead to a diagnosis of anorexia nervosa. A desire to be slim, a wish to diet, and a feeling of being overweight do not in themselves confirm that the young person has anorexia. The diagnosis requires that the young person has a dread of being overweight which is accompanied by an unshakeable belief that she is too large, even if to the objective observer the opposite is true. This distortion of body image is the key element in determining that anorexia nervosa is present. In addition to this key element the young person is usually very thin, and in girls the periods have stopped. In about a third of cases there is also a soft, downy hair on the arms, legs and face, but this is a symptom arising because of the starvation and not a specific feature of anorexia nervosa.

In the midst of the illness the young person diets very severely, and is very knowledgeable about food. It tends to be a constant theme of the young person's conversation. They are often good cooks and take delight in cooking for others, though they maintain a strict dietary regime. Indeed, once established, being able to maintain the strict regime is often a major source of pleasure for the young person, and in more reflective moments he or she may well recount how good it felt to be able to resist a particular food or treat. For some, the diet is not sufficient, and there may also be a punishing exercise regime, which is often justified as part of a health drive. The weight loss may be assisted by taking large quantities of laxatives on a daily basis, or regularly vomiting after meals.

Such dieting may be their only source of self-praise and when considering other aspects of their life they may view themselves with scorn or even disgust. They often stop meeting friends or taking part in social occasions and generally seem more solitary and preoccupied. In day-to-day things they often are more irritable and bad tempered, with an air of gloominess which can lead people to think that they are becoming depressed.

The cessation of menstruation is the first sign of the significant impact which the starvation is having, but if the severe dieting is prolonged, damage can occur to important body organs such as the liver and kidneys. For boys, they tend to develop similar symptoms to girls about eating because of concerns about their body's shape and their weight (Oyebode et al. 1988), but they often prove to have greater underlying psychological problems (Fairburn and Harrison 2003).

Rachel's parents had been concerned about her for many months. They knew that she ate very little, and her mother believed that her periods had stopped at least six months ago. Rachel had refused professional help, but had finally agreed when her favourite aunt, with whom Rachel felt an affinity, insisted that she must see someone. The dietary history Rachel gave indicated that she was eating only 450 calories a day, and when she was weighed it was found that her weight was 40% below the weight that was typical for her height and age. After much discussion she agreed to be admitted to hospital on a voluntary basis, and over the next few days more details of her routines emerged. She had been eating almost nothing but low-fat yoghurt and salad for some months, and over the same period she had been pursuing a very intensive fitness regime which involved jogging daily and swimming four times per week.

Rachel could recite the calorific value of almost every food item, and described her greatest pleasure as cooking Sunday lunch for the family. The ward staff commented that in her first few days in hospital she kept very active, and never seemed to stay still for a moment.

Although finishing meals was expected as part of the programme, increasingly Rachel did not finish her meals when junior nurses supervised them. These nurses said that Rachel had told them how frightened and upset she felt whenever she was expected to eat. They felt sorry for Rachel and felt that they were being cruel in insisting that she ate.

After three weeks Rachel's weight gain was minimal, and a search revealed the remains of meals outside of the room window, and within the room the staff found plastic bags filled with food behind furniture, and even in the springs of a chair.

The causes of anorexia nervosa

As the concerns about anorexia nervosa have grown, so have the attempts to explain why some adolescents develop such a potentially profound problem. Psychological theories tend to suggest the origins of anorexia nervosa are to be found in the young person's own struggle with the pressures of maturity, and their attempts to delay it (Crisp 1980). The cessation of periods, the maintaining of the angularity of youth, and the delay in other secondary sexual characteristics are all certainly consequences of starvation. This type of theory is given added credence because many girls with anorexia nervosa tend to dress in a childish manner. In clinical samples a fear of growing up is certainly a common feature if the anorexia began before fourteen years of age, whereas in older girls it is a desire to be thin which dominates their thinking (Heebink et al. 1995). Such thinking is of course in line with much of modern advertising, and the demand for specific body shape gives a very high rates of anorexia nervosa amongst fashion models, ballerinas, and athletes (Rome 2003).

There has however been a wealth of research exploring other potential explanations. There have been some promising associations found from family and twin studies, but specific genetic links have been difficult to find and research tends to confirm that their influence is relatively small (Scherag et al. 2010). The emergence of anorexia nervosa around the time of puberty has prompted work that explores whether there are differences in the brain's responsiveness to oestrogens in these young people. There do seem to be differences in this, as well as thyroid and steroid sensitivity, but their exact role in the disease is as yet unclear (Young 2010).

Studies on serotonin function within the brain have found significant changes to this brain transmitter, changes which produce a low mood and are eased by limiting carbohydrate ingestion. These changes are evident both during the acute phase of the illness, and persist after recovery, which has led to speculation that these disturbances might predispose to the development of the disorder (Bailer and Kave 2011).

Young people who suffer from anorexia nervosa experience a wide range of additional health problems. There is often a slowed heart rate, low blood pressure and changes to blood chemistry. In the longer term there can be damage to kidneys and liver, and the emergence of osteoporosis at a very young age (Kumar *et al.* 2010).

Intervention

The first stage of any intervention process is to recognise that a problem is developing. With the modern emphasis upon slimness it can be difficult for families, or other concerned adults, to realise that there is a cause for concern. The first worry is usually the marked thinness of the young person, but it can also be concern that the diet seems too severe. Questions asked about eating are usually dismissed, and it is often only when considerable weight has been lost, and there can be no doubt about the matter, that professional help is sought.

The key is to gain an understanding of the history of the problem, the issues which are sustaining it, and then to limit further weight loss. The programme which has traditionally been used for this is based on behavioural principles. The exact make-up of the programme varies depending upon the philosophy of the service, but most would expect that if the young person is 35% below the ideal body weight for height and age, then a hospital admission needs to be seriously considered. If the young person with anorexia nervosa does not wish to be admitted to hospital then if the illness is severe enough they can be compulsorily detained. To do this it has to be evident that the illness is adversely affecting the young person's ability to make rational decisions. It must be remembered, however, that each case is judged on its merits, and diagnosing that someone has anorexia nervosa does not automatically mean that they can be admitted to hospital against their will.

In Britain the National Institute for Clinical Excellence has issued guidance on management which suggests that efforts should be made to treat children and adolescents as outpatients, offering a combination of direct personal and family therapy (Wilson and Shafran 2005). This is because for those in whom the problem started at a young age, family therapy which focuses upon relationships and maturation tends to be most successful, whereas for those in whom the problem started late in adolescence, the best response tends to be achieved by an individual psychotherapy approach (Russell *et al.* 1987). Increasingly this takes the form of cognitive behaviour therapy, which has been viewed as a major element of intervention for some time (Ricca *et al.* 2000).

Whether in hospital or not, the first aim is to bring the body weight back to a more normal level. It is important to have a clear idea of the usual food intake because the new regime must very slowly increase from that level to one which is gradually producing a weight gain. The increase in weight is usually quite frightening to the young person and so the process demands great tact, care and reassurance that they will not be made fat. It is sometimes helpful in these early stages to give a sedative medication, which can help reduce the intense feelings of panic that many feel as the weight chart slowly climbs. This gradual gaining of weight is accompanied by agreed rewards and, supplementing this, there needs to be a continuous educational and support programme to reduce the concern about the steady weight gain.

Anna was treated using a cognitive therapy approach (see Chapter 2). Anna was gradually able to develop new ways of thinking about her weight. Having achieved this it was then possible slowly to change her dietary regime so that it maintained her at a weight appropriate to her height. As part of this programme, she began keeping a diary which listed her positive qualities as well as the nice things which people had said about her on that day. Three times a week she would read recent entries, and over the next few months she confirmed that she was now seeing herself in a different light. Two years on, Anna continues to maintain her weight appropriately, and plays tennis for her university.

In the early stages the young person will usually talk of nothing but food and weight targets, and it is important to establish a sequence of meetings where this is not the focus, but rather it is upon their life and their aspirations for the future. These become the kernel of the individual psychological programme which gathers momentum as the weight concerns reduce.

As already mentioned, the family's role, both in the origin of the difficulties and in their solution, may prove pivotal. Most families find exploration of their intimate workings very difficult, but without major shifts in attitude and approach relapse is very likely. Minuchin and his team (1978) described a pattern in which families were quite overinvolved, with a feeling that the family members were very enmeshed with each other. He also found that conflict between members of the family was avoided, and that if there was marital conflict it was very common for the young person to become caught in the middle of it.

A somewhat similar pattern of findings was noted by Selvini-Palazzoli (1974) in her work with anorexic girls in Italy. Secret alliances between family members were often evident, with a strong expectation that family members would preserve the outward appearance of a settled family life. Although some of the conclusions from such work have been eroded over time, the basic approach to family issues still remains. Understanding the family's functioning remains a fundamental requirement of any intervention programme, especially in the younger patient. The type of family work that is undertaken is largely dictated by the philosophy of the unit treating the young person, but often it has a systems theory basis (see Chapter 2).

Alongside the exploration of family issues, it is important that a consistent approach is agreed with the parents towards eating. In milder weight loss situations this may be the only direct management of the eating, and its success is necessary for any lasting progress. The home regime is based upon agreed menus, and a constant expectation that plates will be cleared. The steady increase in amounts offered is still necessary, and using large dinner plates can help with the illusion that the quantity is small. A single exchange item on each menu is permitted, otherwise the meals are as agreed, and the adults of the family stay with the young person until all is eaten. Resisting excuses and ploys, and maintaining a solid insistence, is not only necessary to maintain the weight, but is often the first indication of a major shift in how the family functions.

Any concerned adult can offer the opportunity to listen to worries or concerns, but if they become food or weight orientated, these discussions should be diverted by saying 'those are issues to discuss with your specialist'. Within school, projects on anorexia may be sought out, and may offer the opportunity to ventilate certain feelings or ideas. It is important that the illness does not become too dominant, however, because maintaining a wide range of interests and having success in different arenas are crucial to the recovery process. Gently steering into new tasks, highlighting success and praising positive progress can all help in reducing the drive to be thinner.

The role of medication in treating anorexia nervosa remains unclear. Certain medications such as the atypical antipsychotics are known to affect weight, and so potentially could be helpful. The research suggests that these medications appear safe and there is some evidence of positive effects on depression, anxiety and core eating disordered psychopathology in patients with anorexia nervosa. However there is no clear evidence that they have a direct beneficial effect upon weight gain (McKnight and Park 2010). Also there may be a role for antidepressants, and dietary supplements such as zinc (Flament *et al.* 2011).

Outcome

Although the general approach to anorexia nervosa has been established for several years, the outcome is still very variable. This is because recovery is determined far more by how successful the psychological efforts have been than whether an appropriate weight was achieved. In general, over half of the girls will achieve a reasonable weight and see their periods restored, but boys have a much poorer course (Steinhausen *et al.* 1991). On average 50% of sufferers take six years or more to recover after their first treatment, while the average for those who also use purgatives can be eleven years (Herzog *et al.* 1997). The likelihood of full recovery diminishes over time, with relapses occurring in 30% of those who do not complete their full treatment programme (Strober *et al.* 1997). Unfortunately, 10–20% of individuals do not improve despite treatment, and they develop a chronic condition which has a continuing negative impact upon both education and work (Byford *et al.* 2007).

It used to be thought that the earlier the illness started the poorer the outcome (Walford and McCune 1991), but it is now clear that the age of onset is not associated with having a more severe illness, or making it more likely to recur (Zipfel *et al.* 2000). Indeed, it appears that developing the disease as an adult is a predictor of much poorer outcome in the longer term (Ratnasuriya *et al.* 1990).

The disruption to the onset of full puberty prompted by the illness does influence the child's physical development (Russell 1985). Although most recover their weight, they are more likely to suffer chronic health problems. No agreement exists on the best management of bone loss. Achieving an appropriate weight seems to help the bones to recover, but there is no evidence that oestrogen replacement is of assistance (Mehler and MacKenzie 2009).

Women who have suffered from anorexia do not find it harder to become pregnant, but they do seem to suffer from a greater frequency of complications with their pregnancy, such as prematurity, or requiring a caesarean section (Bulik *et al.* 1999). There is also sadly a small number of sufferers who die prematurely, though as treatment programmes have improved this has reduced.

Bulimia nervosa

Bulimia nervosa is a variation of anorexia nervosa which was initially distinguished as a separate problem by Russell in 1979. He described a group of girls who had an intense fear of becoming fat but, unlike typical anorexic girls, most of this group were not extremely thin. This group was also distinctive because their dietary routine was not extremely restrictive, but rather had episodes when they would eat a very large quantity of food, and afterwards they would vomit, use large amounts of laxatives, or exercise to an extreme degree to prevent the binge meal causing them to put on weight. It is worth mentioning that eating problems do not always present as clearly anorexic or bulimic, and that this group of atypical eating disorders can be quite challenging to manage because they tend to be severe and long-lasting.

Young people with bulimia still report being dissatisfied with their current body shape, state they would prefer to be thinner, and tend to overestimate their body size. The problem tends to begin well after puberty, and occurs in about 1.5% of girls and 0.5% of boys (Hudson *et al.* 2007). It can occasionally occur in girls before they start their periods, but this is unusual (Schmidt *et al.* 1992).

Amanda was 17 years of age and during a school field trip a teacher became worried because Amanda seemed to spend long periods in the toilet after each meal. The teacher wanted to send Amanda home, but Amanda said that this had been happening for some time and that she had a stomach problem. As the week progressed Amanda began to confide in the teacher and in response to the teacher's obvious concern Amanda confessed that she in fact made herself sick after meals. Amanda considered herself to be ugly, and felt fat. She had tried many types of diet and had had slimming pills from her doctor, but couldn't seem to lose weight.

In the last year she had started to be sick after meals, and felt much happier after she had been sick, because she knew this food would not add to her weight problem. Her family had also noticed that she had stopped eating lunch, and was now often getting up at night to 'have a snack'. After much discussion Amanda agreed to be referred to a specialist clinic.

Initially, Amanda found it hard to talk about her eating problems, but eventually described how upset she was about her appearance, and how desperately she wanted to be thinner. She explained how sometimes the desire to eat became overwhelming, and on these occasions she would literally eat everything in the kitchen. She described how on these occasions she would even eat packets of butter as though they were some sort of ice-cream bar. Afterwards she had to be sick, and then could rest. At other times she felt the need to be sick only after large meals, and said that she was taking thirty laxative tablets a day to help keep her weight down.

There has been no specific cause identified for the onset of bulimia. In most cases there are clear influences from adverse life-events, with a significant minority of the girls who are suffering from bulimia reporting that they have been victims of sexual abuse (Pope and Hudson 1992), and there is a strong link to family substance misuse (Lilenfeld *et al.* 1998). Recent animal studies have investigated the potential role for dopamine mechanisms in sustaining the binge eating and it appears that this, together with other factors such as genetic traits, dietary restraint, stress, etc., results in progressive impairments of dopamine mechanisms, and persistence of the binge eating (Bello and Hajnal 2010).

These young people can often show wider emotional difficulties, such as alcohol and drug misuse (Dansky *et al.* 2000) and self-harming tendencies (Paul *et al.* 2002). The physical effect of repeated vomiting exposes the oesophagus to stomach acid and so is likely to provoke ulcers, and in rare cases it may cause the oesophagus to rupture (Overby and Litt 1988). There is also often a characteristic pattern of enamel erosion on the teeth and enlarged salivary glands in the cheeks, which may be noticed by their dentists.

Intervention

Identifying bulimia nervosa can be very difficult. Hearing someone being sick may be the only clue, because otherwise there are few outward signs to notice. Therefore, it is the young person's declaration that there is a problem which tends to be the first indication. A referral to the local psychiatric services is the usual route of response, but experienced counsellors or community psychiatric nurses may be other avenues of help. In trying to assist young people with bulimia various approaches have been used, with guided self-help being the first stage of treatment for milder forms of the problem.

If unsuccessful, or if the problem is having a significant detrimental impact upon the young person's life then a more intensive therapeutic approach is required. This is usually through cognitive therapy (discussed in Chapter 2) which engages the patient in a careful examination of how the problem is viewed and thought about, as well as trying to understand what prompts specific behaviours, and to seek solutions to them. The exact nature of the programme is tailored to the individual, but focus upon their low self-esteem, issues around their mood, and interpersonal difficulties are often core elements of the programme.

Medication may sometimes also have a part to play. Work in various centres has produced evidence that certain antidepressants can reduce episodes of bulimia and the preoccupation with body size (Goldstein *et al.* 1995). A review of this work concludes that psychological treatment and antidepressants do not differ in remission rates, but dropout rates are lower with psychological treatment. A combination of antidepressants and psychological treatment is increasingly being seen as the best way of intervening with this condition (Flament *et al.* 2011).

The family's role in helping to resolve the problems depends upon whether direct family themes, such as conflict or abuse, are seen to be underlying the behavioural pattern. The use of family therapy can sometimes deal with such issues in a way that allows the young person to escape what feels like an oppressive atmosphere. If such themes are not dominant, then the family role tends to be one of support – both in terms of offering time for quiet reflection, and in terms of routine and structure. If it is clear that the hour after mealtimes is a particularly difficult time, then restructuring routines so that there is no opportunity to vomit can be helpful. This can be achieved by giving chores, playing board games or even taking a walk together. Such plans work best when agreed with sufferers, and this also allows them to be challenged if they try to excuse themselves.

Within other settings, such as school, assistance in breaking patterns is harder to organise. Keeping occupied is the most important requirement: empty time is dangerous time. A routine of going to clubs or assisting with the library can be quite powerful, but direct help means that the problem has to be shared, and that specific things are asked of the adult. It is unusual for school staff even to know that one of their students has bulimia, and so positive help tends to be very uncommon.

Friends can be a great source of help. They can be asked to be vigilant, and close friends can be empowered to be quite forceful in stopping trips to the toilet unaccompanied. These types of intrusion are, however, only of value if the young person wants them, and they are part of a structured plan. As isolated measures they offer little, and if not sought by the sufferer, they can ruin relationships, and make matters worse by deepening the sense of isolation.

Outcome

Bulimia has been identified as a separate condition now for some years, and over this time there has been a steady flow of studies pointing to the value of psychological intervention, particularly cognitive behaviour therapy. However, if this approach fails there are few alternative therapeutic approaches that appear to offer any chance of success (Mitchell *et al.* 2002). After one year about 28% show persistent improvement, but over time there is a continuing rate of improvement, so by ten years as many as 70% report significant improvement in their symptoms (Keel and Brown 2010).

Women with bulimia nervosa tend to recover better the earlier the onset (Lisa *et al.* 2001). It also seems that the seriousness of the initial psychological problems does not help to predict how good the recovery will be (Johnson-Sabine *et al.* 1992), although a history of childhood obesity and complications such as self-harming do (Paul *et al.* 2002). In those who find little benefit from therapy the disorder can have a significant impact on their education, work and social functioning. They are also prone to develop a wide variety of different psychological problems (Collins and King 1994), which perhaps explains the significant risk of suicide that exists for this group (Crowe *et al.* 2009).

Conclusion

Eating is a crucial part of every person's life, and any disruption to it is potentially life-threatening. It is therefore not surprising that disruption to eating, by whatever mechanism, provokes extreme concern from family and professionals alike. The research shows a steady move towards understanding what are the most effective ways to intervene in such situations, which hopefully gives the young person the best chance of minimising the impact of the eating disorder upon future life.

Sources of further help

www.b-eat.co.uk/Home
www.childrenfirst.nhs.uk
www.mentalhealth.org.uk/publications
www.nimh.nih.gov/health/publications/eating-disorders/anorexia-nervosa
www.eating-disorders.org.uk
www.anad.org

References

Ali, M.M., Fang, H. and Rizzo, J.A. (2010). Body weight, self-perception and mental health outcomes among adolescents. *Journal of Mental Health Policy and Economics* 13: 53–63.

Bacaltchuk, J., Hay, P. and Trefiglio, R. (2001). Antidepressants versus psychological treatments and their combination for bulimia nervosa. *Cochrane Database Systematic Review* (4): CD003385.

Bailer, U.F. and Kaye, W.H. (2011). Serotonin: Imaging findings in eating disorders. *Current Topics in Behavioral Neuroscience* 6: 59–79.

Baughcum, A., Powers, S., Johnson, S. *et al.* (2001). Maternal feeding practices and beliefs and their relationships to overweight in early childhood. *Journal of Developmental and Behavioral Pediatrics* 22: 391–408.

Bello, N.T. and Hajnal, A. (2010). Dopamine and binge eating behaviors. *Pharmacology, Biochemistry and Behavior* 97: 25–33.

Bulik, C.M., Sullivan, P.F., Fear, J.L. *et al.* (1999). Fertility and reproduction in women with anorexia nervosa: A controlled study. *Journal of Clinical Psychiatry* 60: 130–5.

Byford, S., Barrett, B., Roberts, C. *et al.* (2007). Economic evaluation of a randomised controlled trial for anorexia nervosa in adolescents. *British Journal of Psychiatry* 191: 436–40.

Collins, S. and King, M. (1994). Ten year follow up of 50 patients with bulimia nervosa. *British Journal of Psychiatry* 164: 80–7.

Crisp, A.H. (1980). *Anorexia Nervosa: Let Me Be*. London: Academic Press.

Crow, S.J., Peterson, C.B., Swanson, S.A. *et al.* (2009). Increased mortality in bulimia nervosa and other eating disorders. *American Journal of Psychiatry* 130: 1342–6.

Dansky, B.S., Brewerton, T.D. and Kilpatrick, D.G. (2000). Comorbidity of bulimia nervosa and alcohol use disorders: Results from the national women's study. *International Journal of Eating Disorders* 27: 180–190.

Dare, C. and Eisler, I. (1992). The family therapy of anorexia nervosa. In P. Cooper and A. Stein (eds) *The Nature and Management of Feeding Problems in Young People*. New York: Harwood Academics.

Darlington, A.S. and Wright, C.M. (2006). The influence of temperament on weight gain in early infancy. *Journal of Developmental and Behavioral Pediatrics* 27: 329–35.

de Moira, A.P., Power, C. and Li, L. (2010). Changing influences on childhood obesity: A study of 2 generations of the 1958 British birth cohort. *American Journal of Epidemiology* 171: 1289–98.

Fagot-Campagna, A. (2010). Emergence of type 2 diabetes mellitus in children: Epidemiological evidence. *Journal of Pediatric Endocrinology and Metabolism* 13 Suppl. 6: 1395–402.

Fairburn, C.G. and Beglin, S.J. (1990). Studies of the epidemiology of bulimia nervosa. *American Journal of Psychiatry* 147: 401–8.

Farrow, C.V. and Blissett, J. (2008). Controlling feeding practices: Cause or consequence of early child weight? *Pediatrics* 121: 164–9.

Flament, M.F., Bissada, H. and Spettigue, W. (2011). Evidence-based pharmacotherapy of eating disorders. *International Journal of Neuropsychopharmacology* 18: 1–19.

Goldstein, D.J., Wilson, M.G. and Thompson, V.L. (1995). Long-term Fluoxetine treatment in bulimia nervosa. *British Journal of Psychiatry* 166: 660–6.

Gull, W.W. (1873). Anorexia hysterica (apepsia hysterica). *British Medical Journal* 2: 527–9.

Heebink, D.M., Sunday, S.R. and Halmi, K.A. (1995). Anorexia nervosa and bulimia nervosa in adolescence: Effects of age and menstrual status on psychological variables. *Journal of the American Academy of Child and Adolescent Psychiatry* 34: 378–82.

Herzog, W., Dorer, D.J., Keel, P.K. *et al.* (1999). Recovery and relapse in anorexia and bulimia nervosa: A 7.5-year follow-up study. *Journal of the American Academy Of Child and Adolescent Psychiatry* 38: 829–37.

Herzog, W., Schellberg, D. and Deter, H.-C. (1997). First recovery of anorexia nervosa patients in the long-term course: A discrete-time survival study. *Journal of Consulting and Clinical Psychology* 65: 169–77.

Hudson, J.I., Hiripi, E., Pope, H.G. *et al.* (2007). The prevalence and correlates of eating disorders in the National Comorbidity Survey Replication. *Biological Psychiatry* 61: 348–58.

Jacobs, B. and Isaacs, S. (1986). Pre-pubertal anorexia nervosa: A retrospective controlled trial. *Journal of Child Psychology and Psychiatry* 27: 237–50.

Janssen, I., Craig, W.M., Boyce, W.F. *et al.* (2004). Associations between overweight and obesity with bullying behaviors in school-aged children. *Pediatrics* 113: 1187–94.

Johnson-Sabine, E., Reiss, D. and Dayson, D. (1992). Bulimia nervosa: A follow up study. *Psychological Medicine* 22: 951–9.

Kaye, W.H., Nagata, T. and Weltzin, T.E. (2001). Double-blind placebo-controlled administration of fluoxetine in restricting- and restricting-purging-type anorexia nervosa. *Biological Psychiatry* 49: 644–52.

Keel, P.K. and Brown, T.A. (2010). Update on course and outcome in eating disorders. *International Journal of Eating Disorders* 43: 195–204.

Kumar, K.K., Tung, S. and Iqbal, J. (2010). Bone loss in anorexia nervosa: Leptin, serotonin and the sympathetic nervous system. *Annals of the New York Academy of Science* 1211: 51–65.

Lilenfeld, L.R., Kaye, W.H. and Greeno, C.G. (1998). A controlled family study of anorexia nervosa and bulimia nervosa: Psychiatric disorders in first-degree relatives and effects of proband comorbidity. *Archives of General Psychiatry* 55: 603–10.

Lucas, A.R., Beard, C.M. and O'Fallon, W.M. (1991). Fifty year trends in the incidence of anorexia nervosa in Rochester, Minnesota: A population-based study. *American Journal of Psychiatry* 148: 917–22.

McKnight, R.F. and Park, R.J.(2010). Atypical antipsychotics and anorexia nervosa: A review. *European Eating Disorders Review* 18: 10–21.

McPherson, K., Brown, M., Marsh, T. *et al.* (2009). *Obesity: Recent Trends in Children Aged 2–11y and 12–18y.* London: National Heart Forum.

Mehler, P.S. and MacKenzie, T.D. (2009). Treatment of osteopenia and osteoporosis in anorexia nervosa: A systematic review of the literature. *International Journal of Eating Disorders* 42: 195–201.

Minuchin, S., Rosman, B. and Baker, L. (1978). *Psychosomatic Families: Anorexia Nervosa in Context.* Cambridge, MA: Harvard University Press.

Mitchell, J.E., Halmi, K. and Wilson, G.T. (2002) A randomized secondary treatment study of women with bulimia nervosa who fail to respond to CBT. *International Journal of Eating Disorders* 32: 271–81.

Montague, C.T. and Farooqi, I.S. (1997). Congenital leptin deficiency is associated with severe early-onset obesity in humans. *Nature* 387: 903–8.

Morris, D. (1967). *The Naked Ape: A Zoologist's Study of the Human Animal.* London: Jonathan Cape.

Overby, K.J. and Litt, I.F. (1988). Mediastinal emphysema in an adolescent with anorexia nervosa and self–induced emesis. *Pediatrics* 81: 134–6.

Oyebode, F., Boodhoo, J.A. and Schapira, K. (1988). Anorexia nervosa in males: Clinical features and outcome. *International Journal of Eating Disorders* 7: 121–4.

Patton, G.C. (1988). Mortality in eating disorders. *Psychological Medicine* 18: 947–51.

Patton, G.C., Carlin, J.B., Shao, Q. *et al.* (1997). Adolescent dieting: Healthy weight control or borderline eating disorder. *Journal of Child Psychology and Psychiatry* 38: 299–306.

Paul, T., Schroeter, K., Dahme, B. *et al.* (2002). Self-injurious behavior in women with eating disorders. *American Journal of Psychiatry* 159: 408–11.

Pope, H. and Hudson, J. (1992). Is childhood sexual abuse a risk factor for bulimia nervosa? *American Journal of Psychiatry* 149: 455–63.

Raghuveer, G. (2010). Lifetime cardiovascular risk of childhood obesity. *American Journal of Clinical Nutrition* 91: 1514S–19S.

Ratnasuriya, R.H., Eisler, I., Szmukler, G.I. *et al.* (1990). Anorexia nervosa: Outcome and prognostic factors after 20 years. *British Journal of Psychiatry* 158: 495–502.

Ricca, V., Mannucci, E., Zucchi, T. *et al.* (2000). Cognitive-behavioural therapy for bulimia nervosa and binge eating disorder: A review. *Psychotherapy and Psychosomatics* 69: 287–95.

Rofey, D.L., Kolko, P.R. and Iosif, A.M. (2009). A longitudinal study of childhood depression and anxiety in relation to weight gain. *Child Psychiatry and Human Development* 40: 517–26.

Rome, E.S. (2003). Eating disorders. *Obstetric and Gynaecological Clinics of North America* 30: 353–77.

Russell, G.F.M. (1985). Premenstrual anorexia nervosa and its sequelae. *Journal of Psychiatric Research* 19: 363–9.

Russell, G.F.M., Szmukler, G.I., Dare, C. *et al.* (1987). An evaluation of family therapy in anorexia nervosa and bulimia nervosa. *Archives of General Psychiatry* 44: 1047–56.

Schmidt, U., Hodes, M. and Treasure, J. (1992). Early onset bulimia nervosa: Who is at risk? *Psychological Medicine* 22: 623–8.

Selvini-Palazzoli, M. (1974). *Self Starvation: From Individual to Family Therapy in the Treatment of Anorexia Nervosa.* New York: Aronson.

Scherag, S., Hebebrand, J. and Hinney, A. (2010). Eating disorders: The current status of molecular genetic research. *European Child and Adolescent Psychiatry* 19: 211–26.

Steinhausen, H.-Ch., Rauss-Mason, C. and Seidel, R. (1991). Follow up studies of anorexia nervosa: A review of four decades of outcome research. *Psychological Medicine* 21: 447–54.

Strober, M., Freeman, R. and Morrell, W. (1997). The long-term course of severe anorexia nervosa in adolescents: Survival analysis of recovery, relapse, and outcome predictors over 10–15 years in a prospective study. *International Journal of Eating Disorders* 22: 339–60.

Walford, G. and McCune, N. (1991). Long term outcome of early onset anorexia nervosa. *British Journal of Psychiatry* 159: 383–9.

Whitaker, A., Johnson, J., Shaffer, D. *et al.* (1990). Uncommon troubles in young people: Prevalence estimates of selected psychiatric disorders in a non-referred psychiatric population. *Archives of General Psychiatry* 47: 487–96.

Williams, K.E., Field, D.G. and Seiverling, L. (2010). Food refusal in children: A review of the literature. *Research in Developmental Disabilities* 31: 625–33.

Wilson, G.T. and Shafran, R. (2005). Eating disorders guidelines from NICE. *Lancet* 365: 79–81.

Young, J.K. (2010). Anorexia nervosa and estrogen: Current status of the hypothesis. *Neuroscience and Biobehavior Review* 34: 1195–200.

Zipfel, S., Lowem, B., Reasm, D.L. *et al.* (2000). Long-term prognosis in anorexia nervosa. *Lancet* 355: 721–2.

Chapter 6

Traumatic and stressful situations

Introduction

It is an interesting observation that while some people can cope with adversity without experiencing great distress, others become stuck in remembrance, misery and fear. There is a growing understanding as to why this should be, and managing adverse life events effectively is important because to fail to do so has a strong association with the development of mental illness both in the immediate aftermath, and sometimes throughout the person's life. The work in this area shows that some children are protected from the harmful effects of negative life events by their own inner strengths, and wider issues, while others can be assisted to develop such resilience through appropriate therapeutic measures (Place *et al.* 2002).

A key factor in trying to predict how a traumatic event might be dealt with is the child's age. At about 2 years of age the toddler can distinguish individuals and begin to recreate experiences in play. This means that at this age a child can't anticipate events or consequences very easily because the context that would act as a warning is missing. By the age of 3 years the child's play is becoming more sophisticated and is starting to become the medium through which the child seeks to gain an understanding of the world. With this development comes a fundamental change of thinking as the child begins to shed the belief that the world is governed solely by their actions.

Around the age of 4 years the child develops the ability to recognise alternative ways of proceeding and can favour one course of action over another, which is the beginning of the child recognising that there can be alternative origins for problems other than their own action. By 6 years of age this ability is so fully developed that the child is able to relate the causes of events to origins beyond their influence. The importance of this developmental sequence is that a child younger than 5 years of age is likely to view any traumatic event as something that they caused. The death of a parent, for instance, will be linked to some earlier fleeting thought about wishing them dead, or a sequence of abuse will be seen by the child as something that they are responsible for. Such an attribution can be a major source of guilt for the child, and act as the stimulus for the development of a variety of psychological difficulties.

Traumatic events and post-traumatic stress disorder

Generally when children are faced with a major traumatic episode they tend to remain quiet, but then show acute distress in the immediate aftermath. Almost immediately they begin to try to think of some reason why this should have happened to them, a process called 'causal attribution' (Joseph *et al.* 1991). This 'search for a reason' can go on for months and, for children who continue to have difficulties after a traumatic event, it is one of the aspects which tends to become a persistent feature of their thinking in later years.

In general, any child over 3 years of age will have good recall of traumatic events unless they were unconscious or concussed. This will not be the case, however, if there were several traumatic events (see the section on being the victim of abuse later in this chapter), or if the single event has a long-lasting effect – such as the death of a parent.

In the days and weeks following the event(s), images associated with the trauma keep recurring either in quiet moments or when any reminder occurs. Fearfulness quickly becomes a feature of the child's functioning – not only a fear that events may be repeated, but of more mundane elements such as being separated from parents, the dark, or the presence of strangers. Sleep is often disturbed by vivid dreams, which are often life-like re-enactments of the events. The child's play becomes dominated by the events, as do their drawings, and they may demonstrate a need to keep recounting the story. The play elements tend to have an obvious link to the trauma, and become quite monotonous in content. This is especially so for children under the age of 3 years who cannot fully verbalise their experiences and so play out their feelings and experiences over and over again. In older children intrusive 'flashbacks' occur, which bring with them not only elements of the events but the emotions which are associated with them. Such emotional intensity is very draining, as well as distressing, and so the person usually tries to avoid being reminded of the event and generally may appear emotionally flat. These features of the general process will show some variation in specifics, depending upon the age of the child.

Within months some of the features, especially the emotional elements such as sleeplessness, irritability and the anxious striving to be close to parents, fade, but the re-enacting of events in play tends to persist. This monotonous preoccupation may cause the child either to become increasingly withdrawn or perhaps to victimise others as they have been victimised. If the symptoms persist for a long period they can profoundly disturb the child's life. They may find it hard to remember positive events in their lives, and have difficulties with concentration and working memory (Vasterling *et al.* 2002). As well as these emotional and cognitive changes they are also at increased risk of having chronic physical illnesses (Berkowitz 2003), as well as developing problems with substance abuse, failing at school, and having poor employment records (Sansone *et al.* 2005). Perhaps most worrying is the strong association which exists between experiencing traumatic events and an increased risk of suicide (Ganz and Sher 2010).

Issues influencing the emergence of post-traumatic stress disorder

For most traumas, the majority of children exposed appear to be unharmed or only transiently affected, but the frequency with which people are seen to suffer from post-traumatic stress disorder (PTSD) has increased as our recognition of the problems grow. For instance with regards to road traffic accidents, as many as 14% of those involved will show symptoms some 9 months after the accident (Stallard et al. 2004). Indeed it has been estimated that 8–9% of individuals may experience symptoms of PTSD at some point in their lives (Yule 2001).

A number of themes and issues have been associated with the development of PTSD including the child's previous trauma experiences and intrinsic methods of coping, the nature of the trauma and any resulting injury the child may have suffered, the responses of the child at the time of trauma, and the family and social support and parental stress reactions (Le Brocque et al. 2010). Whatever their origin, experiencing significantly traumatic events can affect the brain's function in several ways because, for the symptoms to persist, there have to be changes to the brain's functioning.

Investigations into the changes within the brain associated with PTSD have tended to focus on a particular part of the brain called the amygdala, which is a major centre of emotional control. The amygdala is associated with recognising threatening situations, and prompting the body's stress reactions (Bremner et al. 2008). It seems that in PTSD the normal control mechanisms for the amygdala's actions are reduced (Simmons et al. 2008), leaving it to increase anxiety unchecked.

One of the mechanisms that the amygdala influences is the management of cortisol, one of the body's main stress hormones. Research suggests that young people who develop PTSD may have had disturbances to this mechanism prior to the traumatic event, making them more vulnerable to adverse effects from traumatic experiences. What is particularly interesting is that the pattern of changes to the cortisol mechanisms is different in PTSD from those found in stress reactions and depression (Strohle and Holsboer 2003), suggesting this is a unique mechanism rather than a general bodily reaction. The significance of cortisol in establishing and maintaining PTSD is not clear, but it is interesting to note that there are positive changes to the cortisol levels in people who benefit from therapy (Olff et al. 2007), while there is little change to cortisol levels in those for whom the symptoms are persistent (Yehuda et al. 2007).

Treatment avenues

The first few days after traumatic events can be very distressing for all, although helping the child to share their experiences and feelings can prove helpful. However if the distress is quite severe, or the routine of daily life remains disrupted for any length of time, then formal therapeutic intervention is indicated. The evidence suggests that therapies that contain an element of exposure are the most helpful (Institute of Medicine 2008), and the largest body of evidence is in relation to cognitive behaviour therapy, with both individual and group programmes proving effective at decreasing symptoms (Wethington *et al.* 2008). These pro-grammes usually combine direct discussion of the traumatic event with increasing linkage to the emotions associated with it. This is combined with stress manage-ment and relaxation techniques as well as exploring the thoughts and associations that have become associated with the events.

An example of such a programme is Prolonged Exposure (Foa *et al.* 2007), which focuses upon the link between the event and the symptoms, based on the theo-retical stance that the person is still perceiving a dangerous situation even though the event is long past. Within the programme there is a gradual encouragement to remember more vividly the traumatic event(s), and specific encouragement to try to engage emotionally with the memories. The programme then progresses to encouraging changes in thinking about the meaning of the event(s), and the introduction of new activities so that the emotional significance declines, and more positive processes dominate. The process may involve visiting the physical settings that are associated with the trauma. This type of approach has been shown to be quite effective, with up to 86% of patients reporting improvement (Powers *et al.* 2010), and the benefits being such that it is the recommended approach for military veterans (Nemeroff *et al.* 2006).

Eye movement desensitisation and reprocessing (EMDR) has also been increasingly recommended for treatment of PTSD (Feeny *et al.* 2004). In EMDR, patients are asked to recall the traumatic event while following the back-and-forth hand movements of the therapist with their eyes. It has been suggested that the treatment is linking the traumatic memory with new and more positive associa-tions so that the memory no longer prompts significant emotion (Maxfield 2003). While the exact nature of the mechanism is still subject to controversy (Nowill 2010), the therapy has proven to be effective (Bisson *et al.* 2007).

The nature of the distress shown after major traumatic events naturally prompts the desire to bring immediate relief. This can be achieved by medication, but the temptation to ease the immediate distress with anxiolytics such as the benzodi-azepines should be avoided because they are potentially addictive, and their use may actually contribute to the development of PTSD (Berger *et al.* 2009). Anti-depressant medications have tended to be the most commonly used in treating PTSD, but in isolation these have not proved to be very effective. While anti-depressants bring about modification of emotions and moods, the beneficial effects are only maintained for as long as the medication is given. Generally the role of medication is to relieve disabling symptoms and quickly establish a more normal pattern of day-to-day functioning, as well as allow the young person to cope better with the emotionally distressing memories in therapy. Such facilitation hopefully accelerates the recovery process, though there is no strong evidence that this aspect of the medication treatment programme is successful (Hetrick *et al.* 2010).

However there are promising results from medications which have a very dif-ferent form of action. Prazosin (a drug initially developed to treat high blood pressure) is proving useful in dealing with sleep-related PTSD symptoms (Taylor *et al.* 2008). D-cycloserine (initially developed as an antibiotic for treating tuber-culosis) influences the brain chemicals involved in learning (Davis *et al.* 2006), and may eventually have a role in accelerating psychological treatment effects by speeding up the reduction in disturbing memories.

In terms of long-term outcome, it is clear that there are many factors which appear to influence both the degree of initial difficulty and the response to treatment. It appears from one study (Le Brocque *et al.* 2010) that the majority of children can be expected to improve, with perhaps 10% of children having a chronic level of stress symptoms. The outlook for children engaged in treatment is generally encouraging, but it should be noted that the very positive benefits reported in formal clinical trials of interventions such as cognitive behaviour therapy may not be fully translated into effective treatments in clinical settings (Ollendick and Davis 2004).

Preventative strategies

With such potential for long-term emotional difficulties there have been significant efforts made to find interventions that prevent the emergence of PTSD after significant traumatic events. Psychological debriefing is a term sometimes used to describe one type of such work. This consists of encouraging discussion of the traumatic event, exploring the person's reactions to it, helping them to view their reactions as normal, or guiding them towards more positive feelings, as well as helping them find mechanisms to control their reactions. It is not clear that such debriefing has a positive effect (Bisson *et al.* 1997), and indeed it appears to be the presence, or absence, of other factors (such as previous psychological problems and adequate social support) that are more likely to affect the outcome rather than whether early protective intervention occurred (Bisson and Deahl 1994). There is evidence that if early intervention is required then cognitive behaviour therapy is more effective than supportive counselling (Ehlers and Clark 2003). It is therefore important that victims are assessed carefully to identify those who would benefit from early intervention to ensure that the correct approach is adopted for each individual.

More recently, interest has been focused on whether specific medication given immediately after traumatic events can reduce the risk of PTSD occurring. The ß-blocker propranolol (initially developed to treat high blood pressure) has been the focus of much attention because it may interrupt the consolidation of traumatic memories in the brain (Pitman *et al.* 2002). While its value is not fully established, there is recent evidence supporting its use with Prazosin to dampen the emotional content of traumatic memories (Shad *et al.* 2011).

Growing up in a violent household

There is clear evidence that growing up in a violent household has a damaging effect upon a child's development (Sternberg *et al.* 2006). This arises not only because of the direct impact that witnessing or being a victim of violence causes, but also because of the way that the violence prevents effective parenting. A recent survey in the UK found that around one in five children (18.6%) have been severely maltreated, with more than one in eight children (13.4%) having experienced severe maltreatment by a parent or guardian, and one in 14 children (6.9%) having experienced severe physical violence at the hands of an adult (NSPCC 2011).

Exposure to frequent arguments between parents is a damaging experience for children, but witnessing violence between parents is even more so (Martinez-Torteya et al. 2009), and indeed it appears to be as damaging as if the child were the direct victim of the violence themselves (Kitzmann et al. 2003). Research in this field has indicated that physically abused toddlers tend to show far more angry non-compliance than their peers, and are easily frustrated in tasks or games, as well as suffering sleep disturbances and physical complaints such as headaches and stomach aches. Older children tend to show disruptive and aggressive reactions. A particularly interesting observation is that boys who have grown up in violent households appear to become more aroused by angry exchanges than their peers, and perhaps as a consequence are far more likely to involve themselves in these exchanges (Cummings et al. 1994).

Difficulties tend to recur throughout such children's lives, with exposure to violence being associated with a significantly increased risk of alcoholism, illicit drug use, and depression (Widom et al. 2007), and a greater tendency to suicide (Brodsky et al. 2008). They also have more physical disorders such as obesity, diabetes, chronic pain disorders and cardiovascular disease (Anda et al. 2006). However, the most frequent outcome for children from violent households is delinquency (Becker and McCloskey 2002) (see Chapter 4). As adults they are particularly prone to having romantic relationships which are punctuated by violent and abusive episodes (Lavoie et al. 2002), with the risk of such outcomes being some four times greater than the general population (Martinez-Torteya et al. 2009). Finally the quality of care they show their own children is likely to be diminished (Pilyoung et al. 2010), creating the potential for such difficulties to emerge in their offspring.

Cicchetti and Toth (1995) have described how growing up in a violent household, or being the victim of any type of abuse, has the potential to distort four areas of a child's functioning:

- emotional regulation;
- attachment;
- sense of self;
- peer relationships.

Emotional regulation comprises the way the young person copes with feelings and this can result in exaggerated reactions, or responses which are too quick and ill thought out, to situations of potential aggression. In other situations the emotions may be more the expected ones of misery or distress, but prompted by trivial and unrelated situations, which can give the impression that the young person is moody or suffering from a depressive illness when in fact the problem is a distorted regulatory mechanism.

As described in Chapter 4, abused children have more insecure attachments, making it difficult for the toddler to cope with separation, and giving a 'disorganised', disorientated quality to the child's life. Lower levels of attachment to parents increase the risk of the child showing antisocial behaviour (Sousa *et al.* 2011), and having poorer levels of cognitive functioning (Koenen *et al.* 2003). However, if toddlerhood is without major incident, and the negative experiences begin later in life, then the risk of disturbing attachment markedly decreases (Lynch and Cicchetti 1991).

The child's sense of self becomes established by the age of 2 years, and, if there are abusive experiences before this age, then this sense of self is distorted. Such children find it harder to engage in the symbolic play so typical of toddlerhood (Alessandri 1991) and they tend to be more aggressive and less competent with their peers. They also often have low self-esteem, and experience a reduced sense of being able to cope (Cicchetti and Toth 1995).

As has already been pointed out in Chapter 1, establishing effective peer relationships is a key developmental issue for all children. Violent experiences can distort this process because the victims have heightened levels of physical and verbal aggression and may respond violently to friendly overtures or even signs of distress in others (Mueller and Silverman 1989). This often makes it difficult for the children to establish appropriate peer relationships (Koverloa *et al.* 2005), resulting in them gravitating towards other disruptive and aggressive children with similar difficulties (Winstok *et al.* 2004).

Issues influencing the emergence of difficulties

As was discussed in Chapter 4, adverse life events exert their influence most upon children who have a genetic vulnerability. One focus of particular interest in this regard has been the control of monoamine oxidase A (MAOA), an enzyme that destroys amines, hormones that are significant in regulating emotion. Abused children with low MAOA activity have an increased likelihood of antisocial behaviour, and a higher likelihood of being convicted for violent offences than abused children with high MAOA activity (Frazzetto *et al.* 2007). By contrast, in children who are not abused, the presence of low MAOA activity has little effect on behaviour (Kim-Cohen *et al.* 2006). However it is not only the presence of the vulnerability that appears to be important, but also the timing of the abuse, since different emotional effects appear to emerge depending upon the child's age at the time (Andersen and Teicher 2004).

The role of cortisol in managing stressful situations has been discussed above, and variations in the quality of parental care are linked with individual differences in cortisol and amine responses to stress (Teicher *et al.* 2002). It has been shown that when a child is abused this alters specific parts of the brain (Vythilingam *et al.* 2002), and changes the body's management of cortisol (McGowan *et al.* 2009). However the changes tend to be evident only in children who experience physical and sexual abuse at an early age, and there is little change to cortisol mechanisms if the abuse occurs later in childhood (Cicchetti *et al.* 2010). It is also worthy of note that interventions that successfully improve parental care also result in a normalisation of the body's cortisol management (Fisher *et al.* 2000).

Responding to children who are growing up in a violent household

Helping young people who have experienced a violent upbringing has many similarities to the response offered to children who have been the victims of any traumatic event. Again the intervention focuses on three areas, the first of which is the family element. Supportive, responsive parenting can buffer the effects of interparental conflict on children by reducing the child's sense that they are to blame for the parental discord (DeBoard-Lucas *et al.* 2010).

The most consistent evidence of the effectiveness of interventions to improve parenting comes from reviews of the Webster-Stratton's Incredible Years programme (see Chapter 2). This seeks not only to give the parents effective and appropriate management techniques, but also to improve the quality of the emotional climate within the family. However, strengthening attachments between parents and children may not be sufficient to counter the negative impact of earlier violent trauma in children if it was severe (Sousa *et al.* 2011). Wider family difficulties demand a more systemic approach, and such interventions either alone or as part of multimodal programmes have proved to be effective (Carr 2009).

The second element is work with the child. If the young person can feel trust and security within the treatment relationship, then their understanding of their life events can be explored. As the therapeutic process progresses, their expressions of emotion become more marked before a gradual subsidence of the difficulties occurs. It is important to be alert to these changes because good therapy makes things worse before it makes them better.

The last element of an intervention programme focuses on the environment in which the child is living. One aspect of this is clearly to remove the potential for further violence or abuse, but there are also the important themes of maintaining routines and allowing the child to have experiences of success. In addition, positive relationships of all kinds are important in offering alternative experiences to those that are being explored with in the therapeutic alliance.

Multisystemic therapy (see Chapter 2) may also have a place in responding to child abuse and neglect. Results from studies suggest that this is significantly more effective than standard care in reducing the young person's mental health symptoms and improving family functioning (Swenson *et al.* 2010). Sometimes the situation demands a child be removed from the home, and there is evidence that foster care with a treatment focus is effective at helping children achieve a more settled pattern of functioning (Montgomery *et al.* 2009), with reduced symptoms of mental health problems and particularly a reduction in feelings of dissociation (Taussig and Culhane 2010).

Issues of resilience

Some children can survive very traumatic experiences with no major mental health difficulties, and the reason for this resilience has been the focus of intense research over many years. This is increasingly indicating that resilient behaviour represents a distinct, active neurobiological process, and is not simply the absence of vulnerability (Krishnan *et al.* 2007). The work tends to focus upon three areas – the child, the family, and the wider community. Children who show resilience have been found to have a positive and supportive relationship with their parents, to live in a family which offers a structured and warm parenting regime, to have an easy-going temperament, and to have no major cognitive difficulties. In contrast, children who show limited resilience tend to live in stressful households, to have mothers suffering from mental health problems (particularly depression), and to have coping mechanisms which tend to focus on problems rather than ones which are oriented away from the difficulties (Compas *et al.* 2001).

Efforts to improve resilience focus around these three areas, with those directed toward the child seeking to encourage a more optimistic interpretation of life events. They also seek to establish a more problem-solving style of coping as well as helping the child develop a sense of achievement, positive friendship networks, and physical and recreational diversions (Hall and Place 2010).

Being the victim of sexual abuse

Many of the themes relevant to children growing up in a violent household are commonly found in other forms of abusive situation, but being the victim of sexual abuse does bring with it specific issues and reactions which are worthy of separate consideration. Sexual abuse is a term which can encompass a wide range of inappropriate sexual activity from fondling to full intercourse, with about 5% of reported incidents involving penetrative intercourse (Baker and Duncan 1985), though it does appear that the rate of presentation is declining (Finkelhor and Jones 2006). Some 80% of victims are girls (Finkelhor *et al.* 2010), and although the child can be any age, it is most common for it to begin between the ages of 8 and 12 years (Monck *et al.* 1993). Such abuse occurs irrespective of social status or religious persuasion and in many cases the abuse is a repeated act over several years. Most cases are never reported, and it has been estimated that as few as 2% of cases are brought to the attention of the authorities (Russell 1983), with incest with a sibling probably being the most common (Finkelhor 1979), and yet the least reported.

In the immediate aftermath of the abuse, anxiety symptoms tend to be the most evident, frequently taking the form of insomnia, nightmares and somatic complaints, with over 90% reporting stomach aches around the time of the abuse (van Tilburg *et al.* 2010). Most victims of sexual abuse see themselves as 'damaged goods' because of their experiences (Sgroi 1982), and this compounds the feelings of depression and misery that are so common in these children. This is why so many victims have significant emotional difficulties in adult life, most commonly depression, substance abuse, eating disorders, and self-destructive behaviour (Merrill *et al.* 2001). There is also an increased risk of violent and nonviolent criminal behaviour (Becker and McCloskey 2002), with some showing severe post-traumatic stress symptomatology, which at its most extreme can take the form of dissociative disorders, including dissociative identity disorder (Shipman and Taussig 2009). About 16% of children report feelings of arousal within the abusive relationship (Monck *et al.* 1993). The sense of conflict between these feelings and the knowledge of being abused can be a powerful force in creating some of these emotional problems.

One of the most consistent observations is the way that sexually abusive experiences distort the child's own sexual functioning, and this seems especially true if the abuse occurred before the age of 7 years (McClellan *et al.* 1996). Public masturbation and the tendency to repeat sexually abusive experiences are very common patterns (Monck *et al.* 1993). Infants who have been abused find it difficult to distinguish appropriate displays of affection from the episodes of sexual activity, leading to abused toddlers showing quite explicitly sexual behaviour.

Sara was 4 years of age when her nursery became concerned at her sexualised play. She would openly masturbate while playing, and would sit on adults' knees, rocking slowly while making a moaning sound and becoming quite excited. Investigations revealed that Sara had been subjected to repeated sexual abuse from the age of 2 years old, as had her elder sister.

Sexually abused children are often seen within school to be anxious, inattentive and unable to understand classroom expectations. They tend to be unpopular with peers, and show an increased frequency of withdrawal and aggressive outbursts in any interactions they have with them. Typically, they tend to get by because they are highly dependent upon teachers (Erickson *et al.* 1989).

Intervention with children who have been sexually abused

The first requirement for any intervention is to recognise that abuse is occurring. The majority of cases come to light because of a disclosure by the child, and so an essential first principle is to accept the child's statements when first told. Being the victim of abuse can provoke quite significant behavioural difficulties and so it is dangerous to dismiss a child's report of abuse simply because they have been troublesome in the past.

The recipient of a disclosure of any type of abuse should offer a calm and accepting demeanour. Responses should be in a supportive tone, and either a repetition of their last phrase, or simple requests for them to continue. The information must be passed on to the relevant professionals and so any promise to 'keep the secret' must be avoided. Recipients should record as accurately and as soon as possible what was said, and then follow the advice about making a referral that is contained in the relevant Child Protection Procedures manual.

The professional network of social workers and police typically act on the disclosure by carrying out a careful investigation. The first priority is always to ensure that the child is safe from further abuse, and in half of the families, concern about how supportive the family will be is sufficient for the child to be accommodated away from home (Monck *et al.* 1993).

In most cases a variety of approaches is necessary in order to address the various types of difficulty that abuse can cause. The sexualised components are addressed initially by age-appropriate sex education and establishing with the child what are the age-appropriate ways of dealing with sexual needs and urges. Cognitive behaviour therapy (CBT) is now one of the main elements of treatment intervention. It has been shown to significantly improve the associated emotional and behavioural problems, such as deliberate self-harm (Spinhoven *et al.* 2009), rather than the specific issues around being the victim of sexual abuse (Trowler *et al.* 2002). There is also some evidence that adding medication to the treatment programme may improve its impact for this group of children (Cohen *et al.* 2007).

Interpersonal psychotherapy with sexually abused children and adolescents has been shown to have positive benefits both in terms of specific symptoms, and general functioning, though long term benefit is less evident (Harvey and Taylor 2010). Many settings also make use of group therapy, which can involve elements such as psychodrama, but group work does not appear to help with oppositional and conduct difficulties (Avinger and Jones 2007).

It is important within this process not to lose sight of parental distress, since the success of such programmes can be strongly influenced by how well the parents are coping, and there is some evidence that therapy that involves the parent is more effective than treating the child in isolation (Corcoran and Pillai 2008).

Outcome for sexually abused children

The studies carried out among adults reveal the potential that exists for sexually abusive experiences in childhood to prompt major psychiatric difficulties in adult life. It is clear that the present intervention programmes are effective at reducing the symptoms which show themselves after disclosure of abuse (Monck *et al.* 1993), but female sexual abuse victims continue to experience relationship problems and problems in sexual functioning (Rumstein-McKean and Hunsley 2001). Numerous studies have noted that child sexual abuse victims are vulnerable to later sexual re-victimization, as well as being more likely to have multiple sex partners, become pregnant as teenagers, and experience sexual assault as adults (Lalor and McElvaney 2010). By and large, the severity of the abuse, the use of force, and the victim's prior relationship to the perpetrator are linked to a poorer outcome, whilst strong family support and parental monitoring tend to reduce the impact (Tyler 2002). It is also interesting to note that when the victim is a boy, the long-term effects may be more severe and more complex in nature than previously thought, with a high prevalence of dissociative experiences among those with a history of childhood sexual abuse compared with survivors of other forms of trauma (van den Bosch *et al.* 2003).

Even with positive therapeutic intervention more than one-third of women continue to have significant difficulties (Vickerman and Margolin 2009), with the commonest being depression, obesity, autoimmune disorders (e.g. irritable bowel syndrome, asthma, fibromyalgia), eating disorders, and addictions (Wilson 2010). Sadly, it has been found that about 12% of childhood victims of sexual abuse go on to become abusers themselves (Salter *et al.* 2003), with the sexual offending usually beginning in adolescence (Butler and Seto 2002).

Prevention

There have been some efforts to develop programmes within school which will help children protect themselves from becoming the victims of sexual abuse. These have been shown to increase children's awareness of child sexual abuse, but beyond showing a small increase in disclosure of existing abuse, there is little evidence that they offer any protection to children from intra-familial sexual abuse (Barron and Topping 2008).

Coping with parental separation and divorce

Parental separation is one of the most common traumatic events that a child can face. In fact, children who have experienced a separation or divorce are up to three times more likely to have emotional and behavioural difficulties than the average, and show poorer academic achievement, more conduct and psychological adjustment problems, as well as a low self-concept, and poorer social relations than their peers (Amato 2001). However, divorce is very rarely a single event in time for, in the vast majority of cases, there has been an ongoing relationship difficulty between the parents before the specific act of separation occurs.

A sadly common consequence of separation is the pattern of ongoing friction between the parents which, superficially, can be focused upon contact or financial settlements, but in fact is a continuation of their relationship conflict. Within this type of conflict there can be competition for the affection and allegiance of the child which can take many forms, few of which are helpful to the child's development.

Michael was 6 years old when his parents separated. Michael's mother was very bitter at her husband's departure and the way that he had 'deserted the family'. She resisted any idea of ongoing contact between Michael and his father because she feared he would 'pick up his habits and his ways'. The court imposed regular contact at a neutral venue and before each meeting Michael's mother would remind him that his father was 'a bad man'. After the visits she would closely question Michael about his father's present lifestyle, for instance asking whether he had a new partner.

A situation such as this imposes major stress upon the child. Not only is there a need not to upset the parent who looks after you, but any suggestion of liking the other parent is seen as disloyalty. Equally, the contact sessions cannot be enjoyed for their own sake because of the danger of fuelling the battle by some inadvertent comment.

The impacts of ongoing parental conflict upon a child have been discussed above in connection with family violence, but less severe forms can still produce sleep disturbance, and prompt the child to behave more aggressively towards parents, siblings and peers. If the separation occurs during adolescence then this complicates a time when the young person is endeavouring to cope with the emotional turmoil of this stage of development. The additional stress of the separation tends to intensify the existing emotional features and can precipitate the emergence of acting-out behaviour, depression or even suicidal feelings. At this age, the concrete thinking of the child is giving way to a more abstract and complex understanding of situations which can often lead to the adolescent reaching a strongly held view as to how the events leading up to the separation should be interpreted. Although boys tend to fare less well than girls in the aftermath of parental separation, when adolescence is reached girls of separated parents do experience greater difficulty in separating from their mothers.

However, overall, it is how parents cope with the trauma of separation and divorce that is the major determinant of how children will cope (Guidubaldi and Perry 1985). Children whose parents have not coped well with the divorce tend to have more emotional, behavioural, social, and health difficulties than their peers, and also do less well academically (Frisco et al. 2007). Delinquent behaviour tends to be more common in children whose parents are separated or divorced and, in contrast to the general findings that conduct difficulties emerge in children with a genetic vulnerability (see Chapter 4), this association appears to be as the direct result of the experience of parental divorce (Burt et al. 2008).

When they reach adulthood these children have, on average, obtained less education, show lower levels of psychological well-being, and report more problems in their own marriages, with a greater risk of seeing their own marriages end in divorce (Amato and Sobolewski 2001). However, work to maintain positive relationships between a child and their parents has shown improvements in the quality of the mother–child relationship, and helped the child develop more active and effective coping strategies. These improvements have been noted to persist some six years later (Vélez et al. 2011).

Coming to terms with physical illness

In the Western world about 5% of children have a significant, handicapping physical disorder (Pless and Nolan 1991). How such children react to their difficulties is very varied, but generally the more severe the handicap, the greater the risk of the young person developing a psychiatric disorder (Daud et al. 1993). Most young people do cope, and those who seek to cope actively by thinking of other things or using calming self-statements tend to fare much better than those who simply hope things will be all right (Gil et al. 1991). When problems do occur, they tend to show themselves either as emotional symptoms or as disturbances to everyday functions, such as eating and sleeping (Pearson et al. 1991).

Physically disabled preschoolers show a greater frequency of peer rejection and bullying compared with healthy peers, and in later childhood chronic illness is significantly associated with early-onset depressive symptoms and impairment in several social functioning domains, even after accounting for socioeconomic status (Curtis and Luby 2008). Children with chronic illness report having a lower health-related quality of life than their peers (Sawyer *et al.* 2004), with the child's style of coping being perhaps the most significant factor (Peeters *et al.* 2008). Their ability to maintain an average lifestyle, how well they develop and maintain friendships, their attitude to treatment and indeed their relationship to their healthcare professionals all influence the degree of adjustment (Taylor *et al.* 2008).

Although the development of a significant disability obviously has a major impact upon the young person, it is the impact that it has upon the parent which is often the most significant for predicting future psychological difficulties. In coming to terms with their child's disability or illness, the parents may become depressed or overprotective, or lose interest in the child, all of which can have a marked effect upon the child's development. However, if support can be mobilised for the parents through counselling or formal psychiatric help, then the attentiveness to the child can become more normal, leading to the development of a more healthy lifestyle (Reynolds *et al.* 1988).

Illnesses or injuries which involve the brain are particularly problematic. For instance, children with epilepsy may be up to four times more likely to develop psychiatric problems than the general population, particularly if there are other neurological abnormalities (Rutter *et al.* 1970). In some children it is clear that their seizures can be provoked by becoming emotional or feeling stressed. This observation has prompted the development of programmes which look to control seizures using psychological methods, which appear to offer some children a degree of control (Motofsky and Balaschak 1977).

Head injuries may result in some disturbance of brain function, although the vast majority of such injuries cause problems that are transient and quickly resolved. However if the child is injured in a traumatic way, then this significantly increases the risk of post-traumatic stress disorder emerging (Bryant *et al.* 2010). In severe head injuries up to 50% of victims will show long-term psychiatric problems (Max *et al.* 1998), with these most likely in those who had some emotional or behavioural difficulties before the injury occurred. The likelihood of future difficulties can also be predicted by how much of the immediate post-accident events the child can't remember. If there is post–traumatic amnesia more than a week after the accident then psychiatric difficulties are increasingly likely (Chadwick *et al.* 1981).

The degree to which the child can cope with their chronic illness in turn can strongly influence symptoms and illness management. For instance in diabetes, children who show low levels of resilience tend to have poorer diabetic control, and are less able to maintain their self-care behaviours when faced with any upsets or difficulties (Yi *et al.* 2008).

Bereavement

As for all stressful events, the age at which children are asked to cope can have a crucial impact on how they deal with bereavement. About 4 to 7% of children will have mourned the death of a parent before the age of 16 (Ribbens *et al.* 2005), with children under the age of 10 being more vulnerable to enduring upset as a consequence (Melhem *et al.* 2008).

Children younger than 5 years of age see death as reversible and so, for them, the deceased has simply gone somewhere else, and may perhaps return one day. This belief is simultaneously reassuring to the child and disconcerting for adults, who may feel that the child's lack of marked distress is because 'they don't care' or because 'it hasn't sunk in yet'. In fact neither of these is the case – the child simply believes the person is elsewhere, a fact which is not a cause for significant distress.

By the age of 7 years the child can recognise that death is final. As a result, the loss of a loved one can have a major impact, for the child can recognise the loss but does not have the emotional experience or maturity with which to deal with it. In children over seven, therefore, the sense of loss can provoke reactions which approximate to those seen in adults. Immediately upon learning of the loss there is a sense of shock and disbelief. The young person often appears dazed, but in the following days there is the emergence of misery, and possibly an attempt to withdraw from company. There is usually a deterioration in sleep patterns and concentration, and eating habits change.

There are broadly two patterns that young people may display in the weeks following the death of significant figures in their lives. The first is where the child may find it so difficult to come to terms with the loss that he or she tries to retain a 'relationship' in some way. This often takes the form of retaining a keepsake, or sensing that the person is still with them (Silverman *et al.* 1992). Sometimes the child may report seeing or hearing the person, but these events are not of the same quality as the hallucinations seen in major psychotic illnesses. Reunion fantasies are quite common, and this pattern can cause adults to become concerned about the child.

The second type of reaction is typically seen after a traumatic death. Children feel overwhelmed by the distress and so seek to avoid any remembrance of it. They will avoid items, or situations, that could act as reminders, and begin to fear that other significant people may also suddenly be taken from them. This pattern of avoidance and withdrawal can significantly distort the grieving process, and if prolonged may need professional intervention.

Commonly, in the aftermath of a significant bereavement, children will lose motivation to undertake schoolwork, and will often report intrusive thoughts or images associated with the dead person crowding into their minds when they try to study. There may be a sequence of minor illnesses, which can be an effective way of obtaining adult concern and care for a child who does not fully understand that being bereaved prompts support in its own right.

Over the subsequent weeks these intense emotions tend to give way to a more blunted pattern of sadness and irritability, and sometimes there is the emergence of aggression. Gradually these features fade and become less frequent, so that after 18 months most have effectively dealt with their feelings and stopped grieving. Very few young people go on to have adult problems as a result of a bereavement (Fristed *et al.* 1993), with the strongest determinant being the quality of childcare offered in the aftermath of the bereavement (Breier *et al.* 1988). Indeed, some young people take on a more mature perspective as a result of suffering a bereavement, and emerge better equipped to cope with future adversity (Balk 1990).

When children are faced with coping with the loss of a significant adult it is important to consider the child's age. In younger children it is necessary to be prepared for indifference, and perhaps a surprising lack of distress. In older children the first need is to establish a supportive and caring environment. It is important to recognise that the child will have questions and strong emotions that must be dealt with. The child may not feel able, or feel they have permission, to grieve, or may not know how to respond to the emotions that they are experiencing. It is also usually helpful if the child attends the funeral. Most children express a desire to attend the ceremony, and research indicates that attendance is generally beneficial to their ultimate adjustment (Weller *et al.* 1988).

Children may miss out on their own grieving process if their sense of duty prompts them to make efforts to distract their parents from their grief. This often takes the form of misbehaviour, since this is the most potent way of obtaining parental attention, and certainly is capable of demanding a high priority in their parents' concerns.

Alex presented at 8 years of age with a six-month history of being difficult and truculent at home. His mother said he had become defiant and everything had become a battle. Alex's parents saw the behaviour as particularly problematic because their younger child had developed leukaemia some months ago and they felt they had enough worries without having to respond to Alex's tantrums and defiance. When seen alone, Alex quickly became weepy and distressed, saying that he was very concerned about his brother, but since he had developed his illness his parents spent all their spare time with him, and Alex felt he had no time with them. He said of the last few weeks that 'they aren't crying all the time now, they're too busy shouting at me'.

The evidence is clear that the strongest predictor of risk to children from parental loss is the level of adjustment and psychological well-being of the surviving parent (Haine *et al.* 2006). If the parent has been so deeply affected by the loss that their parenting abilities have become blunted, or they have lost the motivation to keep insisting upon good behaviour, then major difficulties can rise.

Work with adolescents suggests that they often feel better if they can talk about their feelings of loss with their peers (Gray 1989), but many worry that their friends will not be able to cope with their emotional distress. This awkwardness and uncertainty tends to drive the young person to withdraw into solitude. This is probably why many teenagers report that their friendships deteriorate in the aftermath of a bereavement (Balk 1990).

If the young person retains good social links and is keeping up with schoolwork, then they are coping well with the situation and do not require outside assistance. However, there are several elements that are worth pursuing after a bereavement:

- Ensure that the child gets information on the illness or circumstances of the death. It is important that they understand the situation properly, and to this end the explanations must be concrete and explicit.
- Most children benefit from being given the opportunity to say 'goodbye' properly. The younger the child the more concrete this expression tends to be – for example, a young child may wish to place a favourite toy upon the grave.
- Correct any misunderstandings or wrong information.
- Give the child explicit permission to grieve, and offer opportunities to do so in a safe environment. In younger children, features of the death may dominate pictures and play for some weeks after, and this should be accepted as normal.
- Give information on how people grieve, in particular confirming that it is appropriate to have a range of feelings, not only sadness at the loss, but anger that they have been deserted.
- Re-establish routines as soon as practicable; returning to the familiar and the predictable helps to minimise fears that the young person's own future is threatened by the loss.
- Help retain peer links by offering opportunities, not by creating any sense of pressure.
- Emphasize the need for parental strength and control, and ensure that rules are still enforced.

These issues also need to be considered if a classmate has a terminal illness. In such a situation it is helpful to prepare the class by giving the information in a structured way, and prompting class members to plan how they will react and respond (Yule and Gold 1993).

In situations where formal therapy is deemed necessary, programmes based around the normal management of bereavement have proved to be the most helpful. The Family Bereavement Program (Sandler *et al.* 2003) has, at its core, elements that seek to normalise the grief process, improve the quality of the relationship between the child and parent, while encouraging the parent to offer effective discipline, and reduce the child's exposure to negative and stressful life events. An element of this programme is to help the child to have more positive thoughts, and to help them recognise what is and is not within their control (Wolchik *et al.* 2008). This programme has proven effective in reducing difficulties for children (Burt 2010), and it has been shown to prevent the development of the disturbed cortisol regulation that is associated with emotional upset (Luecken *et al.* 2010).

Loss and bereavement is a natural part of everyone's life. However, children's mechanisms for coping with this type of emotional upset are immature, and the younger the child the less well developed they are. Sensitivity and awareness of the child's developmental needs will usually give direction to any help or assistance the child might need.

Sources of further help

www.griefencounter.org.uk/
www.childbereavement.org.uk/

http://www.rcpsych.ac.uk/mentalhealthinformation.aspx
http://www.aacap.org/cs/root/facts_for_families/facts_for_families
http://www.nspcc.org.uk/help-and-advice/help_and_advice_hub_wdh71748.html
http://www.domesticviolence.co.uk/

References

Alessandri, S.M. (1991). Play and social behaviours in maltreated pre-schoolers. *Developmental Psychopathology* 3: 191–206.

Amato, P.R. (2001) Children of divorce in the 1990s: An update of the Amato and Keith (1991) meta-analysis. *Journal of Family Psychology* 15: 355–70.

Amato, P.R. and Sobolewski, J.M. (2001).The effects of divorce and marital discord on adult children's psychological well-being. *American Sociological Review* 66: 900–21.

Anda, R.F., Felitti, V.J., Bremner, J.D. *et al.* (2006). The enduring effects of abuse and related adverse experiences in childhood. *European Archives of Psychiatry and Clinical Neuroscience* 256: 174–86.

Andersen, S.L. and Teicher, M.H. (2004). Delayed effects of early stress on hippocampal development. *Neuropsychopharmacology* 29: 1988–93.

Avinger, K.A. and Jones, R.A. (2007). Group treatment of sexually abused adolescent girls: A review of outcome studies. *The American Journal of Family Therapy* 35: 315–26.

Baker, A.W. and Duncan, S.P. (1985). Child sexual abuse: A study of prevalence in Great Britain. *Child Abuse and Neglect* 9: 457–67.

Balk, D.E. (1990). The self-concept of bereaved adolescents: Sibling death and its aftermath. *Journal of Adolescent Research* 5: 112–32.

Barron, I. and Topping, K. (2008) School-based child sexual abuse prevention programmes: The evidence on effectiveness. *Journal of Children's Services* 3: 31–53.

Becker, K.B. and McCloskey, L.A. (2002). Attention and conduct problems in children exposed to family violence. *American Journal of Orthopsychiatry* 72: 83–91.

Berger, W., Mendlowicz, M.V., Marques-Portella, C. *et al.* (2009). Pharmacologic alternatives to antidepressants in posttraumatic stress disorder: A systematic review. *Progress in Neuropsychopharmacology and Biological Psychiatry* 33: 169–80.

Berkowitz, S.J. (2003). Children exposed to community violence: The rationale for early intervention. *Clinical Child and Family Psychology Review* 6: 293–302.

Bisson, J.I. and Deahl, M.P. (1994). Psychological debriefing and prevention of post-traumatic stress. *British Journal of Psychiatry* 165: 717–20.

Bisson, J.I., Jenkins, P.L., Alexander, J. *et al.* (1997). Randomised controlled trial of psychological debriefing for victims of acute burn trauma. *British Journal of Psychiatry* 171: 78–81.

Bisson, J.I., Ehlers, A., Matthews, R. *et al.*(2007) Psychological treatments for chronic post-traumatic stress disorder. Systematic review and meta-analysis. *British Journal of Psychiatry* 190: 97–104.

Breier, A., Kelsoe, J.R., Kirwin, P.D. *et al.* (1988). Early parental loss and development of adult psychopathology. *Archives of General Psychiatry* 45: 987–93.

Bremner, J.D., Elzinga, B., Schmahl, C. *et al.* (2008) Structural and functional plasticity of the human brain in post-traumatic stress disorder. *Progress in Brain Research* 167: 171–86.

Brent, D.A. (2010) The Family Bereavement Program reduces problematic grief in parentally bereaved youths. *Evidence Based Mental Health* 13: 115.

Brodsky, B.S., Mann, J.J., Stanley, B. *et al.* (2008). Familial transmission of suicidal behavior: Factors mediating the relationship between childhood abuse and offspring suicide attempts. *Journal of Clinical Psychiatry* 69: 584–96.

Burt, S.A., Barnes, A.R., McGue, M. *et al.* (2008). Parental divorce and adolescent delinquency: Ruling out the impact of common genes. *Developmental Psychology* 44: 1668–77.

Butler, S.M. and Seto, M.C. (2002) Distinguishing two types of adolescent sex offenders. *Journal of the American Academy of Child Adolescent Psychiatry* 41: 83–90.

Carr, A. (2009). The effectiveness of family therapy and systemic interventions for child-focused problems. *Journal of Family Therapy* 31: 3–45.

Chadwick, O., Rutter, M. and Brown, G. (1981). A prospective study of children with head injuries: II. Cognitive sequelae. *Psychological Medicine* 11: 49–61.

Cicchetti, D. and Toth, S.L. (1995). A developmental psychopathological perspective on child abuse and neglect. *Journal of the American Academy of Child and Adolescent Psychiatry* 34: 541–65.

Cicchetti, D., Rogosch, F.A., Gunnar, M.R. *et al.* (2010). The differential impacts of early physical and sexual abuse and internalizing problems on daytime cortisol rhythm in school-aged children. *Child Development* 81: 252–69.

Cohen, J.A. (2003). Treating acute post-traumatic reactions in children and adolescents. *Biological Psychiatry* 53: 827–33.

Cohen, J., Mannarino, A.P., Perel, J.M. *et al.* (2007). A pilot randomized controlled trial of combined trauma-focused CBT and Sertraline for childhood PTSD symptoms. *Journal of the American Academy of Child and Adolescent Psychiatry* 46: 811–19.

Compas, B.E., Connor-Smith, J.K., Saltzman, H. *et al.* (2001). Coping with stress during childhood and adolescence: Problems, progress, and potential in theory and research. *Psychological Bulletin* 127: 87–127.

Corcoran, J. and Pillai, V. (2008). A meta-analysis of parent-involved treatment for child sexual abuse. *Research on Social Work Practice* 18: 453–64.

Cummings, E.M., Henness, K., Rabideau, G. *et al.* (1994). Responses of physically abused boys to inter-adult anger involving their mothers. *Developmental Psychopathology* 6: 31–42.

Curtis, C.E. and Luby, J.L. (2008). Depression and social functioning among preschool children with chronic medical conditions. *Journal of Pediatrics* 153: 408–13.

Daud, L.R., Garralda, M.E. and David, T.J. (1993). Psychosocial adjustment in pre-school children with atopic eczema. *Archives of Diseases in Childhood* 69: 670–76.

Davis, M., Ressler, K., Rothbaum, B.O. *et al.* (2006). Effects of D-cycloserine on extinction: Translation from preclinical to clinical work. *Biological Psychiatry* 60: 369–75.

DeBoard-Lucas, R.L., Fosco, G.M., Raynor, S.R. *et al.* (2010) Interparental conflict in context: Exploring relations between parenting processes and children's conflict appraisals. *Journal of Clinical Child and Adolescent Psychology* 39: 163–75.

De Young, M. (1984). *Sexual Victimization of Children.* Jefferson, NC: McFarland.

Ehlers, A. and Clark, D. (2003). Early psychological interventions for adult survivors of trauma: A review. *Biological Psychiatry* 53: 817–26.

Feeny, N.C., Foa, E.B., Treadwell, K.R.H. *et al.* (2004). Post-traumatic stress disorder in youth: A critical review of the cognitive and behavioral treatment outcome literature. *Professional Psychology: Research and Practice,* 35: 466–76.

Finkelhor, D. (1986). *Sourcebook on Child Sexual Abuse.* New York: Sage.

Finkelhor, D. and Jones, L. (2006) Why have child maltreatment and child victimization declined? *Journal of Social Issues* 62: 685–716.

Finkelhor, D., Turner, H., Ormrod, R. *et al.* (2010). Trends in childhood violence and abuse exposure: Evidence from two national surveys. *Archives of Pediatric and Adolescent Medicine* 164: 238–42.

Frazzetto, G., Di Lorenzo, G., Carola, V. *et al.* (2007). Early trauma and increased risk for physical aggression during adulthood: The moderating role of MAOA genotype. *PLoS One* 2(5): e486.

Fisher, P.A., Gunnar, M.R., Chamberlain, P. *et al.* (2000). Preventive intervention for maltreated preschool children: Impact on children's behavior, neuroendocrine activity and foster parent functioning. *Journal of the American Academy of Child and Adolescent Psychiatry* 39: 1356–64.

Foa, E., Hembree, E. and Rothbaum, B. (2007). *Prolonged Exposure Therapy for PTSD: Emotional Processing of Traumatic Experiences, Therapist Guide*. Oxford: Oxford University Press.

Frisco, M.L., Muller, C. and Frank, K. (2007). Parents' union dissolution and adolescents' school performance: Comparing methodological approaches. *Journal of Marriage and Family* 66: 721–41.

Fristed, M.A., Jedel, R., Weller, R.A. (1993). Psychosocial functioning in children after the death of a parent. *American Journal of Psychiatry* 150: 511–13.

Ganz, D. and Sher, L. (2010). Suicidal behavior in adolescents with post-traumatic stress disorder. *Minerva Pediatrica* 62: 363–70.

Gil, K.M., Williams, D.A., Thompson, R.J. *et al.* (1991). Sickle cell disease in children and adolescents: The relation of child and parent pain coping strategies to adjustment. *Journal of Pediatric Psychology* 16: 643–63.

Gray, R.E. (1989). Adolescent perceptions of social support after the death of a parent. *Journal of Psychosocial Oncology* 7: 127–44.

Guidubaldi, J. and Perry, J.D. (1985). Divorce and mental health sequelae for children: A two year follow-up of a nationwide sample. *Journal of the American Academy of Child Psychiatry* 24: 531–7.

Haine, R.A., Ayers, T.S., Sandler, I.N. *et al.* (2008). Evidence-based practices for parentally bereaved children and their families. *Professional Psychology: Research and Practice* 39: 113–21.

Hall, B. and Place, M. (2010). Cutting to cope: A modern adolescent phenomenon. *Child: Care, Health and Development* 36: 623–9.

Harvey, S.T. and Taylor, J.E. (2010). A meta-analysis of the effects of psychotherapy with sexually abused children and adolescents. *Clinical Psychology Review* 30: 517–35.

Helzer, J.E., Robins, L.N. and McEvoy, L. (1987). Post-traumatic stress disorder in the general population: Findings of the Epidemiologic Catchment Area Survey. *New England Journal of Medicine* 317: 1630–4.

Hetrick, S.E., Purcell, R., Garner, B. *et al.* (2010). Combined pharmacotherapy and psychological therapies for post-traumatic stress disorder (PTSD). *Cochrane Database Systematic Reviews* (7): CD007316.

Institute of Medicine (2008). *Treatment of Post-traumatic Stress Disorder: An Assessment of the Evidence*. Washington, DC: National Academies Press.

Joseph, S.A., Brewin, C.R. and Yule, W. (1991). Causal attribution and psychiatric symptoms in survivors of the *Herald of Free Enterprise* disaster. *British Journal of Psychiatry* 159: 542–6.

Kim-Cohen, J., Caspi, A., Taylor, A. *et al.* (2006). MAOA, maltreatment, and gene-environment interaction predicting children's mental health: New evidence and a meta-analysis. *Molecular Psychiatry* 11: 903–13.

Kitzmann, K.M., Gaylord, N.K., Holt, A.R. *et al.* (2003). Child witnesses to domestic violence: A meta-analytic review. *Journal of Consulting and Clinical Psychology* 71: 339–52.

Koenen, K.C., Moffitt, T.E., Caspi, E. *et al.* (2003). Domestic violence is associated with environmental suppression of IQ in young children. *Development and Psychopathology* 15: 297–311.

Koverloa, C., Papas, M.A., Pitts, S. *et al.* (2005). Longitudinal investigation of the relationship among maternal victimization, depressive symptoms, social support, and children's behavior and development. *Journal of Interpersonal Violence* 20: 1523–32.

Krishnan, V., Han, M.H., Graham, D.L. *et al.* (2007). Molecular adaptations underlying susceptibility and resistance to social defeat in brain reward regions. *Cell* 131: 391–404.

Lalor, K. and McElvaney, R. (2010) Child sexual abuse, links to later sexual exploitation/ high-risk sexual behavior, and prevention/treatment programs. *Trauma Violence Abuse* 11: 159–77.

Lavoie, F., Hébert, M., Tremblay, R. *et al.* (2002). History of family dysfunction and perpetration of dating violence by adolescent boys: A longitudinal study. *Journal of Adolescent Health* 30: 375–83.

Le Brocque, R.M., Hendrikz, J. and Kenardy, J.A. (2010). The course of post-traumatic stress in children: Examination of recovery trajectories following traumatic injury. *Journal of Pediatric Psychology* 35: 637–45.

Livingstone, R. (1987). Sexually and physically abused children. *Journal of the American Academy of Child and Adolescent Psychiatry* 26: 413–15.

Luecken, L.J., Hagan, M.J., Sandler, I.N. *et al.* (2010) Cortisol levels six years after participation in the Family Bereavement Program. *Psychoneuroendocrinology* 35: 785–9.

Lynch, M. and Cicchetti, D. (1991). Patterns of relatedness in maltreated and non-maltreated children: Connections among multiple representational models. *Developmental Psychopathology* 3: 207–26.

Max, J.E., Koele, S.L. and Smith, W.L. (1998). Psychiatric disorders in children and adolescents after severe traumatic brain injury: A controlled study. *Journal of American Academy Child Adolescent Psychiatry* 37: 832–40.

McClellan, J., McCurry, C., Ronnei, M. *et al.* (1996). Age of onset of sexual abuse: Relationships to sexually inappropriate behaviors. *Journal of the American Academy of Child and Adolescent Psychiatry* 35: 1375–83.

McGowan, P.O., Sasaki, A., D'Alessio, A.C. *et al.* (2009). Epigenetic regulation of the glucocorticoid receptor in human brain associates with childhood abuse. *Nature Neuroscience* 12: 342–8.

Martinez-Torteya, C., Bogat, G., von Eye, A. *et al.* (2009). Resilience among children exposed to domestic violence: The role of risk and protective factors. *Child Development* 80: 562–77.

Melhem, N.M., Walker, M., Moritz, G. *et al.* (2008) Antecedents and sequelae of sudden parental death in offspring and surviving caregivers. *Archives of Pediatric and Adolescent Medicine* 162: 403–10.

Merrill, L.L., Thomsen, C.J., Sinclair, B.B. *et al.* (2001). Predicting the impact of child sexual abuse on women: The role of abuse severity, parental support, and coping strategies. *Journal of Consulting and Clinical Psychology* 69: 992–1006.

Monck, E., Bentovim, A. and Goodall, G. (1993). *Child Sexual Abuse: A Descriptive and Treatment Study*. London: HMSO.

Montgomery, P., Gardner, F., Bjornstad, G. *et al.* (2009). *Systematic Reviews of Interventions Following Physical Abuse: Helping Practitioners and Expert Witnesses Improve the Outcomes of Child Abuse. DCSF-RBX-09-08A*. London: Department for Children, Schools and Families.

Motofsky, D. and Balaschak, B. (1977). Psychological control of seizures. *Psychological Bulletin* 843: 723–7.

Mueller, E. and Silverman, N. (1989). Peer relations in maltreated children. In D. Cicchetti and V. Carlson (eds) *Child Maltreatment: Theory and Research on the Causes and Consequences of Child Abuse and Neglect*. New York: Cambridge University Press.

National Society for the Prevention of Cruelty to Children. (2011). *Child Cruelty in the UK 2011: An NSPCC Study into Childhood Abuse and Neglect over the Past 30 Years*. London: NSPCC.

Nemeroff, C.B., Bremner, J.D., Foa, E.B. *et al.* (2006). Post-traumatic stress disorder: A state-of-the-science review. *Journal of Psychiatric Research* 40: 1–21.

Nowill, J. (2010). A critical review of the controversy surrounding eye movement desensitization and reprocessing. *Counselling Psychology Review* 25: 63–70.

Olff, M., de Vries, G.J., Güzelcan, Y. *et al.* (2007). Changes in cortisol and DHEA plasma levels after psychotherapy for PTSD. *Psychoneuroendocrinology* 32: 619–26.

Ollendick, T.H. and Davis, T.E. (2004). Empirically supported treatments for children and adolescents: Where to from here? *Clinical Psychology: Science and Practice* 11: 289–94.

Pearson, D.A., Pumariega, A.J., Seilheimer, D.K. (1991). The development of psychosomatic symptomatology in parents with cystic fibrosis. *Journal of the American Academy of Child and Adolescent Psychiatry* 30: 290–7.

Peeters, Y., Boersma, S.N. and Koopman, H.M. (2008). Predictors of quality of life: A quantitative investigation of the stress-coping model in children with asthma. *Health and Quality of Life Outcomes* 6: 24.

Pilyoung, K., Leckman, J.F., Mayes, L.C. *et al.* (2010). Perceived quality of maternal care in childhood and structure and function of mothers' brain. *Developmental Science* 13: 662–73.

Pitman, R.K., Sanders, K.M., Zusman, R.M. *et al.* (2002). Pilot study of secondary prevention of post-traumatic stress disorder with propranolol. *Biological Psychiatry* 51: 189–92.

Place, M., Reynolds, J., Cousins, A. *et al.* (2002). Developing a resilience package for vulnerable children. *Child and Adolescent Mental Health* 7: 162–7.

Pless, I.B. and Nolan, T. (1991). Revision, replication and neglect: Research on maladjustment in chronic illness. *Journal of Child Psychology and Psychiatry* 22: 347–65.

Powers, M., Halpern JM, Ferenschak MP. *et al.* (2010). A meta-analytic review of prolonged exposure for post-traumatic stress disorder. *Clinical Psychology Review* 30: 635–41.

Reynolds, J.M., Garralda, M.E. and Jameson, R.A. (1988). How parents and families cope with chronic renal failure. *Archives of Diseases in Childhood* 63: 821–6.

Ribbens McCarthy, J. and Jessop, J. (2005) *Young People, Bereavement and Loss: Disruptive Transitions*. London: NCB Books.

Roberts, N.P., Kitchiner, N.J., Kenardy, J. *et al.*(2009). Systematic review and meta-analysis of multiple-session early interventions following traumatic events. *American Journal of Psychiatry* 166: 293–301.

Rogers, C.N. and Terry, T. (1984). Clinical intervention with boy victims of sexual abuse. In I.R. Stuart and J.R. Greer (eds) *Victims of Sexual Aggression: Treatment of Children, Women, and Men*. New York: Van Nostrand Reinhold.

Rumstein-McKean, O. and Hunsley, J. (2001). Interpersonal and family functioning of female survivors of childhood sexual abuse. *Clinical Psychology Review* 21: 471–90.

Russell, D.E. (1983). The incidence and prevalence of intrafamilial and extrafamilial sexual abuse of female children. *Child Abuse and Neglect* 7: 133–46.

Rutter, M., Graham, P. and Yule, W. (1970). *A Neuropsychiatric Study in Childhood* (Clinics in Developmental Medicine 35/36). London: Heinemann.

Sandler, I.N., Ayers, T.S., Wolchik, S.A.. *et al.* (2003). The Family Bereavement Program: Efficacy evaluation of a theory-based prevention program for parentally bereaved children and adolescents. *Journal of Consulting and Clinical Psychology* 71: 587–600.

Sansone, R.A., Dakroub, H., Pole, M. *et al.* (2005). Childhood trauma and employment disability. *International Journal of Psychiatry Medicine* 35: 395–404.

Sawyer, M.G., Reynolds, K.E., Couper, J.J. *et al.* (2004). Health-related quality of life of children and adolescents with chronic illness: A two year prospective study. *Quality of Life Research* 13: 1309–19.

Sgroi, S. (1982). *Handbook of Clinical Intervention in Child Sexual Abuse.* Lexington, MA: Lexington Books.

Shad, M.U., Suris, A.M., North, C.S. (2011). Novel combination strategy to optimize treatment for PTSD. *Human Psychopharmacology* 26: 4–11.

Shipman, K. and Taussig, H. (2009) Mental health treatment of child abuse and neglect: The promise of evidence-based practice. *Pediatric Clinics of North America* 56: 417–28.

Silverman, P.R., Nickman, S., Worden, J.W. (1992). Detachment revisited: The child's reconstruction of a dead parent. *American Journal of Orthopsychiatry* 62: 494–503.

Simmons, A., Paulus, M.P., Thorp, S.R. *et al.* (2008). Functional activation and neural networks in women with post-traumatic stress disorder related to intimate partner violence. *Biological Psychiatry* 64: 681–90.

Sousa, C., Herrenkohl, T.I., Moylan, C.A. *et al.* (2011). Longitudinal study on the effects of child abuse and children's exposure to domestic violence, parent-child attachments, and antisocial behavior in adolescence. *Journal of Interpersonal Violence* 26: 111–36.

Spinhoven, P., Slee, N., Garnefski, N. *et al.* (2009) Childhood sexual abuse differentially predicts outcome of cognitive-behavioral therapy for deliberate self-harm. *Journal of Nervous and Mental Diseases* 197: 455–7.

Sroufe, L.A. and Fleeson, J. (1986). Attachment and the construction of relationships. In W. Hartup and Z. Rubin (eds) *Relationships and Development.* Hillsdale, NJ: Erlbaum.

Stallard, P., Salter, E. and Velleman, R. (2004). Post-traumatic stress disorder following road traffic accidents: A second prospective study. *European Child and Adolescent Psychiatry* 13: 172–8.

Stallard, P., Velleman, R., Salter, E. *et al.* (2005). A randomised controlled trial to determine the effectiveness of an early psychological intervention with children involved in road traffic accidents. *Journal of Child Psychology and Psychiatry* 47: 127–34.

Sternberg, K.J., Baradaran, L.P.., Abbott, C.B. *et al.* (2006). Type of violence, age, and gender differences in the effects of family violence on children's behavior problems: A mega-analysis. *Developmental Review* 26: 89–112.

Strohle, A. and Holsboer, F. (2003). Stress responsive neurohormones in depression and anxiety. *Pharmacopsychiatry* 36: S207–14.

Swenson, C.C., Schaeffer, C.M., Henggeler, S.W. *et al.*(2010) Multisystemic therapy for child abuse and neglect: A randomized effectiveness trial. *Journal of Family Psychology* 24: 497–507.

Taussig, H. and Culhane, S. (2010) Impact of a mentoring and skills group program on mental health outcomes for maltreated children in foster care. *Archives of Pediatric and Adolescent Medicine* 164: 739–46.

Taylor, F.B., Martin, P., Thompson, C. *et al.* (2008). Prazosin effects on objective sleep measures and clinical symptoms in civilian trauma post-traumatic stress disorder: A placebo-controlled study. *Biological Psychiatry* 63: 629–32.

Taylor, R.M., Gibson, F., Franck, L.S. (2008). The experience of living with a chronic illness during adolescence: A critical review of the literature. *Journal of Clinical Nursing* 17: 3083–91.

Teicher, M.H., Andersen, S.L., Polcari, A. *et al.* (2002). Developmental neurobiology of childhood stress and trauma. *Psychiatric Clinics of North America* 25: 397–426.

Trowler, J., Kolvin, I., Weeramanthri, T. *et al.* (2002). Psychotherapy for sexually abused girls: Psychopathological outcome findings and patterns of change. *British Journal of Psychiatry* 160: 234–47.

Tyler, T.A. (2002). Social and emotional outcomes of childhood sexual abuse: A review of recent research. *Aggression and Violent Behavior* 7: 567–89.

van den Bosch, L.M.C., Verheul, R., Langwland, W. *et al.* (2003). Trauma, dissociation, and post-traumatic stress disorder in female borderline patients with and without substance abuse problems. *Australian and New Zealand Journal of Psychiatry* 37: 549–55.

van Tilburg, M.A.L., Runyan, D.K., Zolotor, A.J. *et al.* (2010). Unexplained gastrointestinal symptoms after abuse in a prospective study of children at risk for abuse and neglect. *Annals of Family Medicine* 8: 134–40.

Vasterling, J.J., Duke, L.M., Brailey, K. *et al.* (2002). Attention, learning, and memory performances and intellectual resources in Vietnam veterans: PTSD and no disorder comparisons. *Neuropsychology* 16: 5–14.

Vélez, C.E., Wolchik, S.A., Tein, J.Y. *et al.* (2011). Protecting children from the consequences of divorce: A longitudinal study of the effects of parenting on children's coping processes. *Child Development* 82: 244–57.

Vickerman, K.A. and Margolin, G. (2009) Rape treatment outcome research: Empirical findings and state of the literature. *Clinical Psychology Review* 29: 431–48.

Vythilingam, M., Heim, C., Newport, J. *et al.* (2002). Childhood trauma associated with smaller hippocampal volume in women with major depression. *American Journal of Psychiatry* 159: 2072–80.

Wethington, H.R., Hahn, R.A., Fuqua-Whitley, D.S. *et al.* (2008). The effectiveness of interventions to reduce psychological harm from traumatic events among children and adolescents: A systematic review. *American Journal of Preventive Medicine* 35: 287–313.

Widom, C.S., DuMont, K. and Czaja, S.J. (2007). A prospective investigation of major depressive disorder and comorbidity in abused and neglected children grown up. *Archives of General Psychiatry,* 64: 49–56.

Wilson, D.R. (2010). Health consequences of childhood sexual abuse. *Perspectives on Psychiatric Care* 46: 56–64.

Winstok, Z., Eisikovits, Z. and Karnieli-Miller, O. (2004). The impact of father-to-mother aggression on the structure and content of adolescents' perceptions of themselves and their parents. *Violence Against Women* 10: 1036–42.

Weller, E.B., Weller, R.A. and Fristad, M.A. (1988). Should children attend their parent's funeral? *Journal of the American Academy of Child and Adolescent Psychiatry* 22: 559–62.

Wolchik, S., Ma, Y., Tein, J. *et al.* (2008). Parentally bereaved children's grief: Self-system beliefs as mediators of the relations between grief and stressors and caregiver-child relationship quality. *Death Studies* 32: 597–620.

Yehuda, R., Morris, A., Labinsky, E. *et al.* (2007). Ten year follow-up study of cortisol levels in aging Holocaust survivors with and without PTSD. *Journal of Trauma and Stress* 20: 757–61.

Yi, J.P., Vitaliano, P.P., Smith, R.E. *et al.* (2008). The role of resilience on psychological adjustment and physical health in patients with diabetes. *British Journal of Health Psychology* 13: 311–25.

Yule, W. (2001). Post-traumatic stress disorder in the general population and in children. *Journal of Clinical Psychiatry* 62: 23–8.

Yule, W. and Gold, A. (1993). *Wise Before the Event: Coping with Crisis in Schools.* London: Calouste Gulbenkian Foundation.

Chapter 7

Neurodevelopmental disorders

Introduction

The term 'neurodevelopmental disorder' is used to describe conditions which are caused by problems in the growth or development of the brain. They tend to have their origin very early in a child's life, and by their nature usually have an enduring quality. The group includes disorders of intellectual development and communication as well as specific learning difficulties. Autistic spectrum disorder, attention deficit hyperactivity disorder (ADHD), and motor disorders such as Tourette's syndrome fall within this classification. Obsessional compulsive disorder is traditionally considered to be part of the anxiety disorder group, but the qualities that it shares with Tourette's syndrome, as well as the emerging evidence about its origins make this an appropriate place for it to be considered.

Autistic spectrum disorders

In 1943 Leo Kanner described eleven children who showed a pattern of behaviour which he described as autistic (Kanner 1943). The following year Hans Asperger described a similar disorder (Asperger 1944) and these descriptions form the basis of what is now commonly called autistic spectrum disorders. At the core of this disorder are significant social difficulties, together with impairments in two other domains, communication and behaviour (Dover and Le Couteur 2007). It is now accepted that autistic spectrum disorder is a neurodevelopmental condition with a biological basis, and there has been intense research interest around both its nature and origin.

The difficulties that are seen within autistic spectrum disorders are on a continuum rather than being discrete disorders, and subgroup differences tend to be based on symptom severity rather than different symptom profiles (Wiggins *et al.* 2011).

If there are concerns that a child has autistic features then a comprehensive diagnostic assessment is needed. These assessments are usually undertaken by a group of clinicians who are able to assess any difficulties the child might show with cognition, language and motor skills as well as considering the issues that would support the diagnosis.

Reaching a diagnosis

Historically, autism was only recognised in individuals with severe impairment and learning disabilities, but more recently about half of the cases show average intellectual ability (Plauché *et al.* 2007). This dramatic change has come about in part because the diagnostic criteria for autistic spectrum disorders have been widened (Mandy and Skuse 2008), which has resulted in children with much higher functioning being diagnosed with the disorder. Traditionally there were three diagnostic groups − classical autism, Asperger's syndrome and in cases where some features were present but the diagnosis could not be clearly made, the classification was pervasive developmental disorder not otherwise specified (PDD-NOS).

Asperger's syndrome shows clear similarities with autism, but the predominant domain of difficulty is with social understanding and interpersonal interaction. There are fewer problems with speech, though the language often shows strange syntax and construction, and the children often have average, or above average, intelligence.

The diagnosis of PDD-NOS has also been the focus of considerable research, with evidence that almost all of these children show a distinct symptom pattern, namely impairments in social reciprocity and communication, but without significant repetitive and stereotyped behaviours, and there are far fewer feeding and visuo-spatial problems (Mandy *et al.* 2011).

Tim was a difficult boy from birth. He did not settle when comforted by his mother and as a toddler preferred to play by himself, and would become aggressive if other children attempted to join his play. He enjoyed collecting toy dinosaurs and would spend long periods lining them up according to colour and size, but did not use them in imaginative play. If out shopping he would become extremely distressed if there were dinosaurs in the shop and his mother would not obtain them for him.

When Tim commenced school he proved to be a very able pupil, but became easily distressed if corrected in his work, and at break times did not play with the other children, preferring to stand at the fence and look out on the empty playing field. His interest had changed from dinosaurs to metal chains, and in his bedroom he had many examples of different sizes and metals, and would not go to school without a small piece of chain in his pocket. The promise of a visit to the hardware store was able to settle his behaviour when in public, but the family could never eat in restaurants because Tim insisted on specific items of food which had to be presented on his own plate from home, and with none of the items touching each other.

Tim had no friends within school, and was never invited to birthday parties because he refused to participate in any of the shared activities, and he was very likely to become aggressive if the others did not fully comply with his wishes or expectations.

Given that the symptoms of autistic spectrum disorders fall upon a continuum, determining whether a disorder is present becomes a matter of clinical judgement. There have been efforts to bring greater objectivity to the process of diagnosis by the development of structured assessment tools. Perhaps the best known of the validated interview scales is the Revised Autism Diagnostic Interview (ADI-R) (Le Couteur *et al.* 1989) and more recently the Developmental, Diagnostic and Dimensional Interview (3di) (Skuse *et al.* 2004).

It is common for the information drawn from parents to be supplemented by direct assessment of the child. The commonest instrument for this is the Autism Diagnostic Observation Schedule (ADOS) (Lord *et al.* 2000), which is a play- and activity-based assessment that provides a standard context within which to examine the child's social behaviour, communication and play.

Although there are clear difficulties around the issue of diagnosis, it is important that an accurate conclusion is achieved because of the implications for the child's future functioning, educational provision, and also the family's peace of mind. Families do not tend to see a difference between different aspects of the disorder, but find a diagnosis helpful because it not only increases their understanding of their child but tends to bring practical support.

Prevalence

The changes in the diagnostic criteria over time have led to a significant increase in prevalence since the 1960s, with currently rates being estimated at 30 per 10,000 for core autism and up to 1 in 100 for the full spectrum of disorders (Baird *et al.* 2006). It is predominantly a disorder of boys, being four times more common in boys than girls (Giarelli *et al.* 2010).

Impact of the disorder

Around the second year of life every child begins to show a variety of rituals, habits, routines and preferences, some of which resemble the behaviours associated with autistic spectrum disorders. This behaviour reaches its peak around 3 years of age and then gradually reduces. In children with autistic spectrum difficulties these features are more pronounced, and do not fade, rather do they become quite a dominant feature of the child and the family's life.

Severe learning difficulties are present in a significant proportion of cases (Chakrabarti and Fombonne 2005), and there can also be challenging behaviours such as stereotypies, self-injury, and aggressive outbursts. The resistance to changes of routine can produce quite marked non-compliance, and in the more severely afflicted there are often very limited self-help skills. The ability to discern emotion from facial expressions is essential for successful social interaction, and successful social interaction helps to develop accuracy in understanding the meaning of facial expressions (Leppanen and Nelson 2006). Studies of children with autistic spectrum disorders have shown impairments in face processing (Hubl *et al.* 2003), and these difficulties markedly increase the social difficulties of the child.

The impact upon the family can be quite profound, with increased levels of parental stress and mental health problems being quite common as the family struggle to cope with the child's behavioural problems, and their poor social and communication skills (Lecavalier *et al.* 2006). There can also be changes within the family's functioning, with parents reporting reduced marital happiness, and family life showing less adaptability and cohesion (Higgins *et al.* 2005). These stresses can magnify if the family have other children presenting difficulties, and in this regard the relative risk of a second child having this diagnosis is 20–50 times higher than the general population (O'Roak and State 2008).

Causes

Given the profound nature of the difficulties, there has been an intense research effort to understand the origins of the disorder. The nature of the social difficulties has prompted particular focus upon deficits the child may have in their 'theory of mind'. Theory of mind is the ability to attribute beliefs, intentions, desires, etc. to yourself and others and to understand that others have beliefs, desires and intentions that are different from your own. It has been seen as a mechanism that can explain the behavioural difficulties that children with autism show (Sodian and Thoermer 2008). The non-social features such as the restricted interests and the need for sameness, appear to be efforts by the child to identify the rules that govern the world around them in order to predict reactions (Baron-Cohen 2009).

There have been attempts to find physical causes for autism, and perhaps the best-known of these is the suggested link between the MMR vaccine and autism, which after considerable public interest has now been discredited (Deer 2011). Other physical and environmental causes have been found to have very limited association.

The genetic heritability of core autism has been found to be approximately 90% (Rutter 2005). The relative risk to siblings of developing autism is approximately 2% to 8%, a much higher rate than is found in the general population (Muhle *et al.* 2004).

This high degree of heritability has prompted considerable research efforts to identify the genetic origins of autism, but this has proved very difficult because only perhaps 10% of autism cases are due to specific gene variations (Weiss *et al.* 2009). The exact processes remain unclear, but it is probably mediated through epigenetic processes, as described in Chapter 1 (Nagarajan *et al.* 2006).

There is no single target for these processes, and it seems probable that a variety of disturbances to various mechanisms result in the pattern of difficulties which these children show. For instance, research has shown that oxytocin, a hormone which has a major role in emotional bonding is also significant in influencing social behaviour (Tost *et al.* 2010), and study suggests that changes to the regulation of oxytocin may be one of the mechanisms involved in the emergence of autism (Gregory *et al.* 2009). Disturbance of other brain transmitters such as serotonin have been found to have an association with autism (Goddard *et al.* 2008).

As well as studying the chemical processes within the brain there has been considerable work looking at its physical make-up, and the interconnection between various parts. It has been found that children with autism have an accelerated post-natal growth in defined brain regions compared with controls (Courchesne *et al.* 2007), and there are increases in late development in the critical parts of the brain associated with autistic symptoms (Herbert *et al.* 2004). Alterations at the synaptic level are also associated with developing autistic spectrum disorder (van Spronsen and Hoogenraad 2010).

Together, results of clinical, neuroimaging, neuropathological and neurochemical studies show that the autistic spectrum disorders are disorders of neuronal-cortical organisation that cause deficits in information processing in the nervous system, ranging from synaptic organisation to connectivity and brain structure. These changes probably alter the developmental trajectory of social communication and seem to be affected by genetic and environmental factors (Pardo and Eberhart 2007).

Associations with other disorders

Comorbid behavioural or developmental disorders are common in children with autistic spectrum disorder. These can take the form of intellectual delays, behaviours such as aggression, affective difficulties such as depression or anxiety, sleep disruption, and sensory difficulties (Simonoff *et al.* 2008). There is also a high prevalence of medical conditions such as tics, and as many as 30% of children have seizures (Tuchman *et al.* 2010).

There is a significant prevalence of ADHD complicating autism, though some-times this diagnosis is not recognised because the symptoms are assumed to originate from the autism. Between 20% and 50% of children with ADHD met criteria for autistic spectrum disorder, and between 30% and 80% of children with autism meet criteria for ADHD (Rommelse *et al.* 2011). Family and twin studies suggest that the association is probably arising from common aetiological factors (Ronald and Hoekstra 2011), and studies looking at executive functioning found common neuropsychological traits between the two disorders (Geurts *et al.* 2009).

Intervention

From its initial recognition there have been intense efforts to develop interventions which will improve a child's functioning and moderate the emotional and behav-ioural difficulties. Much of this effort has been focused upon programmes to be delivered either within the school or at home and many have a very strong behav-ioural component.

Psychological approaches

The generic behaviourally oriented parent training packages can be effective for parents of children with autistic spectrum disorders. Parents tend to report that the elements that they find of particular value are advice about delivering time-out, physical guidance and blocking (Whittingham *et al.* 2009), but the best results are achieved if the programmes are adapted to meet the specific needs of this client group (Matson et al. 2009).

There are also several programmes which have been specifically developed to meet the needs of children with autistic spectrum disorders, and the most researched are structured programmes which seek to teach appropriate behavioural responses through behaviour modification (Rogers and Vismara 2008). Perhaps one of the best-known is Applied Behavioural Analysis (ABA) (Lovaas 1987) which focuses upon reducing stereotypical autistic behaviours through extinction, and seeks to provide the child with socially acceptable alternatives to self-stimulatory behaviours. It is a popular approach in several settings, and its intensive and prolonged nature appears to improve some of the core symptoms of autistic spectrum disorder (ASD) compared to special education (Ospina et al. 2008).

There have also been attempts to develop this type of programme in a time-limited format. The Group Intensive Family Therapy (GIFT) is a 12-week programme delivered for 3 hours each weekday. It is designed for preschoolers with ASD, and it aims to teach parents how to deliver applications of applied behavioural analysis. Although it is a much shorter programme, review suggests that it is still able to improve the child's cognitive and adaptive functioning (Anan et al. 2008).

In the UK, the National Autistic Society has developed a package focused on young children which combines weekly group training sessions for parents with individualised home visits. Over a 3-month period the aim is to help parents understand autism, learn to communicate more effectively with their children, and to develop positive behaviour management strategies (Shields 2001).

Evidence from the wealth of studies suggests that, in general, parent training leads to improved child communicative behaviour, increased maternal knowledge of autism, enhanced maternal communication style and parent–child interaction, and reduced maternal depression (McConachie and Diggle 2007). Whatever the approach, the degree of parental involvement is very significant in their overall effectiveness (Schieve et al. 2007).

Medication

To date no medicine has been identified which can materially alter the core difficulties found in autistic spectrum disorder. Medication has therefore tended to focus upon specific psychiatric symptoms. Targets generally include hyperactivity, inattention, repetitive thoughts and behaviour, self-injurious behaviour and aggression (Bryson et al. 2003).

Atypical antipsychotics such as risperidone help moderate symptoms to a degree, and are most useful in reducing aggression (Findling 2005). This type of medication appears to be better tolerated and have less risk of extrapyramidal effects compared with the older neuroleptics.

Serotonin selective reuptake inhibitors (SSRIs) have been found to be effective in treating anxiety and obsessive-compulsive behaviour. They are an appropriate treatment for coexisting depression, and can help reduce repetitive behaviours (Kolevzon et al. 2006). Although some practitioners recommend early treatment with medication such as SSRIs in order to capitalise on early neural plasticity (Chugani 2005), the research suggests that SSRIs may be less well tolerated and not as effective in younger children with autism compared to adolescents and adults.

Most medication interventions are indicated by specific difficulties within the individual. For instance sleep difficulties are a common problem, and may be helped by medication. However there is interest in developing treatments which have a more general focus, and there is some interesting work on medications that influence social and language functioning that may in the future prove to be significant (Posey et al. 2008).

Outcome

Some young children with a diagnosis of autism can show a surprising increase in language and intellectual functioning between 6 and 10 years of age (Sigman et al. 2005), and some will show a better understanding of emotional issues as they mature. Within the individual there is also likely to be shifting patterns of pre-occupation, and changes to the areas where they demand sameness. However overall significant difficulties will persist, and the degree to which these will hamper their future functioning depends upon the severity of the young person's behavioural difficulties, their cognitive abilities and the degree to which they have useful speech.

Mental health problems are quite common, with perhaps 70% of young people with Asperger's syndrome experiencing at least one episode of major depression, and up to 50% suffering from recurrent episodes. Anxiety disorders are also common, but psychotic disorders and substance-induced disorders are not (Lugnegård et al. 2011). Gender plays no part in the probability of developing such difficulties, and it is important that those involved with their care maintain a high degree of vigilance to ensure that any mood disorders are detected quickly and treated.

Obsessive-compulsive disorder

Although it is not traditionally classified as a neurodevelopmental disorder, as the understanding of the nature and origins of obsessive-compulsive disorder (OCD) increases, there are arguments that it should be considered to be more organic in origin (Maia et al. 2008). It is characterised by the presence of either obsessions (worries) or compulsions (the need to carry out rituals). Common obsessions in children include preoccupations with contamination, fear they will harm themselves or others, a preoccupation with symmetry (such as the need for an even number of chips on the plate), as well as fear that a bad outcome will occur if a ritual is not completed in just the right way. The most common compulsions in children include washing, checking, counting, and putting items in order or rank. These are often repeated a set number of times, but also may be repeated until the person feels 'just right'. This disorder is considered to be a member of the group of anxiety disorders, and occurs on a continuum of severity.

Reaching a diagnosis

Features of OCD are present in many people, and the symptoms show an increase in adolescence as one of the coping mechanisms for dealing with the issues of puberty. It becomes a disorder when the symptoms begin to intrude or disrupt the routine of daily life. When the disorder begins in childhood the symptoms tend to occur more often in boys, at a ratio of 3:1. The symptoms emerge at around 8 years of age, and gradually increase through puberty, showing a degree of decline late in adolescence. Adult onset OCD is said to start after puberty, and tends to occur a little more frequently in girls (Castle *et al.* 1995).

The Children's Yale-Brown Obsessive Compulsive Scale (Scahill *et al.* 1997) is a semi-structured interview which asks about OCD symptoms and their severity over the previous week, and is the standard assessment instrument for this disorder.

Prevalence

Because the symptoms form a continuum with normal functioning the prevalence of OCD is difficult to determine, but it is suggested to affect 1–2% of the population, with a point prevalence of 0.25% (Heyman *et al.* 2003).

Impact of the disorder

Individuals with OCD typically recognise the senseless nature of their obsessions and compulsions, but feel powerless to stop them, and indeed are fearful of the consequences if they should try. Sometimes the actions blur into tics or other motor habits, and there are usually features of other mental health difficulties such as mood disorders. The symptoms need to disrupt daily life to prompt the diagnosis, and sometimes such disruption can be quite severe.

James had always been concerned about infection and germs, and at the age of 13 became particularly concerned about cleanliness. He would shower three times a day and change his clothes on several occasions through the day. He then became concerned that his clothes were not remaining clean, and began to wash his hands between putting on each item of clothing. Over the subsequent weeks it took him longer and longer to get ready for school, and eventually he could not leave the house.

As well as the direct effect there is commonly the presence of other emotional or behavioural difficulties, and a deterioration in school performance. Some sufferers have significant difficulties with working memory, particularly visual memory, and if these are present this predicts a poorer outcome (Bloch *et al.* 2011).

Causes

The origins of OCD are not fully understood, but a genetic contribution to the development of OCD is suggested by the significant familial associations that have been found (Hanna *et al.* 2005), and from these it has been calculated that the risk of first-degree relatives developing OCD is some 12% (Nestadt *et al.* 2000). There are significant changes to brain structure (Tiago *et al.* 2008), and an increase in brain chemistry activity when the symptoms are pronounced (Grant *et al.* 2007) which fades with successful treatment.

The role of infection in prompting the emergence of the disorder has received considerable interest, with paediatric autoimmune neuropsychiatric disorder associated with streptococcal infections (PANDAS) being the most well established (Swedo *et al.* 1998). Children with PANDAS-prompted OCD may also show tics, and there are abrupt exacerbations associated with symptoms of infection.

This origin of OCD appears to be strongly inherited and generally has a better prognosis. It most commonly occurs at around 6 years of age, and is associated with choreiform movements (quick jerky movements of the feet or hands) (95%), emotional lability (66%), school performance changes (60%), personality changes (54%), bedtime fears (50%), fidgetiness (50%), separation fears (40%), sensory defensiveness (40%), irritability (40%), and impulsivity and distraction (38%) (Kalra and Swedo 2009).

In this variation, the OCD symptoms arise when the child has a streptococcal bacterial infection and the mechanism that the body uses to fight the infection, the immunological system, responds abnormally in these children.

No matter what the origin, parents of children with OCD are often highly involved in their child's rituals. For example, they might help their child in avoiding certain situations or stimuli, or provide items to help them complete the ritual. This is an important element in maintaining the symptoms, and if persistent it predicts a poor outcome. In addition, symptoms tend to increase in emotionally charged atmospheres, and these can render treatment programmes less effective. This means that understanding the wider family dynamics, and intervening with issues where necessary can be a significant element in improving the child's response to therapy.

Associations with other disorders

The most common comorbidities in children with OCD are ADHD (34–51%), depression (33–39%), specific developmental disabilities (24%), Tourette's Syndrome (18–25%), oppositional defiant disorder (17–51%), and anxiety (16%) (Geller 2006). It is also increasingly clear that the earlier the onset of the OCD symptoms the greater the risk of ADHD or other anxiety disorders being evident. There can also be autistic behavioural traits. The repetitive behaviours and compulsions seen in autism appear identical to those of OCD.

Up to 80% of children with Tourette's syndrome reporting obsessive-compulsive symptoms (Leckman *et al.* 1997), and nearly two-thirds of children with OCD have some form of tic disorder also (Leonard *et al.* 1992). Indeed distinguishing between tics and the compulsive component of OCD is particularly difficult when the rituals are simple, repetitive movements such as tapping and touching. As a consequence there continues to be debate in some quarters as to whether this type of symptom is more correctly diagnosed as Tourette's syndrome rather than OCD (Leckman *et al.* 2003).

Intervention

As with many disorders and difficulties in childhood, the response of the family, and the degree to which they are involved in the child's treatment, can exert a strong influence on outcome. In OCD poor parental responses can maintain the symptoms (Storch *et al.* 2007a), and if they are very emotional about the difficulties, this can increase them. Therefore, providing parents with as much information as possible about OCD, and helping them understand how best to respond is an important element of any treatment programme.

Similarly, if the symptoms are evident within school then advising about the best type of management is important to maintain a settled atmosphere in this important area of a child's life. This becomes essential if the child also has a significant tic disorder (see below).

Psychological therapies

The most established treatment for OCD is exposure and response prevention (ERP) (Foa *et al.* 1984) which involves confronting feared situations and resisting the urge to perform a compulsion. As exposure to the feared situation is repeated, anxiety diminishes and eventually anxiety extinguishes altogether. These programmes can be quite difficult for the child to undertake, and CBT which focuses upon cognitive restructuring rather than anxiety habituation is now the first-line treatment in most cases (Krebs and Heyman 2010). This type of intervention has been shown to be effective whether delivered intensively or on a more structured basis (Storch *et al.* 2007b).

Adding medication to the CBT can improve the outcome in some cases (Walkup *et al.* 2008), and this is seen as the optimum treatment approach for childhood-onset OCD by some specialist groups (Pediatric OCD Treatment Study Team 2004), and is recommended as the treatment for individuals with severe functional impairment by the National Institute for Health and Clinical Excellence (2005).

Medication

Medication has been, and remains, a major method of intervention in this disorder. Preparations that increase the concentration of serotonin in the brain synapse have been used as a treatment option for some time, and currently it is the SSRIs that are the main medications used, with about 70% responding positively (Geller 2006). If the symptoms do not ease sufficiently then adding a low-dose of an atypical antipsychotic such as risperidone to the SSRI may be helpful, and this is especially true if the child is also suffering from tics (McDougle *et al.* 2000).

However these medication approaches still obtain only modest benefit (Foa *et al.* 2005), and so there have been a variety of other compounds examined, many of which are known to influence the brain chemical glutamate, which is associated with emotional learning and fear extinction. The most studied of these is d-cycloserine, which is believed to consolidate the learning that occurs during exposure to anxiety-provoking situations (Ledgerwood *et al.* 2003). In young people, combining this with CBT does show modest benefit, and perhaps its value may ultimately prove to be increasing the speed and efficiency of exposure treatment (Norberg *et al.* 2008).

Outcome

Childhood-onset OCD is a chronic disabling disorder, but the long-term prognosis is improving as knowledge and treatments improve. Many children see their symptoms reduce significantly through late adolescence and early adulthood. Developing the symptoms early, having symptoms that have a religious or sexual focus, and experiencing other mental health problems, such as depression, tend to predict a poorer outcome (Mancuso *et al.* 2010). In these cases peer problems, poor educational progress and troubled employment history tend to be relatively common elements of their difficulties later in life.

Tics and Tourette's syndrome

Tics are involuntary and purposeless movements which may consist of mild facial spasms or blinking with the eyes, or involve jerks in other parts of the body, sometimes in quite a violent fashion. They are repetitive and can be deliberately suppressed for short periods. The child usually is aware that the movement is going to happen because they feel uncomfortable, or have a strange sensation, but feel incapable of preventing it.

The most distinctive, and perhaps most disabling variation of tic disorder, is that described by Georges Gilles de la Tourette in 1885. The syndrome that bears his name is an inheritable, childhood-onset neurological disorder marked by persistent multiple motor tics and at least one vocal tic. The vocal tics that are most intrusive can be the shouting of obscenities (called 'coprolalia') but may be grunts or noisy clearing of the throat. There can also be involuntary obscene gestures (called 'copropraxia'), or the copying of other people's sounds or gestures.

Reaching a diagnosis

From the age of 6, Michael had an increasing tendency to blink his eyes and wrinkle his nose as though trying to stop it itching. His family were not particularly concerned about this, but over the next three years he began to shrug one shoulder in a frequent pattern which sometimes was quite lengthy. This behaviour particularly irritated his father who would shout at him to stop, though this tended to increase the amount of movement.

There gradually began to emerge grunts and squeaks which were associated with the movements, and over a period of nine months these became louder, and gradually the family recognised them to be swear words. The extended family frequently told the parents they considered Michael very rude for swearing so much, and all family outings and trips needed to be planned carefully, so that Michael would not embarrass them.

Within school Michael progressed well academically, and initially had friends that he could play with, but as the rude words emerged more clearly the other children tended to not want to play with him. In primary school his teacher understood the origins of the difficulty, but when a new teacher came he was frequently removed from the class for disrupting it, and one or two parents began complaining to the headteacher that their children were being upset by Michael's constant swearing.

The average age of onset for tic disorder is 5–7 years, and the course is often insidious. The symptoms tend to reach their peak between ages 10 and 12, with the symptoms then subsiding to a variable degree. In Tourette's syndrome the vocal component usually emerges around 11 years of age. Typically, tics occur many times a day, nearly every day, with a pattern of waxing and waning over time.

The vocal noises are necessary for the diagnosis of Tourette's syndrome, but in only about a third of cases that attend clinics are these clearly recognisable as obscenities, in most cases being grunts or coughs. The symptoms tend to be more severe the earlier the onset (Khalifa and von Knorring 2005).

Prevalence

The prevalence for children and adolescents between 5 and 18 years old is approximately 1% (Cavanna *et al.* 2009), and it is much more common in children who attend special educational settings (Kurlan *et al.* 2001). In childhood the male-to-female prevalence ratio for Tourette's syndrome is about 4:1 (Khalifa and von Knorring 2003), which reduces to 2:1 when the symptoms emerge in teenage years.

Impact of the disorder

The quality of life of young people with tic disorders is significantly worse than their peers across all areas of their life, particularly in respect of academic and work performance, as well as family and peer relationships (Khalifa and von Knorring 2003). Generally there is no change to cognitive functioning or working memory (Cavanna 2009). However if the child is also suffering from ADHD then difficulties with working memory are present (Verte *et al.* 2005).

Causes

The evidence indicates that Tourette's syndrome has a strong genetic origin, especially if the symptoms emerge at a young age (Rosario-Campos *et al.* 2005). Brain scans have shown that the disorder is associated with changes to the part of the brain known as the basal ganglia (Frey and Albin 2006), which is associated with the control of motor functions. The age of onset, and the timing of this in terms of the brain's development, appear to have a significant impact upon the degree of difficulty that the child experiences (Plessen *et al.* 2009).

Associations with other disorders

Among children diagnosed with Tourette's syndrome about 79% also have at least one co-occurring mental health or neurodevelopmental condition (Scahill *et al.* 2009), the most common of which are obsessive-compulsive disorder (OCD) and attention deficit hyperactivity disorder (ADHD) (Cavanna *et al.* 2009). Although OCD and ADHD occur very frequently together, it appears that they are two separate conditions, with any aggression or conduct difficulties arising from the ADHD component (Sukhodolsky *et al.* 2003).

Children with OCD commonly show features which are similar to, and may even be mistaken for, tic disorder. There is a growing suggestion that they are in fact related disorders because there appears to be a genetic link between them (Pauls *et al.* 1986), but careful analysis can usually distinguish uncomplicated OCD from Tourette's syndrome (Mula *et al.* 2008).

Given the nature and distress that the symptoms can cause, and the bullying they may experience because of their tics, it is not surprising that depression is commonly found in young people with tic disorder (Robertson 2006a). However in about 12% of children with Tourette's syndrome there are no other emotional or behavioural difficulties (Freeman *et al.* 2000), and these children show an average pattern of development.

Intervention

The majority of treatment options for tics are pharmacological. Although the diagnosis of Tourette's syndrome does not require evidence of significant disruption to daily functioning, treatment with medication should not be commenced unless the symptoms are causing significant problems in school or in social relationships. The most commonly prescribed drugs are atypical antipsychotics (e.g. risperidone). In general, the more potent the medication the more effective it is in ameliorating tics (Scahill *et al.* 2006), with risperidone improving symptoms in 30–62% of cases (Bruggeman *et al.* 2001).

Aripiprazole, another atypical antipsychotic, is becoming the first choice treatment for treating tic disorder. It works on a different part of the nerves that have dopamine-mediated synapses, and not only is effective at reducing tics, but it also has a positive effect upon any behavioural symptoms, and causes few side-effect problems for these young people (Eddy *et al.* 2011). Another medication which has proved helpful in the treatment of tic disorder is clonidine, and indeed it has been recommended as a first choice, in combination with methylphenidate, when the symptoms coincide with ADHD (Tourette's Syndrome Study Group 2002).

Psychological and other approaches

Several other types of treatment have been shown to be beneficial, of which the most closely studied is habit reversal (Himle *et al.* 2006). The initial element of habit reversal is to help the child to become aware of what is occurring just before the tic happens and then encouraging them to undertake an action that is incompatible with the tic. Other behavioural approaches have also been found to help, such as exposure therapy (Verdellen *et al.* 2007), but there is some concern that these interventions can simply move the tics from one part of the body to another. In view of the significant impact the tic can have upon the child's wider functioning, there is value in also addressing issues around education and the school as well as the family's understanding and responses.

Outcome

Tic disorders tend to be persistent, with an early onset predicting the more chronic course. In children with tic disorder who also have ADHD it is important to intervene with both disorders because the combination tends to predict a poorer school performance (Robertson 2006b). If the tics are significant and persist into adult life then anxiety and depressive symptoms may well emerge (Lewin *et al.* 2011).

Attention deficit hyperactivity disorder and similar difficulties

Children who present with difficult and disruptive behaviour are a major concern both to parents and schools. A subgroup of these children will also be restless and fidgety, find it difficult to settle to tasks, and have poor impulse control. For some years this group of children have been distinguished as perhaps presenting a different problem from that of merely poor behaviour, and are now described as having attention deficit hyperactivity disorder (ADHD). It is a lifelong developmental disorder which has its roots in genetic and early life experiences and its clinical manifestations often persist into adolescence and adulthood (Vaughan *et al.* 2008).

Reaching a diagnosis

The features that permit the diagnosis of ADHD are set out in Figure 7.1. Often children with concentration problems have in their history elements suggesting developmental delay or birth difficulties, and it should also be borne in mind that physical problems, such as epilepsy or thyroid problems, can prompt children to present as being restless and having poor concentration. If any such elements are suspected, then a medical opinion should be sought.

Assessment of behavioural difficulties requires careful assessment of all the elements that might be contributing to the pattern of difficulties. Probably the commonest reason for children to present with restless, inattentive behaviour is weakness in the parenting regime. Such difficulties usually arise when the child shows a great deal of wilfulness, and the parental response has been inconsistent, or simply been one of 'giving in for a quiet life'. This type of presentation requires a different type of approach (see Chapter 4).

The assessment of ADHD requires information about the child's functioning in several settings. In addition to the elements of the comprehensive assessment described in Chapter 2, there will also be information gathered from home and

A *EITHER* Six (or more) of the following symptoms of *inattention* have persisted for at least six months to a degree that is maladaptive and inconsistent with developmental level:

- often fails to give close attention to details or makes careless mistakes in schoolwork, work or other activities
- often has difficulty sustaining attention in tasks or play activities
- often does not seem to listen when spoken to directly
- often does not follow through on instructions and fails to finish schoolwork, or chores (not due to oppositional behaviour or failure to understand instructions)
- often has difficulty organising tasks and activities
- often avoids, dislikes or is reluctant to engage in tasks that require sustained mental effort (such as schoolwork or homework)
- often loses things necessary for tasks or activities (e.g. toys, schoolwork, pencils, books)
- is often easily distracted by extraneous stimuli
- is often forgetful in daily activities.

OR

Six (or more) of the following symptoms of *hyperactivity/impulsivity* have persisted for at least six months to a degree that is maladaptive and inconsistent with developmental level:

- often fidgets with hands or feet or squirms in seat
- often leaves seat in classroom or in other situations in which remaining seated is expected
- often runs about or climbs excessively in situations in which it is inappropriate (in adolescents this may be subjective feelings of restlessness)
- often has difficulty playing or engaging in leisure activities quietly
- is often 'on the go' or often acts as if 'driven by a motor'
- often talks excessively
- often blurts out answers before questions have been completed
- often has difficulty waiting turn
- often interrupts or intrudes on others (e.g. butts into conversations or games).

B Some hyperactive-impulsive or inattentive symptoms that caused impairment were present before seven years of age.

C Some impairment from the symptoms is present in two or more settings.

D There must be clear evidence of clinically significant impairment in social or academic functioning.

E The symptoms do not occur exclusively during the course of another condition.

Figure 7.1 Attention deficit disorder (DSM-IV)

school through questionnaires which ask about specific behaviours, and periods of observation. There are many such instruments available, with perhaps the ones in most common use being Conners Rating Scale – Revised (Conners 1998), and the SNAP IV (Swanson 1992). However the choice of questionnaire tends to be dictated by local preference since the vast majority of the assessment questionnaires available have good sensitivity to rapidly identify potential cases (Collett *et al.* 2003), though the SNAP IV has the advantage of being free (obtainable at www.adhd.net).

Physical assessment and other evaluations should also form part of the process, with evaluation of the child's executive functioning and working memory being seen as increasingly important because of its implications for academic functioning. There are no specific diagnostic tests for ADHD that will uniquely confirm the diagnosis, but executive function (Holmes *et al.* 2010a), working memory assessment (Holmes *et al.* 2010b) and the Continuous Performance Test are helpful in distinguishing the disorder (Riccio *et al.* 2001). The Continuous Performance Test measures vigilance, specifically the ability to sustain attention when faced with long sequences of repetitive stimuli. Sustained attention can also be measured by the Test of Everyday Attention for Children (TEA-Ch) (Manly *et al.* 2001).

Prevalence

Differences in diagnostic criteria have slowly narrowed, and the prevalence of the disorder has become consistently estimated to be 3–5%, with these rates being relatively similar in most countries of the world (Polanczyk et al. 2007). The other major shift in the understanding of prevalence is to do with gender. In younger children ADHD is four times more likely in boys, but studies in adolescence show a more equal ratio (Cohen *et al.* 1993). It is now recognised that this discrepancy emerges because the girls tend not to show the markedly disruptive behaviour which brings the boys to professional attention. In adulthood the ratio continues to be equal (Rucklidge 2010). This pattern is prompting the diagnostic criteria to be re-examined, and it is increasingly likely that in women at least the diagnosis may be made in adulthood.

Impact of the disorder

The very large body of work which has been undertaken with children who have ADHD has demonstrated that they can experience significant problems in many areas. For instance, they have difficulties with response inhibition, vigilance, verbal and spatial working memory, and planning (Willcutt *et al.* 2005), and these give them major difficulties in school. Children with ADHD are four to five times more likely to need special educational services (Jensen *et al.* 2004), and their academic difficulties begin early in life, generally being evident by 3 years of age. By adolescence they often have an established pattern of achieving below expected marks in all school subjects and performing poorly on standardised academic achievement tests (Massetti *et al.* 2008). Also, these children are much more prone to experience exclusions, and even expulsion from school, or to simply drop out of education completely (Bagwell *et al.* 2001).

Perhaps increasing these difficulties is the fact that they tend not to complete homework, and that their handwriting is poor (Racine *et al.* 2008). These academic difficulties are cross-cultural and not specific to the Western countries (Norvilitis *et al.* 2010).

The inattentive symptoms of ADHD show a clear relationship to the learning problems, but the poor level of academic achievement may also be due to the presence of subtle neurocognitive impairments characterised by elements such as daydreaming, becoming easily confused, and lacking mental alertness, which are the outward features of working memory and executive function deficits (Holmes *et al.* 2010a).

The impulsive aspects of the behaviour these children show often prompt them to indulge in risky or even dangerous activities, and parents often say that they 'have no fear'. These behaviours are evident from a very early age (Angold and Egger 2007), and by teenage years they are often well-known to the local casualty departments. The degree of hyperactive and impulsive behaviour tends to predict the development of later oppositional behaviours and conduct problems among boys (Pardini and Fite 2010). They are often in conflict with peers, and tend to gravitate to the children who are also disruptive and marginalised.

Causes

Family, twin and adoption studies show that ADHD is a familial disorder with high heritability, indicating that a significant genetic component influences the risk of developing the disorder, with as much as 76% of the risk being due to genetic factors (Faraone *et al.* 2005). However no single genetic profile has been found to account for the development of ADHD, rather is the pattern one of statistically significant association with a variety of genes that are associated with the dopamine system. The most persistent associations are found with the dopamine genes DRD4 and DRD5 (Li *et al.* 2006), and the dopamine transporter gene (DAT1) (Kuntsi *et al.* 2006).

These may exert their influence on epigenetic mechanisms (see Chapter 1). For instance, smoking during pregnancy increases the risk if the mother has the DRD4 7-repeat allele which is associated with ADHD (Pluess *et al.* 2009). Risks are also increased if there is prenatal exposure to alcohol and recreational drugs (Accornero *et al.* 2007).

The changes to the dopamine network within the brain of these children shows some paradoxical patterns (Konrad and Eickhoff 2010), and there is also a significant decrease in cortical folding bilaterally (Wolosin *et al.* 2009). Interestingly these changes are specific to boys, with no volume or shape differences being evident in girls with ADHD (Qui *et al.* 2009), a finding which may be associated with the late emergence of difficulties in girls, when brain structures are relatively settled.

As well as these genetic and physical factors there are features within the environment which can influence the disorder. Severe deprivation can prompt ADHD symptoms, and it is worth mentioning that there has been a steady pattern of evidence that hypersensitivity to specific foods can prompt or provoke ADHD symptoms (Pelsser *et al.* 2009).

Associations with other disorders

As many as 65% of children with ADHD have one or more comorbid conditions, the most common of which are oppositional defiant and conduct disorder, anxiety and mood disorders, tics or Tourette's syndrome, learning disorders and autistic spectrum disorders (Biederman 2005). Of these, it is the oppositional defiance and conduct difficulties which have consistently been the most studied.

Oppositional defiance is characterised by resistance to authority, with conduct problems being characterised by a pattern of antisocial behaviour where there may be episodes of stealing, lying and truanting (see Chapter 4). Of course there are many reasons for the emergence of conduct problems, the most established of which is persisting family difficulties (Loeber and Stouthamer-Loeber 1986). However, the frequency with which attention problems and conduct disorder occur together has prompted much research into whether there is a link between the two.

It is now clear that ADHD does not cause conduct disorder, but facilitates its emergence if there is a vulnerability to this behaviour (Schachar and Tannock 1995). Also it is the conduct disorder and not the presence of ADHD that predicts adult criminality (Mordre *et al.* 2011).

Martin was a 7-year-old boy presenting with violent outbursts towards his younger sister and a continuous refusal to comply with his mother's wishes. In the evenings she found it hard to prevent him destroying toys, which he did when he became frustrated in any way. Martin was always difficult to settle to bed, constantly demanding his mother's attendance, and the routine had therefore become that Martin would sleep in his mother's bed. The day was always punctuated with battles – over dressing, washing, what to have for breakfast, and so on. This picture contrasted starkly with that seen in school where Martin was settled, performing well, and presenting no behavioural difficulties to the staff.

Such a sharp contrast between two environments points to a problem within relationships, and it became evident over time that Martin's mother was struggling with a significant depressive illness which had prevented her from establishing a clear and consistent pattern of management with him. Treatment of this depressive illness, and a series of sessions focusing upon management, allowed Martin's mother to establish a clear and decisive parenting approach. With its introduction Martin said he now felt happier, and that he could cope with no longer being allowed to sleep in his mother's bed.

Martin's case illustrates the importance of assessing a child's behaviour in several settings. A pattern of behaviour problems specific to one area is a strong indication not of attention deficit but that there are issues within that setting that the child is reacting to.

The second comorbidity that is worth consideration is autistic spectrum disorder (ASD). The diagnostic guidelines for ADHD have traditionally prevented making a comorbid diagnosis with ASD, based on the rationale that ADHD symptoms in patients with ASD are primarily attributable to the ASD diagnosis. However between 20% and 50% of children with ADHD meet the criteria for ASD, and between 30% and 80% of children with ASD meet the criteria for ADHD. This has led to the proposal that ASD and ADHD partly share aetiological, particularly genetic factors (Rommelse et al. 2011), and the diagnostic criteria are increasingly permitting both diagnoses to be made.

It is worth pointing out that although there appear to be genetic and neuro-logical links between ADHD and ASD, executive functioning does distinguish the disorders. Children with ADHD display difficulties with sustained attention, while having relatively little problem with planning or cognitive flexibility, whereas children with autism have little problem with inhibition.

In recent years there has been a growing tendency to try to distinguish children with severe ADHD from those that are showing features of bipolar disorder. Bipolar disorder is a significant mental illness which is becoming quite an acceptable diagnosis as various celebrities attribute their personal difficulties to its presence. It is often episodic in nature, with individuals switching from distinct episodes of depression to overactive periods of mania, accompanied by distortions of ideas, often with periods of settled mood in between. It used to be considered very rare in children, but it shares several symptoms with ADHD – excessive talking, increased activity, inappropriate responses in social situations, lack of inhibition, and distractibility. The diagnosis in children remains controversial, but despite this it is still considered to be a valid one (Youngstrom et al. 2008) because, as with autism and ADHD, there are differences in the executive function profiles between bipolar disorder and ADHD. Children with bipolar disorder tend to show impair-ments in interference control, planning and set-shifting, whereas impairments in verbal and spatial working memory and phonemic verbal fluency appear specific to ADHD (Walshaw et al. 2010).

Intervention

Medication: stimulants

Medication, and in particular the use of central nervous system stimulants, has been the treatment method which has received the most research attention over the recent past. The most commonly used is methylphenidate, but dexamfetamine is also sometimes prescribed. These drugs, which are part of the amphetamine family, change the level of brain chemicals, particularly dopamine, and have been clearly demonstrated to help children to concentrate, improve their vigilance, and reduce their tendency to be distracted (Peterson et al. 2009). This tends to improve overall classroom performance (Du Paul et al. 1994) and, in addition, many children report an improvement in their social interaction, especially with peers.

A particular concern for this class of medication is the fact that it is part of a family of drugs which are known to be drugs of abuse, and addictive (see Chapter 9). However, there is no evidence that children prescribed these medications develop addiction to them (Spencer et al. 1996). It is also clear that although part of this family, methyphenidate is a relatively poor source of feeling euphoric, especially if taken orally (Volkow and Swanson 2003).

As with all drugs, the stimulant medications do have side-effects. Children almost always report a significant drop in appetite, especially at lunchtime, and there is often some difficulty with sleep. For a small minority the medication makes them more irritable and restless. For a time there was concern that if the drug was taken for a long period it might interfere with a child's growth, but it is now clear that the medication has no enduring impact upon a child's height or weight (Biederman et al. 2010b).

Other medications

The main alternative to stimulant medication is atomoxetine. This is a medication which has a specific impact upon the noradrenaline transmitter in the brain, and studies have shown it to be an effective treatment option (Spencer et al. 2002). It does not cause appetite reduction, and there is a lower incidence of insomnia. However it is not as effective as the stimulants, having an effect size of 0.57, compared to 0.99 for immediate release stimulants, and 0.95 for slow-release preparations (Faraone 2009).

A type of antidepressant, Bupropion, has also been shown to be effective for ADHD in children (Daviss et al. 2001). Better known perhaps as an aid to stop smoking, it appears as effective as methylphenidate, but again tends to be suggested when stimulants are inappropriate.

In addition to these medications, it is sometimes helpful to target specific symptoms, such as aggression, directly (Connor et al. 2009). Methylphenidate can be effective if these aggressive elements are driven by impulsivity, but if not then the addition of an atypical antipsychotic medication may be appropriate (Schur et al. 2003).

However, although stimulants are able to produce improvement in many areas of the child's functioning, they do not produce a normalisation of skills in the domain of learning and applying knowledge, because even with medication the academic performance of children with attention deficit disorder is some 10% poorer than predicted (Gualtieri and Johnson 2008). Improving the children's working memory increases academic achievement, a gain which shows persistence over time (Holmes et al. 2010b). This offers an additional avenue of intervention which has the potential to help children achieve closer to their natural potential.

Behavioural techniques

Behavioural techniques have a part to play in helping a young person attend to tasks, and gradually increase the period that attention can be sustained. They are also helpful in curbing some of the conduct elements which may be part of the picture. The principles outlined in Chapter 4 would apply equally to this type of problem. However, the emphasis here is upon trying to improve attention and to increase the child's general sense of self-esteem and self-worth. It is also worth remembering that such young people often don't fully register instructions, or information generally. It is therefore important that instructions and information are regularly repeated, with information being given in various ways, such as saying it, writing it down, and perhaps using diagrams or pictures.

Children with attention deficit need structure and routine. They should be helped to make schedules and break assignments down into small tasks to be performed one at a time. It may be necessary to ask them repeatedly what they have just done, how they might have acted differently, and why others react as they do. Especially when young, these children often respond well to the strict application of clear and consistent rules, and so parenting packages can be effective in helping families achieve this.

Behavioural strategies are complex and time-consuming to implement, and typically less effective at reducing core symptoms of ADHD than medication (Antshel and Barkley 2008). It should also be borne in mind that parent training has been found to be less beneficial for children whose parents demonstrate ADHD symptoms (Sonuga-Barke *et al.* 2006).

More specific psychological interventions have been explored, with CBT showing an impact upon behavioural and social maladjustment, but making only marginal change to the core symptoms of ADHD (Durlak *et al.* 1991). The frequent problems with interpersonal difficulties and impaired social functioning have been tackled by programmes that use social skills training. These aim to improve the child's social skills and teach them to behave in a more socially acceptable manner, but such programmes only appear to be helpful when part of a more comprehensive treatment approach (Gol and Jarus 2005).

Family conflict is one of the most troublesome consequences of attention deficit. Parents blame themselves, each other, and the child for the difficulties. As they become angrier and impose more punishment, the child becomes more defiant and alienated. A father or mother with adult attention deficit sometimes compounds the problem (Minde *et al.* 2003). To avoid constant family warfare, parents need to learn to distinguish behaviour with a biological origin from other, more oppositionally driven behaviours, and develop a strong parenting regime.

The best type of intervention typically combines medication with family therapy or parent training, coping-skills training for the child, and school-based behavioural programmes. Ensuring that the school is offering appropriate management, and that there is good communication between school and family is very important. Most children with attention deficit are taught in the regular classroom, but their pattern of difficulties presents a challenge to the teachers who work with them because they often need some special approaches to help them learn.

For example, it is helpful if the teacher seats the child in an area with few distractions, and provides an area where the child can move around and release excess energy, as well as establishing a clear set of rules and rewards for appropriate behaviour. The regular repetition of instructions, or writing instructions on the board, can be helpful, as can closely monitoring the child's own recording, and offering quiet study areas.

Rewards for success are key, and they may be something as simple as the opportunity to run around for five minutes – which is not only a reward but also a release that will help the child settle to the next segment. Gradually extending the time of each segment shapes the young person's behaviour, and begins to create a more durable concentration span.

Finally it is worth considering for a moment the value of diet. There is clear evidence that colourings and preservatives have some effect upon the behaviour of children whether they have ADHD or not, but no evidence that they are causative (McCann *et al.* 2007).

There is a small group of children who show a hypersensitivity to certain foods, and for this group a specifically designed elimination diet that is rigorously followed has been shown to be helpful. For instance, in one study such a diet reduced both ADHD and oppositional defiant symptoms in 60% of cases where such food hypersensitivity had been identified (Pelsser *et al.* 2011).

There has been great interest in whether supplementing children's diet with omega-3 fatty acid could improve their behaviour, and in particular whether it exerts a positive impact upon the core symptoms of ADHD. The research evidence suggests a very modest impact at best (Soh *et al.* 2009), and this may be in part because the science suggests that it is only the long chain omega-3 that comes from fish that is helpful (Richardson 2007).

On a more general note, it has been found that children who do not eat breakfast show reduced attention in class (Wesnes *et al.* 2003), though there is no evidence that sugar in the diet influences cognition or behaviour (Wolraich *et al.* 1995).

Outcome

For some time ADHD was thought to fade in adolescence, but it is now clear that in the majority of cases the symptoms of ADHD persist into adult life (Kooij *et al.* 2010), with up to 60% continuing to have clinically significant symptoms of ADHD as adults (Kessler *et al.* 2005). Persistence of ADHD is also associated with higher rates of psychiatric comorbidity, as well as higher levels of educational and interpersonal difficulties (Biederman *et al.* 2010a). Children with ADHD are more prone to heavy nicotine use in adolescence, and drug misuse as adults (Wilens 2007). Treatment does offer some protection, with young people treated with stimulants being significantly less likely to develop depressive and anxiety disorders, less troubled with disruptive behaviour, and less likely to fail academically as they move into adulthood (Biederman *et al.* 2009).

As adults, the symptom profile is somewhat different, with sufferers reporting less actual hyperactivity but having feelings of inner restlessness, inability to relax, or over-talkativeness (Kessler *et al.* 2010). Impulsivity can still be problematic and this can prompt behaviour that may get them into trouble with the law, with up to 40% of the long-term prison population having ADHD (Ginsberg *et al.* 2010).

They may have persistent problems in their relationships, and with depression and mood lability (Skirrow *et al.* 2009), as well as struggling with the parenting of their own children (Minde *et al.* 2003). They often have a poor work record, and frequently have problems with driving (Fischer *et al.* 2007). Treatment helps to moderate the psychosocial impairment that results as a consequence of 'core' ADHD symptoms, but these difficulties are likely to be especially evident if the ADHD has not been treated (Able *et al.* 2007).

Conclusion

There has been a vast amount of effort put into understanding ADHD, and it is becoming clear that the core problem is a chronic disorder that is genetically influenced. The fact that other disorders mimic the symptomatology has, until recently, tended to confuse the picture. The condition remains very important to understand because as well as the concentration difficulties, these young people are very prone to have conduct problems and experience educational failure. Alternatively, providing interventions which assist with the difficulties offers a degree of protection to future functioning and helps to provide better parenting for the next generation.

Sources of further help

www.autism.org.uk
www.mencap.org.uk/families
www.autismresearchcentre.com
www.ninds.nih.gov/disorders/
www.childrenfirst.nhs.uk/families/az_child_health/a/autism.html
www.gosh.nhs.uk/gosh_families/information_sheets
www.kidshealth.org/kid/health_problems
www.tskids4.tripod.com
www.nlm.nih.gov/medlineplus/attentiondeficithyperactivitydisorder.html
www.addiss.co.uk
www.mentalhealth.org.uk/help-information/mental-health-a-z/A/attention-deficit/
www.incredibleyears.com
www.rcpsych.ac.uk/mentalhealthinfo/mentalhealthandgrowingup/behaviouralproblems
www.nlm.nih.gov/medlineplus/childbehaviordisorders.html
www.aacap.org/galleries/eAACAP.ResourceCenters/ODD_guide.pdf
www.nimh.nih.gov/publicat/adhdqa.cfm
www.nimh.nih.gov/publicat/autismmenu.cfm

References

Able, S.L., Johnston, J.A., Adler, L.A. *et al.* (2007). Functional and psychosocial impairment in adults with undiagnosed ADHD. *Psychological Medicine* 37: 1–11.

Accornero, V.H., Amado, A.J., Morrow, C.E. *et al.* (2007). Impact of prenatal cocaine exposure on attention and response inhibition as assessed by continuous performance tests. *Journal of Developmental and Behavioral Pediatrics* 28: 195–205.

Anan, R.M., Warner, L.J., McGillivary, J.E. *et al.*(2008). Group Intensive Family Training (GIFT) for pre-schoolers with autism spectrum disorders. *Behavioral Interventions* 23: 165–80.

Angold, A. and Egger, H.L. (2007). Preschool psychopathology: Lessons for the lifespan. *Journal of Child Psychology and Psychiatry* 48: 961–6.

Antshel, K.M. *and* Barkley, R. (2008). Psychosocial interventions in attention deficit hyperactivity disorder. *Child and Adolescent Psychiatric Clinics of North America* 17: 421–37.

Asperger, H. (1944). 'Autistic psychopathy' in childhood. In Frith U. (ed.) *Autism and Asperger Syndrome*. Cambridge: Cambridge University Press.

Baird, G., Simonoff, E., Pickles, A. *et al.* (2006). Prevalence of disorders of the autism spectrum in a population cohort of children in South Thames: The Special Needs and Autism Project (SNAP). *Lancet* 368: 210–15.

Baron-Cohen, S. (2009) Autism: The Empathizing-Systemizing (E-S) Theory. *Annals of the New York Academy of Science* 1156: 68–80.

Biederman, J. (2005). Attention-deficit/hyperactivity disorder: A selective overview. *Biological Psychiatry* 57: 1215–20.

Biederman, J., Monuteaux, M.C., Spencer, T. *et al.* (2009). Do stimulants protect against psychiatric disorders in youth with ADHD? A 10-year follow-up study. *Pediatrics* 124: 71–8.

Biederman, J., Petty, C.R., Evans, M. *et al.* (2010a). How persistent is ADHD? A controlled 10-year follow-up study of boys with ADHD. *Psychiatry Research* 177: 299–304.

Biederman, J., Spencer, T.J., Monuteaux, M.C. *et al.* (2010b). A naturalistic 10-year prospective study of height and weight in children with attention-deficit hyperactivity disorder grown up: Sex and treatment effects. *Journal of Pediatrics* 157: 635–40.

Bloch, M.H., Sukhodolsky, D.G., Dombrowski, P.A. *et al.* (2011). Poor fine-motor and visuospatial skills predict persistence of pediatric-onset obsessive-compulsive disorder into adulthood. *Journal of Child Psychology and Psychiatry* 52: 974–83.

Bruggeman, R., Van der Linden, C., Buitelaar, J.K. *et al.* (2001) Risperidone versus pimozide in Tourette's disorder: A comparative double blind parallel group study. *Journal of Clinical Psychiatry* 62: 50–6.

Castle, D.J., Deale, A., Marks, I.M. (1995). Gender differences in obsessive compulsive disorder. *Australian and New Zealand Journal of Psychiatry* 29: 114–17.

Cavanna, A.E. (2009). Cognitive functioning in Tourette syndrome. *Discovery Medicine* 8: 191–5.

Cavanna, A.E., Servo, S., Monaco, F. *et al.* (2009) The behavioral spectrum of Gilles de la Tourette syndrome. *Journal of Neuropsychiatry and Clinical Neuroscience* 21: 13–23.

Chakrabarti, S. and Fombonne, E. (2005). Pervasive developmental disorders in preschool children: Confirmation of high prevalence. *American Journal of Psychiatry* 162: 1133–41.

Chugani, D.C. (2005). Pharmacologic intervention in autism: Targeting critical periods of brain development. *Clinical Neuropsychiatry* 2: 346–53.

Cohen, P., Cohen, J. and Kasen, S. (1993). An epidemiological study of disorders in late childhood and adolescence: I. Age and gender-specific prevalence. *Journal of Child Psychology and Psychiatry* 34: 851–67.

Collett, B.R., Ohan, J.L. and Myers, K.M. (2003). Ten-year review of rating scales: V. Scales assessing attention-deficit/hyperactivity disorder. *Journal of the American Academy of Child and Adolescent Psychiatry* 42: 1015–37.

Conners, C.K. (1998). Rating scales in attention-deficit/hyperactivity disorder: use in assessment and treatment monitoring. *Journal of Clinical Psychiatry* 59: 24–30.

Connor, D.F., Chartier, K.G., Preen, E.C. *et al.* (2010). Impulsive aggression in attention-deficit-hyperactivity disorder: Symptom severity, comorbidity, and attention-deficit-hyperactivity disorder subtype. *Journal of Child and Adolescent Psychopharmacology* 20: 119–26.

Courchesne, E., Pierce, K., Schumann, C.M. *et al.* (2007). Mapping early brain development in autism. *Neuron* 56: 399–413.

Daviss, W.B., Bentivoglio, P., Racusin, R. (2001). Bupropion sustained release in adolescents with comorbid attention-deficit/hyperactivity disorder and depression. *Journal of the American Academy of Child Adolescent Psychiatry* 40: 307–14.

Deer, B. (2011). How the case against the MMR vaccine was fixed. *BMJ* 342: c5347.

Dover, C.J. and Le Couteur, A. (2007). How to diagnose autism. *Archives of Disease in Childhood* 92: 540–5.

Du Paul, G.J., Barkley, R. and McMurray, M. (1994). Response of children with ADHD to methylphenidate: Interaction with internalizing symptoms. *Journal of the American Academy of Child and Adolescent Psychiatry* 33: 894–903.

Durlak, J., Fuhrman, T. and Lampman, C. (1991). The effectiveness of cognitive-behavior therapy for maladaptive children: A meta-analysis. *Psychological Bulletin* 110: 204–14.

Eddy, C.M., Rickards, H.E. and Cavanna, A.E. (2011). Treatment strategies for tics in Tourette syndrome. *Therapeutic Advances in Neurological Disorders* 4: 25–45.

Faraone, S.V. (2009). Using meta-analysis to compare the efficacy of medications for attention-deficit/hyperactivity disorder in youths. *P&T* 34: 678–94.

Faraone, S.V., Perlis, R.H., Doyle, A.E. *et al.* (2005). Molecular genetics of attention-deficit/hyperactivity disorder. *Biological Psychiatry* 57: 1313–23.

Findling, R.L. (2005). Pharmacologic treatment of behavioral symptoms in autism and pervasive developmental disorders. *Journal of Clinical Psychiatry* 66(Suppl. 10): 26–31.

Fischer, M., Barkley, R.A., Smallish, L. *et al.* (2007). Hyperactive children as young adults: Driving abilities, safe driving behavior, and adverse driving outcomes. *Accident; Analysis and Prevention* 39: 94–105.

Foa, E.B., Steketee, G., Grayson, J.B. *et al.* (1984). Deliberate exposure and blocking of obsessive-compulsive rituals: Immediate and long-term effects. *Behavior Therapy* 15: 450–72.

Foa, E.B., Liebowitz, M.R., Kozak, M.J. *et al.* (2005). Randomized, placebo-controlled trial of exposure and ritual prevention, clomipramine, and their combination in the treatment of obsessive-compulsive disorder. *American Journal of Psychiatry* 162: 151–61.

Freeman, R.D., Fast, D.K., Burd, L. *et al.* (2000). An international perspective on Tourette's syndrome: Selected findings from 3,500 individuals in 22 countries. *Developmental Medicine and Child Neurology* 42: 436–47.

Frey, K.A. and Albin, R.L. (2006). Neuroimaging of Tourette's syndrome. *Journal of Child Neurology* 21: 672–7.

Gargaro, B.A., Rinehart, N.J., Bradshaw, J.L. *et al.* (2011). Autism and ADHD: How far have we come in the comorbidity debate? *Neuroscience and Biobehavioral Reviews* 35: 1081–8.

Geller, D.A. (2006). Obsessive-compulsive and spectrum disorders in children and adolescents. *Psychiatric Clinics of North America* 29: 353–70.

Geurts, H.M., Corbett, B. and Solomon, M. (2009). The paradox of cognitive flexibility in autism, *Trends in Cognitive Science* 13: 74–82.

Giarelli, E., Wiggins, L.D., Rice, C.E. *et al.* (2010). Sex differences in the evaluation and diagnosis of autism spectrum disorders among children. *Disability and Health Journal* 3: 107–16.

Ginsberg, Y., Hirvikoski, T. and Lindefors, N. (2010). Attention deficit hyperactivity disorder (ADHD) among longer-term prison inmates is a prevalent, persistent and disabling disorder. *BMC Psychiatry* 10: 112.

Goddard, A.W., Shekhar, A., Whiteman, A.F. *et al.* (2008). Serotoninergic mechanisms in the treatment of obsessive-compulsive disorder. *Drug Discovery Today* 13: 325–32.

Gol, D. and Jarus, T. (2005). Effect of a social skills training group on everyday activities of children with attention deficit–hyperactivity disorder. *Developmental Medicine and Child Neurology* 47: 539–45.

Gregory, S.G., Connelly, J.J., Towers, A.J. *et al.* (2009). Genomic and epigenetic evidence for oxytocin receptor deficiency in autism. *BMC Medicine* 7: 62.

Gualtieri, C.T. and Johnson, L.G. (2008). Medications do not necessarily normalize cognition in ADHD patients. *Journal of Attentional Disorders* 11: 459–69.

Hanna, G., Himle, J.A., Curtis, G.C. *et al.* (2005). A family study of obsessive- compulsive disorder with pediatric probands. *American Journal of Medical Genetics: Part B Neuropsychiatric Genetics* 134: 13–19.

Herbert, M.R., Ziegler, D.A., Makris, N. *et al.* (2004). Localization of white matter volume increase in autism and developmental language disorder. *Annals of Neurology* 55: 530–40.

Heyman, I., Fombonne, E., Simmons, H. *et al.* (2003). Prevalence of obsessive-compulsive disorder in the British nationwide survey of child mental health. *International Review of Psychiatry* 15: 178–84.

Higgins, D.J., Bailey, S.R. and Pearce, J.C. (2005). Factors associated with functioning style and coping strategies of families with a child with an autism spectrum disorder. *Autism* 9: 125–37.

Himle, M.B., Woods, D.W., Piacentini, J.C. *et al.* (2006) Brief review of habit reversal training for Tourette syndrome. *Journal of Child Neurology* 21: 719–25.

Holmes, J., Gathercole, S.E., Place, M. *et al.* (2010a). An assessment of the diagnostic utility of executive function assessments in the identification of ADHD in children. *Child and Adolescent Mental Health* 15: 37–43.

Holmes, J., Gathercole, S.E., Place, M. *et al.* (2010b) Working memory deficits can be overcome: Impacts of training and medication on working memory in children with ADHD. *Applied Cognitive Psychology* 24: 827–36.

Hubl, D., Bolte, S., Feineis-Matthews, S. *et al.* (2003). Functional imbalance of visual pathways indicates alternative face processing strategies in autism. *Neurology* 61: 1232–7.

Jensen, P.S., Hoagwood, K.E., Roper, M. *et al.* (2004). The services for children and adolescents-parent interview: Development and performance characteristics. *Journal of the American Academy of Child Adolescent Psychiatry* 43: 1334–44.

Kalra, S.K. and Swedo, S.E. (2009). Children with obsessive-compulsive disorder: Are they just 'little adults'? *Journal of Clinical Investigation* 119: 737–46.

Kanner, L. (1943). Autistic disturbances of affective contact. *Nervous Child* 2: 217–50.

Kessler, R.C., Adler, L.A., Barkley, R. *et al.* (2005) Patterns and predictors of ADHD persistence into adulthood: Results from the National Comorbidity Survey Replication. *Biological Psychiatry* 57: 1442–51.

Kessler, R.C., Green, J.G., Adler, L.A. *et al.* (2010). Structure and diagnosis of adult attention-deficit/hyperactivity disorder: Analysis of expanded symptom criteria from the Adult ADHD Clinical Diagnostic Scale. *Archives of General Psychiatry* 67: 1168–78.

Khalifa, N. and von Knorring. A.L. (2005). Prevalence of tic disorders and Tourette syndrome in a Swedish school population. *Developmental Medicine and Child Neurology* 45: 315–19.

Kolevzon, A., Mathewson, K.A., Hollander, E. (2006). Selective serotonin reuptake inhibitors in autism: A review of efficacy and tolerability. *Journal of Clinical Psychiatry* 67: 407–14.

Konrad, K. and Eickhoff, S.B. (2010). Is the ADHD brain wired differently? A review on structural and functional connectivity in attention deficit hyperactivity disorder, *Human Brain Mapping* 31: 904–16.

Kooij, S.J.J., Bejerot, S., Blackwell, A. *et al.* (2010). European consensus statement on diagnosis and treatment of adult ADHD: The European Network Adult ADHD. *BMC Psychiatry* 10: 67.

Krebs, G. and Heyman, I. (2010). Treatment-resistant obsessive-compulsive disorder in young people: Assessment and treatment strategies. *Child and Adolescent Mental Health* 15: 2–11.

Kuntsi, J., Neale, B.M., Chen, W. *et al.* (2006). The IMAGE project: Methodological issues for the molecular genetic analysis of ADHD. *Behavior and Brain Function* 2: 27.

Kurlan, R., McDermott, M.P., Deeley, C. *et al.* (2001). Prevalence of tics in school-children and association with placement in special education. *Neurology* 57: 1383–8.

Laugeson, E.A., Frankel, F., Mogil, C. *et al.* (2009). Parent-assisted social skills training to improve friendships in teens with autism spectrum disorders. *Journal of Autism and Developmental Disorders* 39: 596–606.

Lecavalier, L., Leone, S. and Wiltz, J. (2006). The impact of behaviour problems on caregiver stress in young people with autism spectrum disorders. *Journal of Intellectual Disability Research* 50: 172–83.

Le Couteur, A., Rutter, M., Lord, C. *et al.* (1989) Autism Diagnostic Interview: a standardized investigator-based instrument. *Journal of Autism and Developmental Disorders* 19: 363–87.

Ledgerwood, L., Richardson, R. and Cranney, J. (2003). Effects of D-cycloserine on extinction of conditioned freezing. *Behavioral Neuroscience* 117: 341–9.

Leonard, H.L., Lenane, M.C., Swedo, S.E. *et al.* (1992) Tics and Tourette's disorder: a 2- to 7-year follow-up of 54 obsessive-compulsive children. *American Journal of Psychiatry* 149: 1244–51.

Leppanen, J.M. and Nelson, C.A. (2006). The development and neural bases of facial emotion recognition. *Advances in Child Development and Behavior* 34: 207–46.

Lewin, A.B., Storch, E.A., Conelea, C.A. *et al.* (2011). The roles of anxiety and depression in connecting tic severity and functional impairment. *Journal of Anxiety Disorders* 25: 164–8.

Li, D., Sham, P.C., Owen, M.J. *et al.* (2006) Meta-analysis shows significant association between dopamine system genes and attention deficit hyperactivity disorder (ADHD). *Human Molecular Genetics* 15: 2276–84.

Loeber, R. and Stouthamer-Loeber, M. (1986). Family factors as correlates and predictors of juvenile conduct problems and delinquency. In M. Tonry and N. Morris (eds) *Crime and Justice: An Annual Review of Research*, vol. VII. Chicago: University of Chicago Press.

Lord, C., Risi, S., Lambrecht, L. *et al.* (2000). The Autism Diagnostic Observation Schedule – Generic: A standard measure of social and communication deficits associated with the spectrum of autism. *Journal of Autism and Developmental Disorders* 30: 205–23.

Lovaas, O.I. (1987). Behavioral treatment and normal educational and intellectual functioning in young autistic children. *Journal of Consulting and Clinical Psychology* 55: 3–9.

Lugnegård, T., Hallerbäck, M.U. and Gillberg, C. (2011). Psychiatric comorbidity in young adults with a clinical diagnosis of Asperger syndrome. *Research in Developmental Disabilities* 32: 1910–17.

Maia, T.V., Cooney, R.E. and Peterson, B.S. (2008). The neural bases of obsessive-compulsive disorder in children and adults. *Developmental Psychopathology* 20: 1251–83.

Mancuso, E., Faro, A., Joshi, G. *et al.* (2010).Treatment of pediatric obsessive-compulsive disorder: A review. *Journal of Child and Adolescent Psychopharmacology* 20: 299–308.

Mandy, W.P. and Skuse, D.H. (2008). Research review: What is the association between the social-communication element of autism and repetitive interests, behaviours and activities? *Journal of Child Psychology and Psychiatry* 49: 795–808.

Mandy, W., Charman, T., Gilmour, J. *et al.* (2011). Toward specifying pervasive developmental disorder – not otherwise specified. *Autism Research* 4: 121–31.

Manly, T., Anderson, V., Nimmo-Smith, I. *et al.* (2001). The differential assessment of children's attention: The test of everyday attention for children (TEA-Ch), normative sample and ADHD performance, *Journal of Child Psychology and Psychiatry* 42: 1065–81.

Massetti, G.M., Lahey, B.B., Pelham, W.E. *et al.* (2007). Academic achievement over 8 years among children who met modified criteria for attention-deficit/hyperactivity disorder at 4–6 years of age. *Journal of Abnormal Child Psychology* 36: 399–410.

Matson, M.L., Mahan, S. and Matson, J.L. (2009). Parent training: A review of methods for children with autism spectrum disorders. *Research in Autism Spectrum Disorders* 3: 868–75.

McCann, D., Barrett, A., Cooper, A. *et al.* (2007). Food additives and hyperactive behaviour in 3-year-old and 8/9-year-old children in the community: A randomised, double-blinded, placebo-controlled trial. *Lancet* 370: 1560–67.

McConachie, H. and Diggle, T. (2007). Parent implemented early intervention for young children with autism spectrum disorder: A systematic review. *Journal of Evaluation and Clinical Practice* 13: 120–9.

McDougle, C.J., Epperson, C.N., Pelton, G.H. *et al.* (2000). A double-blind, placebo-controlled study of risperidone addition in serotonin reuptake inhibitor-refractory obsessive-compulsive disorder. *Archives of General Psychiatry* 57: 794–801.

Minde, K., Eakin, L., Hechtman, L. *et al.* (2003). The psychosocial functioning of children and spouses of adults with ADHD. *Journal of Child Psychology and Psychiatry* 44: 637–46.

Mordre, M., Groholt, B., Kjelsberg, E. *et al.* (2011). The impact of ADHD and conduct disorder in childhood on adult delinquency. A 30 years follow-up study using official crime records. *BMC Psychiatry* 11.

Muhle, R., Trentacoste, S.V. and Rapin, I. (2004). The genetics of autism. *Pediatrics* 113: 472–86.

Mula, M., Cavanna, A.E., Critchley, H.D. *et al.* (2008). Phenomenology of obsessive compulsive disorder in patients with temporal lobe epilepsy and Gilles de la Tourette syndrome. *Journal of Neuropsychiatry and Clinical Neurosciences* 20: 223–6.

Murphy, D., Pelham, W. and Lang, A. (1992). Aggression in boys with ADHD: Methylphenidate effects on naturalistically observed aggression, response to provocation and social information processing. *Journal of Abnormal Child Psychology* 20: 451–66.

Nagarajan, R.P., Hogart, A.R., Gwye, Y. *et al.* (2006). Reduced MeCP2 expression is frequent in autism frontal cortex and correlates with aberrant MECP2 promoter methylation. *Epigenetics* 1: 1–11.

National Institute for Health and Clinical Excellence (2005). *Obsessive-compulsive disorder: Core interventions in the treatment of obsessive-compulsive disorder and body dysmorphic disorder.* London: NICE.

Nestadt, G., Samuels, J., Bienvenu, J.O. *et al.* (2000). A family study of obsessive compulsive disorder. *Archives of General Psychiatry* 57: 358–63.

Norberg, M.M., Krystal, J.H. and Tolin, D.F. (2008). A meta-analysis of D-cycloserine and the facilitation of fear extinction and exposure therapy. *Biological Psychiatry* 63: 1118–26.

Norvilitis, J.M., Sun, L. and Zhang, J. (2010). ADHD symptomatology and adjustment to college in China and the United States. *Journal of Learning Disability* 43: 86–94.

O'Roak, B.J. and State, M.W. (2008). Autism genetics: Strategies, challenges, and opportunities. *Autism Research* 1: 4–17.

Ospina, M.B., Krebs, S.J., Clark, B. *et al.* (2008) Behavioural and developmental interventions for autism spectrum disorder: A clinical systematic review. *PLoS ONE* 3: e3755.

Pardini, D.A. and Fite, P.J. (2010). Symptoms of conduct disorder, oppositional defiant disorder, attention-deficit/hyperactivity disorder, and callous–unemotional traits as unique predictors of psychosocial maladjustment in boys: Advancing an evidence base for DSM-V. *Journal of the American Academy of Child and Adolescent Psychiatry* 49: 1134–44.

Pardo, C.A. and Eberhart, C.G. (2007). The neurobiology of autism. *Brain Pathology* 17: 434–47.

Pauls, D.L, Leckman, J., Towbin, K.E. *et al.* (1986). A possible genetic relationship exists between Tourette's syndrome and obsessive-compulsive disorder. *Psychopharmacology Bulletin* 22: 730–33.

Pediatric OCD Treatment Study Team. (2004). Cognitive-behavior therapy, sertraline, and their combination for children and adolescents with Obsessive-Compulsive Disorder. *Journal of the American Medical Association* 292: 1969–76.

Pelsser, L.M., Buitelaar, J.K. and Savelkoul, H.F. (2009). ADHD as a (non) allergic hypersensitivity disorder: A hypothesis. *Pediatric Allergy and Immunology* 20: 107–12.

Pelsser, L.M., Frankena, K., Toorman, J. *et al.* (2011). Effects of a restricted elimination diet on the behaviour of children with attention-deficit hyperactivity disorder (INCA study): A randomised controlled trial. *Lancet* 377: 494–503.

Peterson, B.S., Potenza, M.N., Wang, Z. *et al.* (2009). An fMRI study of the effects of psychostimulants on default-mode processing during stroop task performance in youths with ADHD. *American Journal of Psychiatry* 166: 1286–94.

Plauché Johnson, C. and Myers, S.M. (2007). Council on Children with Disabilities: Identification and evaluation of children with autism spectrum disorders. *Pediatrics* 120: 1183–215.

Plessen, K.J., Bansal, R. and Peterson, B.S. (2009). Imaging evidence for anatomical disturbances and neuroplastic compensation in persons with Tourette syndrome. *Journal of Psychosomatic Research* 67: 559–73.

Pluess, M., Belsky, J. and Neuman, R.J. (2009). Prenatal smoking and attention-deficit/ hyperactivity disorder: DRD4-7R as a plasticity gene. *Biological Psychiatry* 66: 5–6.

Polanczyk, G., de Lima, M.S., Horta, B.L. *et al.* (2007) The worldwide prevalence of ADHD: A systematic review and meta-regression analysis. *American Journal of Psychiatry* 164: 942–8.

Posey, D.J., Erickson, C.A. and McDougle, C.J. (2008). Developing drugs for core social and communication impairment in autism. *Child and Adolescent Psychiatric Clinics of North America* 17: 787–801.

Qiu, A., Crocetti, D., Adler, M. *et al.* (2009). Basal ganglia volume and shape in children with attention deficit hyperactivity disorder. *American Journal of Psychiatry* 166: 74–82.

Racine, M.B., Majnemer, A., Shevell, M. *et al.* (2008) Handwriting performance in children with attention deficit hyperactivity disorder (ADHD*). Journal of Child Neurology* 23: 399–406.

Riccio, C.A., Reynolds, C.R. and Lowe, P.A. (2001). Diagnostic efficacy of CPTs for disorders usually first evident in childhood or adolescence. In *Clinical Applications of Continuous Performance Tests*. New York: Wiley.

Richardson, A.J. (2007). N-3 fatty acids and mood: The devil is in the detail. *British Journal of Nutrition* 99: 221–3.

Robertson, M.M. (2006a). Mood disorders and Gilles de la Tourette syndrome: An update on prevalence, etiology, comorbidity, clinical associations, and implications. *Journal of Psychosomatic Research* 61: 349–58.

Robertson, M.M. (2006b). Attention deficit hyperactivity disorder, tics and Tourette's syndrome: The relationship and treatment implications. *European Child and Adolescent Psychiatry* 15: 1–11.

Rommelse, N.N.J., Geurts, H.M., Franke, B. *et al.* (2011). A review on cognitive and brain endophenotypes that may be common in autism spectrum disorder and attention-deficit/hyperactivity disorder and facilitate the search for pleiotropic genes. *Neuroscience and Biobehavioral Reviews* 35: 1363–96.

Rogers, S. and Vismara, L. (2008). Evidence-based comprehensive treatments for early autism. *Journal of Clinical Child and Adolescent Psychology* 37: 8–38.

Ronald, A. and Hoekstra, R.A. (2011). Autism spectrum disorders and autistic traits: A decade of new twin studies, *American Journal of Medical Genetics: Part B Neuropsychiatric Genetics* 156: 255–74.

Rucklidge, J.J. (2010) Gender differences in attention-deficit/hyperactivity disorder. *Psychiatric Clinics of North America* 33: 357–73.

Rutter, M. (2005). Aetiology of autism: Findings and questions. *Journal of Intellectual and Disability Research* 49: 231–8.

Schachar, R. and Tannock, R. (1995). Test of four hypotheses for the comorbidity of attention deficit hyperactivity disorder and conduct disorder. *Journal of the American Academy of Child and Adolescent Psychiatry* 34: 639–48.

Scahill, L., Riddle, M.A., McSwiggin-Hardin, M. *et al.* (1997). Children's Yale-Brown Obsessive Compulsive Scale: Reliability and validity. *Journal of the American Academy of Child and Adolescent Psychiatry* 36: 844–52.

Scahill, L., Erenberg, G., Berlin, C.M. *et al.* (2006). Contemporary assessment and pharmacotherapy of Tourette syndrome. *NeuroRx: Journal of the American Society of Experimental Neurotherapeutics* 3: 192–206.

Scahill, L., Bitsko, R.H., Visser, S.N. *et al.* (2009). Prevalence of diagnosed Tourette Syndrome in persons aged 6–17 years, United States, 2007. *Morbidity and Mortality Weekly Report* 58: 581–5.

Schieve, L.A., Blumberg, S.J., Rice, C. *et al.* (2007). The relationship between autism and parenting stress. *Paediatrics* 119: S114–S121.

Schur, S.B., Sikich, L., Findling, R.L. *et al.* (2003). Treatment recommendations for the use of antipsychotics for aggressive youth (TRAAY): Part I. A review. *Journal of the American Academy of Child and Adolescent Psychiatry* 42: 132–44.

Shields, J. (2001). The NAS EarlyBird Programme: Partnership with parents in early intervention. *Autism* 5: 49–56.

Sigman, M. and McGovern, C.W. (2005). Improvement in cognitive and language skills from preschool to adolescence in autism. *Journal of autism and developmental disorders* 35: 15–23.

Simonoff, E., Pickles, A., Charman, T. *et al.* (2008). Psychiatric disorders in children with autism spectrum disorders: Prevalence, comorbidity, and associated factors in a population-derived sample. *Journal of the American Academy of Child and Adolescent Psychiatry* 47: 921–9.

Skirrow, C., McLoughlin, G., Kuntsi, J. *et al.* (2009). Behavioral, neurocognitive and treatment overlap between attention-deficit/hyperactivity disorder and mood instability. *Expert Review of Neurotherapeutics* 9: 489–503.

Skuse, D., Warrington, R., Bishop, D. *et al.* (2004). The Developmental, Diagnostic and Dimensional Interview (3di): A novel computerised assessment for autism spectrum disorders. *Journal of the Academy of Child and Adolescent Psychiatry* 43: 548–58.

Sodian, B. and Thoermer, C. (2008). Precursors to a theory of mind in infancy: Perspectives for research on autism. *The Quarterly Journal of Experimental Psychology*, 61: 27–39.

Soh, N., Walter, G., Baur, L. *et al.* (2009). Nutrition, mood and behaviour: A review. *Acta Neuropsychiatrica* 21: 214–27.

Sonuga-Barke, E.J., Thompson, M., Abikoff, H. *et al.* (2006). Nonpharmacological interventions for preschoolers with ADHD. *Infants and Young Children* 19: 142–53.

Spencer, T., Biederman, J., Wilens, T. *et al.* (1996). Pharmacology of ADHD across the life cycle. *Journal of the American Academy of Child and Adolescent Psychiatry* 35: 409–32.

Spencer, T., Heiligenstein, J.H. and Biederman, J. (2002). Results from 2 proof-of-concept, placebo-controlled studies of atomoxetine in children with attention deficit/hyperactivity disorder. *Journal of Clinical Psychiatry* 63: 1140–7.

Storch, E.A., Geffken, G.R., Merlo, L.J. *et al.* (2007a). Family accommodation in pediatric obsessive-compulsive disorder. *Journal of Clinical Child and Adolescent Psychiatry* 36: 207–16.

Storch, E.A., Geffken, G.R., Merlo, L.J. *et al.* (2007b). Family-based cognitive-behavioral therapy for pediatric obsessive-compulsive disorder: Comparison of intensive and weekly approaches. *Journal of the American Academy of Child and Adolescent Psychiatry* 46: 469–78.

Sukhodolsky, D.G., Scahill, L., Zhang, H. *et al.* (2003). Disruptive behavior in children with Tourette's syndrome: Association with ADHD comorbidity, tic severity, and functional impairment. *Journal of the American Academy of Child and Adolescent Psychiatry* 42: 98–105.

Swanson, J.M. (1992). *School-Based Assessments and Intervention for ADD Students*. Irvine: KC Publishing.

Swedo, S.E., Leonard, H.L., Garvey, M. *et al.* (1998). Pediatric autoimmune neuro-psychiatric disorders associated with streptococcal infections: Clinical description of the first 50 cases. *American Journal of Psychiatry* 155: 264–71.

Tost, H., Kolachana, B., Hakimi, S. *et al.* (2010) A common allele in the oxytocin receptor gene (OXTR) impacts prosocial temperament and human hypothalamic-limbic structure and function. *Proceedings of the National Academy of Science USA*. 107: 13936–41.

Tourette's Syndrome Study Group. (2002) Treatment of ADHD in children with tics: A randomized controlled trial. *Neurology* 58: 527–36.

Tuchman, R., Alessandri, M. and Cuccaro, M. (2010) Autism spectrum disorders and epilepsy: Moving towards a comprehensive approach to treatment. *Brain and Development* 32: 719–30.

van Spronsen, M. and Hoogenraad, C.C. (2010). Synapse pathology in psychiatric and neurologic disease. *Current Neurology and Neuroscience Reports* 10: 207–14.

Vaughan, B.S., Wetzel, M,W. and Kratochvil, C.J. (2008). Beyond the 'typical' patient: Treating attention-deficit/hyperactivity disorder in preschoolers and adults. *International Review of Psychiatry* 20: 143–9.

Verdellen, C.W., Hoogduin, C.A. and Keijsers, G.P. (2007). Tic suppression in the treatment of Tourette's syndrome with exposure therapy: The rebound phenomenon reconsidered. *Movement Disorders* 22: 1601–6.

Verte, S., Geurts, H.M., Roeyers, H. *et al.* (2005). Executive functioning in children with autism and Tourette's syndrome. *Developmental Psychopathology* 17: 415–45.

Volkow, N.D. and Swanson, J.M. (2003). Variables that affect the clinical use and abuse of methylphenidate in the treatment of ADHD. *American Journal of Psychiatry* 160: 1909–18.

Walkup, J.T., Albano, A.M., Piacentini, J. *et al.* (2008). Cognitive behavioral therapy, sertraline, or a combination in childhood anxiety. *New England Journal of Medicine* 359: 2753–66.

Walshaw, P.D., Alloy, L.B. and Sabb, F.W. (2010). Executive function in pediatric bipolar disorder and attention-deficit hyperactivity disorder: In search of distinct phenotypic profiles. *Neuropsychology Review* 20: 103–20.

Weiss, L.A., Arking, D.E. and the Gene Discovery Project of Johns Hopkins Autism Consortium (2009). A genome-wide linkage and association scan reveals novel loci for autism. *Nature* 461: 802–8.

Wesnes, K.A, Pincock, C., Richardson, D. *et al.* (2003) Breakfast reduces declines in attention and memory over the morning in schoolchildren. *Appetite* 41: 329–31.

Whittingham, K., Sofronoff, K., Sheffield, J. *et al.* (2009). Do parental attributions affect treatment outcome in a parenting program? An exploration of the effects of parental attributions in an RCT of Stepping Stones Triple P for the ASD population. *Research in Autism Spectrum Disorders* 3: 129–44.

Wiggins, L.D., Robins, D.L., Adamson, L.B. *et al.* (2011). Support for a dimensional view of autism spectrum disorders in toddlers. *Journal of Autism and Developmental Disorders* 11: 1230–40.

Wilens, T.E. (2007). The nature of the relationship between attention-deficit/hyperactivity disorder and substance use. *Journal of Clinical Psychiatry* 68: 4–8.

Willcutt, E.G., Doyle, A.E., Nigg, J.T. *et al.* (2005). Validity of the executive function theory of attention-deficit/hyperactivity disorder: A meta-analytic review. *Biological Psychiatry* 57: 1336–46.

Wolraich, M.L., Wilson, D.B. and White, J.W. (1995). The effect of sugar on behaviour or cognition in children: A meta-analysis. *Journal of the American Medical Association* 274: 1617–21.

Wolraich, M.L., Hannah, J.N., Pinnock, T.Y. *et al.* (1996). Comparison of diagnostic criteria for attention-deficit hyperactivity disorder in a county-wide sample. *Journal of the American Academy of Child and Adolescent Psychiatry* 35: 319–24.

Wolosin, S.M., Richardson, M.E., Hennessey, J.G. *et al.* (2009). Abnormal cerebral cortex structure in children with ADHD. *Human Brain Mapping* 30: 175–84.

Youngstrom, E.A., Birmaher, B. and Findling, R.L. (2008). Pediatric bipolar disorder: Validity, phenomenology, and recommendations for diagnosis. *Bipolar Disorders* 10: 194–214.

Chapter 8

Disruptiveness and challenging behaviour in schools and classrooms

Introduction

> Most pupils believe that they and their teachers have different interests. In their view, it is his business to exact of them hard service, theirs to escape from it; it is his privilege to make laws; theirs to evade them. He is benefited by their industry, they by their indolence; he is honoured by their obedience, they by their independence. From the infant school to the professional seminary this moral warfare exists.
>
> (*English Journal of Education* 1858; cited in Furlong 1985: 1)

Historical accounts of childhood misbehaviour in school (Pearson 1983) remind us that problem behaviour is no recent phenomenon. Nevertheless, concern about rising misbehaviour in school is currently a worldwide concern, perhaps reflecting globalising trends towards greater personal autonomy and the rejection of traditional authority (Inglehart and Welzel 2005; Elliott 2009).

Although labels such as 'social, emotional and behavioural difficulties' and 'disruptive' may be helpful to educationalists in accessing specialist provision for children whose behaviour disrupts classes, it is important to note that such terms are largely subjective and often do not clearly relate to specific behaviours. In many cases such labels are reflections of a teacher's mounting concern or anxiety about the impact of a child's behaviour upon others. Although labelling may be directly related to the freeing of additional resources, in seeking to prevent or reduce classroom misbehaviour it is rarely helpful to concern oneself overly with psychological classifications or diagnoses. Rather, it is more important to consider what approaches can be introduced to alleviate or resolve the situation. Such considerations involve a close examination of many factors operating at three different levels. These, and the approaches associated with them, form the basis of this chapter.

Levels of analysis

When asked to consider the reasons for a child's misbehaviour, many teachers and parents will understandably point to aspects of the child's environment, history or psychological make-up (Miller *et al.* 2002). Environmental factors that are often employed to account for misbehaviour include disruption to family life, poor parenting, socio-economic hardship and physical or sexual abuse. Psychological accounts may focus upon such factors as the child's personality, attitudes, temperament and interpersonal style. In such accounts, the prime focus usually involves 'within-child' analyses where the source of the problem is located within the child. The child enters the school each day, along with his or her problems, and the clashes with teachers and other children are an inevitable consequence. As, in such analyses, the origin of the child's problems is perceived to be located outside of the school gates, it is not surprising that schools can feel unsure how best to respond. Often the 'answer' is seen as remedying the child's home circumstances, transferring the child to alternative educational provision, or providing some form of psychological therapy.

It is universally accepted, however, that for the majority of children, classroom behaviour may vary considerably, depending upon who is teaching them at any given time. Although 'within-child' analyses can provide an indication as to why an individual child has a *propensity* to exhibit problem behaviour in school, these are insufficient as a comprehensive explanation for disruptiveness. A focus on the background and interpersonal dynamics of an individual child neglects the importance of the impact of the teacher in determining what *actually transpires*. While research has shown that poorly behaved children at age 5 tend to continue to be a challenge to teachers many years later in secondary school (Houts *et al.* 2010), the effects of individual differences in professional skill upon children's conduct are still very significant. The expert teacher may often be able to secure a settled, industrious classroom despite the fact that many of the children have the potential to be extremely challenging. In contrast, a less skilled teacher may be confronted with major disruption even by children who can usually be relied upon to conduct themselves admirably.

During the final decades of the twentieth century, attention shifted somewhat from the impact of *individual teachers* upon children's behaviour to that of the influence of *schools* as complex social organisations. Unlike studies conducted during the 1960s that appeared to suggest that differences between schools made little or no impact upon student behaviour and attainment, research during the 1970s (Reynolds *et al.* 1976; Rutter *et al.* 1979) began to suggest that the impact of individual schools as social organisations upon children's general level of performance was significant. It is not simply that the classroom skills of the child's teachers may differ from one school to another but, rather, that the overall general ethos or social climate of each school communicates different messages to the child. This work resulted in the burgeoning school effectiveness literature. Interestingly, this was found not to translate easily into prescription for school improvement, perhaps because attempts were often underpinned by a simplistic belief that it was possible to identify discrete factors independent of culture and context (Alexander 2000).

Intervention at the within-child level

The major ways of tackling problems at the within-child level involve a variety of forms of counselling or behavioural techniques. These approaches, of course, have long been misguidedly perceived by some teachers as 'a good talking to' and 'rewards and punishment' respectively. Misunderstanding of the precise nature of counselling and behavioural approaches and their potential for teachers has arguably reduced their impact and, in extreme cases, resulted in their being dismissed as of little value for school contexts.

At the simplest level, counselling attempts to enable the individual to gain a clearer understanding of his or her attitudes, beliefs, attributions, expectations and values, the impact of others upon his/her behaviour, the nature and impact of his/her behaviour upon others and the relationship of these to one's psychological and social functioning. In the specific context of challenging behaviour in school, it is generally hoped by school staff that the outcome of counselling will be that the child gains greater self-understanding and that this will lead to a change of behaviour. Behavioural approaches, in contrast, make rather fewer demands upon the child's ability to reason and ultimately determine what should be their preferred pattern of behaviour (see Chapter 2). Their focus is primarily upon observable behaviour rather than inferred cognition. With regard to disruptiveness in school, the most widely used technique is contingency contracting. This involves establishing a programme that systematically provides rewards and sanctions that are demonstrably contingent upon behaviour. The desired behaviours are described, negotiated, and, ideally, agreed with the child and his or her parents or carers. Positive or negative outcomes directly related to these specific behaviours are made explicit and a system of close monitoring and evaluation is established. Although it is common for both counselling and behavioural approaches to be employed in combination, within the context of school, it is the latter approach that often sits more easily within the prevailing power structures.

Counselling, and other forms of talking therapy, are generally based upon the premise that the client recognises that he/she has a problem and wishes to work with another in order to derive a solution. Where children have problems that do not directly intrude upon the smooth running of school (e.g. anxiety about peer relationships, grief concerning the loss of a loved family member) the practice of counselling is unlikely to lead to role conflict for the teacher concerned. Many young people who engage in disruptive behaviour in school, however, do not actively seek, or wish to enter into, a counselling relationship, nor do they necessarily want to reflect upon or change their present circumstances, for often their disruptiveness is proving reinforcing to them. In such cases, it is fair to say that it is the teacher or school, rather than the child, that perceives a problem.

Although a vast array of differing models of counselling exist, they have in common a general principle that it is the client who has ultimate control, freedom and responsibility to choose what he or she feels is the most effective way forward. The counsellor's task is to help the child gain greater understanding of relevant issues and to empower him/her to decide on a course of action. The decision taken should be accepted and valued by the counsellor. This raises the important question of who in the school can and should engage in the counselling process.

During the 1960s, the notion of the school counsellor, already a fully qualified teacher, who could be non-judgemental and non-authoritarian, gained a degree of popularity. Following the model of the school-based guidance counsellor in the USA, it was anticipated by many that each secondary school would employ a counsellor who would help the child with social, educational and vocational issues. Although the child might be referred by school staff, there would be no doubt that the client was the child rather than the school. In such cases, counsellors would not necessarily see a resolution of those difficulties that have been identified by schools as the central goal of their work.

As educational resources declined and conceptions of the role of the teacher changed to incorporate views of teaching the 'whole child', the notion of the teacher as counsellor gained in popularity. Heads of year or house were increasingly expected to engage in counselling children with a variety of personal and social, as well as educational, problems. Gradually this role was also taken up by class-teachers, and skills of counselling (e.g. active listening, reflecting, clarifying and summarising) were widely taught by means of in-service training and published materials (e.g. Langham and Parker 1989).

The value of teachers having basic counselling skills in working with colleagues, young people and their parents has now become widely accepted although an important distinction should be drawn between the operation of such skills in day-to-day school life and the employment by teachers of counselling as the primary strategy in work with a highly challenging individual.

In contrast with the school counsellor, the teacher's perceived task in 'counselling' challenging children is often to ensure that they are persuaded to change their behaviour in a desired fashion. In such circumstances all of the adult's skills of persuasion may be brought to this task, and existing power differentials are likely to be exploited. In such circumstances one may query whether counselling is appropriate. Consider, for example, the child who is refusing to wear school uniform and is summoned to the head of year to be 'counselled'. Does the description of the ensuing exchange as counselling mean that the child has a real freedom to make a decision? If the child chooses not to act in accordance with the requirements of the school, is the head of year in a position to accept and value the child's decision? To suggest, as is often the case, that a disinterested head of year is merely helping the child to understand the consequences of continued non-acquiescence, that the child is free to make up his or her own mind in the full knowledge of the likely outcomes, is to debase the notion of what true counselling sets out to achieve. In such situations, and however justifiable it may be, the process is not counselling but exhortation, persuasion and/or threat.

> Counselling is about change – personal change – and as such we cannot, and should not, talk in terms of enforcing counselling on others. It is almost impossible to make people change the more fundamental aspects of themselves *unless they want to*. It is also unethical to try to impose such changes on another

person. This is allied at worst to brainwashing or intimidation, and at best to social control.

(Cowie and Pecherek 1994: 55; emphasis in original)

Such a difficulty, albeit to a lesser extent, may also be encountered by other professionals whose responsibility is to provide support to children with behavioural difficulties. Thus, a degree of concern has been expressed about the roles, functions and appropriate focus of salaried and school mentors (Jones *et al.* 2009) with uncertainties as to whether this should involve mentoring, coaching, tutoring or counselling (Napper and Keane 2004). All too easily these can become confused and the counselling role can be underpinned by the need for institutional control (Colley 2003), a pressure that may be particularly felt by salaried mentors (Rose and Jones 2007). Similar dilemmas can be experienced by other education professionals. The educational psychologist or behaviour support teacher, although freed from the day-to-day pressure that a child may exert on the classteacher or school management, is still likely to feel a degree of pressure to effect the desired change in the client, to encourage the child to respond in ways which responsible adults in the education system might find desirable. This is not, of course, to suggest that the interests of the child are overlooked but, rather, that it may become apparent that these are best served by ensuring that problem behaviour is reduced. In many circumstances, therefore, it is not clear whether a professional is actually engaging in counselling as understood by the professional literature or is actually guiding the child to behave in a desired fashion. To illustrate this dilemma, consider the example of Colin.

Colin, aged 14, was becoming an increasing problem for his teachers. Although not aggressive or directly challenging to teachers, his continual use of argument, name-calling and general banter towards peers was becoming increasingly disruptive and undermining the quality of many lessons. Colin was somewhat overweight and had a marked physical resemblance to a famous comedian. This attracted risible comment from peers to which he would reply in kind.

At his first interview with the educational psychologist, Colin professed unhappiness at his circumstances and a strong desire that those who were provoking him should be silenced. He agreed to meet with the psychologist over a period of weeks in the hope that ways forward might be deduced.

At an early stage in their sessions, the educational psychologist considered Colin to be locked in a spiral of peer antagonism. As a result, the boy appeared to be unthinkingly engaged in a series of self-defeating behaviours that met neither his needs nor those of others. For this reason, it was considered that counselling should focus upon events in school and Colin would be asked to explore what happened and determine whether he wished change to take place. It was anticipated that Colin's generally good-natured disposition and his obvious desire for a comfortable existence, together with a greater understanding of his own role in provoking conflict, would result in a desire and an ability to modify his behaviour.

Over a number of counselling sessions, Colin's behaviour in school was examined and analysed. Events antecedent to conflict were identified and, using flowcharts on large sheets of paper, Colin was shown how his reactions would often maintain difficulties for himself. Over time, Colin appeared to have much greater insight into the dynamics of his classroom setting and the ways by which he interacted with others.

Once a degree of insight was gained, Colin was reminded that he had earlier expressed a desire to change his circumstances. He was asked what would have to change in order that the verbal aggression and ensuing classroom disruption might be reduced. Colin persisted in his argument that it was his peers, not he, who would have to change, even though he clearly understood his impact upon them. (This is a common feature of work with children where highly contradictory perceptions can be held simultaneously, the less desirable of which may often be maintained by a powerful need to attribute blame to a third party.) During the course of further sessions, Colin came to accept that meaningful change would be likely to take place only if he were to change his normal pattern of classroom behaviour. At this point he announced that he enjoyed the classroom banter – it alleviated the tedium of lessons – and that he had made a decision that he did not want his present circumstances to change. This position was maintained during further follow-up sessions.

The educational psychologist was now in a difficult situation. Within the counselling relationship it had been suggested that Colin should come to his own decisions about future action, based upon the insights and understandings obtained during the sessions. The boy had, however, chosen an unwelcome path that placed him in direct conflict with the school. If he did not change it was clear that a likely outcome would be exclusion followed by an enforced transfer to a disruptive unit. In the opinion of the psychologist this was a highly undesirable placement, given Colin's circumstances. To what extent, therefore, could the psychologist seek to place greater pressure upon Colin to change his behaviour? The use of behavioural techniques, family controls and school sanctions could be integrated into a programme that might be able to enforce compliance, yet would this indicate that the pose adopted in the counselling interview was little more than a sham, that freedom of choice for the child existed only in so far as this represented the desired outcomes of others? On the other hand, was it sufficient for the psychologist to inform the school and local authority that he had done his best but, unfortunately, Colin did not wish to change and thus the case would be closed? The pressure upon local authorities to provide services perceived by schools to be 'effective' might further reduce the appeal of the latter alternative.

In the final analysis it was considered that the risks to Colin of permanent exclusion were so great that the employment of a behaviour modification pro-gramme geared to reducing his disruptive behaviour was the most appropriate course of action. Such a programme was subsequently established. This involved itemising and agreeing desired behaviours with Colin, his teachers and his parents. After each lesson his teachers provided him with a score which was recorded on a form. His total daily score was then used to establish the extent to which he would receive a variety of rewards such as pocket money and television.

This programme proved highly effective and, despite his initial reluctance, Colin soon became an enthusiastic participant. One is left to consider, however, whether this satisfactory end justified the action taken – was it right to take control from the child once he had refused to change in the desired fashion? Despite the fact that Colin appeared not to recognise the contradictions above, it is likely that, with hindsight, the psychologist would have specified the limitations upon the boy's freedom to choose.

It is important to note that fairly intrusive behavioural techniques were required to help Colin to change. While it is widely accepted that the *skills* of counselling are of value to teachers in working with child, parents and colleagues, counselling as a *therapeutic process* is only rarely an effective and sufficient technique for teachers confronted by acts of major indiscipline.

Behavioural approaches, in contrast to counselling, have as their primary focus observable behaviours and how these may be modified or shaped (see Chapter 2) with particular stress placed upon the relationship between behaviours and their consequences. Put simply, behaviour followed by a positive experience is more likely to recur. Behaviour that has no 'pay-off' or, alternatively, is followed by an adverse consequence is less likely to recur. This very simple maxim, stemming originally from work with animals, becomes somewhat problematic, however, when applied to complex social situations such as classrooms or playgrounds.

Unlike animals in experimental situations, humans engage in complex social behaviours and experience positive and negative results in ways that are not easily reducible to simple cause and effect. The sources of perceived outcomes are similarly many, and the ability of those in authority to control these is comparatively limited. For example, for many adolescents, peer approval is a significantly more powerful factor than any reinforcer (tangible or intangible) which may be at the teacher's disposal.

Behavioural techniques tend to be most effective in settings where the ability to control rewards and sanctions in a consistent and uniform fashion is at its greatest. For this reason, such approaches have become particularly popular in secure settings for children who present with highly complex and challenging behaviour. Institutional contexts of this kind typically provide high levels of control over the child's environment and, thus, can regulate and manage many primary forms of reinforcement. Although similar programmes can be found in day and residential special schools for children with behavioural difficulties, the control over reinforcement here is harder to maintain. Clearly, such a high degree of control over reinforcement is impossible (and, for many people undesirable) in mainstream schools.

These settings can usually offer only a very restricted range of rewards and sanctions, and, given the length of the school day, are able to exert a direct influence for only six hours on five days a week.

To illustrate, consider the case of Mary, aged 14, who is proving to be highly disruptive in her classes. You, as one of her teachers, wish to encourage her to become more responsive to you by relating such desired behaviour to positive outcomes. What rewards (reinforcements) are open to you? The list is likely to be limited and involve few items that will be perceived as particularly attractive by Mary. Now consider likely rewards that result directly from her disruptiveness. These may include peer approval, amusement at the teacher's discomfort, an escape from perceived boredom, an opportunity to take out her anger towards someone else (a parent, sibling, boyfriend?) on a 'safe' target, an opportunity to mask her insecurities about academic work, the opportunity to exert power/control over another. Where Mary is struggling with major unresolved issues (parental separation, an abusive family, social isolation, low self-esteem) the power of such reinforcers may often be greater than those which can be provided by teachers or parents.

Furthermore, you are in contact with Mary for only a fraction of her time in school. Although she appears to be presenting a number of challenges in other lessons, her behaviour does seem inconsistent and clearly differs from one teacher to another. To what extent could you rely upon your colleagues to support you by following the behavioural programme, even if you could persuade senior management to establish one? How could you be certain that whatever is set up will not be undermined by Mary's parents, relatives or friends?

The establishment of a behavioural programme for a highly challenging child in a school setting will usually involve close collaboration between teachers, senior management, parents and, in many cases, an external consultant such as an educational psychologist or behaviour support teacher. In drawing up a behavioural programme the following issues will need to be clearly specified:

- a clear definition of the behaviours which are giving cause for concern: information will be required concerning their nature, frequency, intensity, the settings in which they occur – in particular, the extent to which they are situation- or person-specific – which usually requires the establishment of a detailed system of measuring and recording to provide a pre-intervention baseline and demonstrate what gains, if any, are made subsequently;
- precipitating factors which appear to trigger the behaviour and the usual consequences for the child of the behaviour;
- the present and potential range of rewards and sanctions that can be applied at home and at school;
- factors which may undermine the operation of the programme and the means by which these may be overcome;
- complementary ways by which the behaviour difficulties can be addressed (e.g. use of counselling, peer support, amendments to timetabling/curriculum content and delivery);

- the clear commitment to the programme of all those involved in its operation;
- roles and responsibilities for all those involved in operating and monitoring the programme.

Many attempts to operate individual behavioural programmes founder because there is insufficient attention to detail, progress is not monitored closely and those involved do not adhere closely to agreed action in response to the child's behaviour. Where such failings are not in evidence, behavioural programmes can be very successful. One example, that of Carl, is illustrated below.

Carl, aged 9, attended Hilltown primary school. Located in a highly socially disadvantaged urban area, the school was very experienced in dealing with disaffected, volatile and aggressive children, and its teachers were generally highly competent and confident in tackling misbehaviour. Carl, however, was proving too taxing and was at severe risk of being permanently excluded.

Carl could be a pleasant and amiable boy, yet he was prone to become defiant and aggressive to adults in authority. When asked to engage in class-room tasks he would often refuse outright and seek to amuse himself by taunting other children or playing with equipment/toys. When confronted by his teacher, he would rapidly become verbally aggressive and begin to shout that no one was going to tell him what to do. If his teacher persisted in demanding that he should acquiesce, Carl would hurl materials around the room prior to running out of school. Although Carl had experienced some difficulties during his infant education, the intensity and frequency of his recent classroom outbursts were not in keeping with his earlier behaviour.

Within the peer group, Carl was perceived as a leader who, through his physical prowess and personal qualities, could control the behaviour of the other members of class. He was skilled in his interactions with peers and appeared to enjoy his influential position. When he wished, he appeared able to relate well to adults. Carl's academic ability was not perceived as prob-lematic, although his behaviour was resulting in underachievement.

Carl was the oldest of three children living at home with their divorced mother. Although Carl's mother was highly concerned about her son's behav-iour in school, her attempts to reason with him had proven to be ineffective and she was at a loss to know how to proceed. On occasions, she had stopped him playing out with his friends in the evening or had stopped his pocket money but this 'had not taught him a lesson' and his behaviour had continued unabated.

In his interviews with all concerned, the educational psychologist built up a picture of a boy who had a clear grasp of the nature of his behaviour and its effect upon others. Unlike some children with emotional and behavioural difficulties, Carl appeared not to be overwhelmed by inner tensions, not to have confused attributions as to the intentions of others, did not demonstrate an inability to tolerate perceived provocation or experience an incapacity to maintain acceptable control of his emotions. Rather, it seemed that he enjoyed the exercise of power and found his behaviour in class to be rewarding both in offering him prestige and status and in providing him with opportunities to avoid undesirable tasks. As Carl's influence with peers grew, and as he passed through to the junior section of the school, he appeared to have gained in confidence to a level that he was now more prepared to challenge school in an outright, defiant fashion. A series of short-term exclusions had made no impact upon his behaviour and it appeared that an inevitable outcome of continued misbehaviour would be permanent exclusion. In such circumstances it appeared essential that Carl should come to recognise the authority of his parents and teachers and be encouraged to participate fully in his education.

In discussions with Carl's mother and teachers, it was agreed that a behavioural programme would be established. This would make highly explicit to Carl exactly what was desired behaviour in school and how this would be related to the exercise of privileges at home. Carl's mother proved highly willing to ensure that agreed outcomes were effected and demonstrated her conviction that she was able to ensure that Carl could not subvert these. (Note: this is an essential element in the operation of such programmes and a lack of parental resolve in carrying out agreed action is often a reason for failure.)

It was decided that the key behaviour to tackle was Carl's propensity to temper tantrums in class and his tendency to storm out of the room. It was explained to him that he would receive a coloured sticker each day if he were able to avoid such responses. If he received a sticker he would be awarded points based upon his behaviour; these would be directly related to pocket money. Stickers and points were entered each day on a chart held by his teachers which would be taken home to be scrutinised by his mother each evening.

In the operation of such programmes, it is important that the child is made aware that privileges such as pocket money, sweets and treats are not always an automatic right. Rewards for desired behaviour, therefore, would normally tend to total little more than those which are already being made available; the key issue is that they are now contingent upon the child's actions. Such a stance helps to reduce the possibility that the child is seen as being rewarded for poor behaviour, or that rewards are perceived as bribes.

Carl's mother wished to add a sanction for severe misbehaviour (i.e. when the sticker was not awarded) and after discussion it was decided that in such cases he would be put into his pyjamas and kept in the house after tea. As Carl enjoyed playing out most evenings, it was clear that he would find this undesirable.

Extensive discussion took place between the educational psychologist, Carl, his mother and teachers in order to ensure that the procedures were fully understood. These were also set out in a letter (see Figure 8.1). Figure 8.2 provides an example of the daily record form.

In these cases a common pattern involves the child obtaining scores which are initially high (a honeymoon period), often followed by a sudden deterioration in behaviour. At such a time, it is easy for the adults concerned to become disheartened and to give up. It is important, therefore, to ensure that everyone concerned adheres closely to the agreed procedures and the child recognises that, unlike many other past attempts to tackle his or her behaviour, the present intervention will be maintained in a consistent and sustained fashion. Such a procedure took place with Carl.

Dear Mrs X,

Following our discussion at Hilltown School on 26 March, I thought it would be helpful to make a note of what we agreed about Carl's home–school programme.

1   Carl will be responsible for bringing the form home each evening and returning it to school the following day.
2   The sticker will be necessary each day for Carl to receive any treats that same evening. Should he fail to receive the sticker, he will be sent to his room after tea.
3   When he is successful in obtaining the sticker, Carl may be rewarded with the agreed treats. To receive these, however, he must also obtain a total of nine points for that day.
4   When Carl receives at least nine points he will:
    •   be allowed to watch television
    •   be permitted to play outside with his friends (if such circumstances as the weather etc. are favourable)
    •   receive £1.00 pocket money
    •   receive 50 pence for his savings account.
5   We agreed that we should stress to Carl that this sum reflects the amount he currently receives and by no means should it be perceived as an *additional* incentive or a bribe to be well behaved. I understand that if Carl succeeds in saving enough money, you are prepared to take him on a shopping trip in order that he might buy some football boots.
6   Any further allowances and treats which you provide will depend upon Carl scoring highly on his weekly total. Attempts will be made, wherever possible, however, to limit the availability of money, sweets, treats and the like from other sources (e.g. relatives, friends), as these will reduce the effectiveness of the programme.
7   Carl will not attempt to influence his teachers by entering into negotiation with them. If this does transpire, his teachers have been asked to place a zero on the record form.
8   Carl's teacher, Mrs Wright, will total the points scored each day and return it to him. You have kindly indicated your willingness to sign the form each evening so that she will be aware that you have seen it.
9   If Carl fails to bring the form home, it should be assumed that he has not behaved appropriately that day and, therefore, the agreed rewards will not follow.
10 I have explained the system to Carl and he appears to understand how it will work.
11 Finally, may I stress again the importance of focusing upon good behaviour and using praise as an important added reward.

I hope that you will feel that this letter represents an accurate account of our agreement. Please contact me as soon as possible if you feel that any changes are needed. If not, we shall aim to start the programme from the beginning of the new term.
    We are grateful for your support and obvious commitment to helping Carl make the most of his education.

Figure 8.1 Letter from the educational psychologist to Carl's mother

Unlike many children, Carl very quickly reneged on his agreement to maintain a more desirable pattern of behaviour in class. Although day one had witnessed major improvement in his usual behaviour, on the second day he returned to his former behaviour of shouting out, picking arguments with others and refusing to undertake any work. As his teacher attempted to address the situation, Carl threw his books across the room and ran out swearing. Carl did not receive his sticker.

Consequently, that evening the educational psychologist visited Carl's home. Carl was asked to discuss the events of the day and consider the

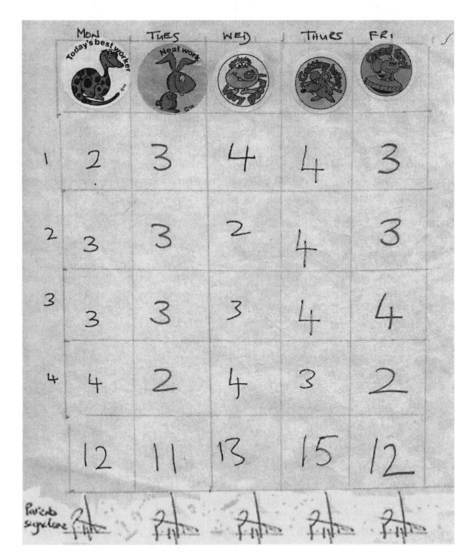

Figure 8.2 A completed record form employed for Carl

outcomes of his behaviour. He seemed surprised that his mother had stuck to the agreement as in the past she had often been inconsistent in seeing through her threats. As the educational psychologist spoke with Carl and his mother and arranged a home visit later that week from an educational social worker, it would have become clear to Carl that this intervention was not going to go away. Carl's behaviour was subsequently transformed and, during the time that the programme operated (ten weeks), there was no recurrence of such extreme behaviour.

Often behaviour scores are placed on a graph. This helps the practitioner to track changes in behaviour over time. Visual representation of progress can also be highly motivating for all those involved as the child's progress can be made visible and thus provides frequent opportunities for praise and congratulations. In Carl's case, the graph proved highly reinforcing.

It should be recognised that such programmes generally set out to reduce extreme behaviours, to make what are perceived to be intolerable situations manageable. In many cases one would expect children's behaviour to regress after completion of the programme. In successful interventions, however, they do not regress to the former level of severity, intensity or frequency. Although, after the programme was terminated, Carl continued to have problems in school from time to time, he was no longer perceived to be particularly difficult, nor did his behaviour warrant further referral to external support agencies.

Factors which reduce the likelihood of effective intervention

It is important to recognise that the successful outcome of the above intervention is not a feature of all behavioural programmes. In the experience of the writers the following factors, if present, greatly reduce the likelihood of a successful home–school behavioural programme:

- The child's behaviour is the result of major emotional confusion and/or a manifestation of severe psychological trauma.
- The child does not have a clear understanding of exactly which behaviours are being addressed and how these will relate to subsequent outcomes.
- The child does not consider that he/she is working with all parties to effect a change in behaviour which is perceived to be helpful for him/her. A strong desire to subvert the programme is clear from the outset.
- Parents are unable or unwilling to suggest rewards which can be made available for desirable behaviour.
- Parents are ambivalent about following through the agreed procedures because they lack the authority or mechanisms of control or because they are concerned that the child will think 'that I don't love him/her any more'.
- Parents do not consider that the behaviour is sufficiently problematic to warrant such concerted intervention.

- Parents are preoccupied with other concerns to an extent that they have insufficient energy/motivation to address the needs of their child.
- Teachers do not have a clear understanding about exactly which behaviours are being addressed. Other issues (e.g. homework completion, where this is not part of the programme) are allowed to affect scores.
- Teachers do not ensure that the monitoring of the scheme is tightly managed. The child's performance is not checked and, where appropriate, praised each day. In secondary schools one member of staff does not assume responsibility for keeping an overview of the programme and addressing weaknesses.
- Teachers fail to appreciate that the programme must be underpinned by skilled and sensitive classroom management.
- External agencies, where these have established the programme, do not maintain an active involvement. As a result, child, parents and teachers may consider that interest in the programme has decreased.
- Regular case discussions are not held and attended by all parties concerned with the operation of the programme.

Intervention at the level of teacher–pupil interaction

It is a truism that, however difficult the child in class, his or her behaviour is determined, to a significant extent, by the effectiveness of the teacher (Cooper 2011). While few would dispute that at the heart of good teaching is the ability to develop and sustain relationships underpinned by caring and respect (Cothran *et al.* 2003), such statements offer little practical guidance to those teachers who may find themselves in potentially challenging situations. Beyond the Rogerian qualities of empathy, warmth, genuineness and unconditional positive regard, essential to many relationships, lies a range of interpersonal behaviours and skills that are common to highly skilled teachers.

Key to achieving the correct sort of relationship between teacher and students is the thorny issue of authority.

> Teachers . . . must assert their dominance over students. But their dominance is never ensured, because conflict and resistance are always lying in wait, ready to spring. Authority relations between teachers and students are thus unstable and exist in a 'quivering' balance that may be upset at any moment.
>
> (Pace and Hemmings 2007: 4)

Pace and Hemmings (2007) note that there are several sources of teacher authority. That which was traditionally given to the teacher by society, 'formal authority', in which children accepted the teacher's authority purely because of their role, is no longer highly evident in many schools, particularly those in Western societies where individual freedoms and personal autonomy are highly valued (Pace 2003; Elliott and Tudge 2007). Another form of authority, 'bureaucratic', involves emphasising regulations and responsibilities in written format. In education, this typically takes the form of school rules, student behaviour reports, and home–school contracts.

While such documents may be helpful for managing cases of severe challenge, the most important form of authority is that which results from the exercise of the teacher's own professional expertise. The expert teacher, operating at the highest level, both in terms of pedagogy and interpersonal dynamics, is one who is less likely to encounter challenges to their authority (Elliott 2009). However, less skilled professionals, conditioned by the mantra, 'Don't smile until Christmas', can easily confuse the demonstration of teacher authority with a lack of warmth, sternness or even a degree of hostility (Balli 2011). The reality is that the more authority the teacher exhibits the more harmonious will typically be the classroom environment.

The seminal work of Kounin (1970) in the United States suggested that those teachers who were considered to be superior in their management of classroom situations differed from their less effective colleagues not in their response to major acts of indiscipline but, rather, in their ability to prevent difficulties from occurring in the first instance. Kounin's work pointed to the importance of teacher vigilance (or 'withitness'), the need to manage effectively the many events taking place in the classroom ('overlapping'), and the skills involved in keeping children alert and free from distraction.

There are several reasons why teachers fail to be as vigilant as is desirable. In a few cases, some are simply unaware of its importance. More often, in circumstances where much effort and concentration is being put into the delivery of complex ideas, or great care is being taken to ensure that the message conveyed is appropriate, teachers, like public speakers more generally, may avoid engaging directly with their audience in order that 'cognitive load' can be reduced (Feldon 2007). The demands involved when scanning the classroom environment, thinking about what they are seeing and hearing and considering how they should best respond, while also concentrating upon the content and nature of their delivery, can be highly problematic, particularly for less experienced teachers or those under stress. Such multi-tasking activity also makes significant demands upon teachers' energy levels and can be particularly difficult to maintain when illness or weariness intrude. More worryingly, some teachers reduce their levels of vigilance in circumstances where they have lost confidence in their capacity to prevent or deal with classroom misbehaviour. As a result, a form of 'selective myopia' can result whereby the teacher seemingly stops noticing what is happening and has a reduced classroom presence. This can create a vacuum, leading to increased dominant or disruptive behaviour on the part of influential members of the student group.

Skilled teachers tend to be able to deal with multiple events in a smooth and authoritative fashion, a skill that was termed 'overlapping' by Kounin. Not only can expert teachers ensure that the classroom runs smoothly, rather like a conductor in an orchestra, they also do not allow intrusive events, such as a wasp flying around the classroom, a child falling off a chair, or the unexpected failure of electronic equipment, to undermine the overarching sense of order. In dealing with overlapping events, such teachers are essentially proactive rather than reactive, and endeavour to convey an impression of quiet confidence whatever the adversity.

In Britain, the work of Robertson (1990) built upon American studies. This work emphasised the nature of teacher authority and how this was signalled through a range of highly subtle verbal and non-verbal cues. From the first meeting of teacher and child, such communication serves to increase or decrease the likelihood of a challenge to the teacher's authority. Many teachers, particularly the less experienced, are unaware of the subtle ways by which children may test them out and only become aware of the potential threat to their authority at a later time. Key non-verbal and verbal behaviours, which add to or diminish the teacher's air of authority, include:

- eye contact (scanning groups of children);
- one-to-one eye contact;
- rate of speech;
- volume and pitch of speech;
- rhythm, fluency and intonation in delivery;
- pitch of voice;
- body posture and kinaesthetics;
- use of territory/space.

Eye contact

Eye contact is an important element in maintaining alertness, holding the listener's concentration and signalling vigilance. Some speakers have a tendency to focus on objects immediately in front of them or to stare blankly out into space. Others address one part of the audience (usually those in the central region) and appear to ignore the others. It is widely accepted that in addressing any group it is important to suggest to each individual that it is he or she to whom the message is being communicated. For teachers, the ability to sweep the classroom visually and give the impression to each child that it is to him or her that the message is being addressed signals a capacity for vigilance, alertness and a grasp of a professional skill that will be perceived even by very young children.

The individual who controls eye contact in an interaction is generally perceived to be the dominant partner. In their dealings with teachers and other authority figures, the nature of children's eye contact in any given situation will signal important messages. Eyes downcast are usually understood to represent submission or deference to authority; a gaze away, often in a slightly upward direction, suggests that while the child accepts the requirement to remain in the teacher's presence, he or she wishes to signal an unwillingness to listen to, or heed, what is being said; a fixed and intense stare, often allied to a rigid posture and a reduction of physical distance, may signal an overt and direct challenge to the teacher's authority and be associated with a degree of physical threat.

It is important to note that these behaviours are conditioned significantly by age, gender and cultural factors. Although enraged infants may stare in a hostile, albeit brief, fashion at the objects of their anger, young children seeking challenge are more likely to employ indirect methods such as averting their eyes and refusing to take notice of the adult. Adolescent girls who wish to signal defiance may similarly avert their gaze while feigning an air of indifference or boredom. The more confrontational 'locked-gaze' behaviours, in a school context, are usually the product of male teacher–male adolescent interactions. Such a situation can be particularly problematic and may quickly escalate into physical confrontation. It is important to note, however, that for children from some non-Western cultures, avoiding eye contact when being chastised is a sign of respect. A failure to recognise cultural differences may increase the likelihood of communication breakdown and possible conflict. The skilled teacher reads such signals and draws upon a range of other contextual and interpersonal cues to determine how best to respond, whether to attempt to establish authority in an overt fashion, for example, by saying, 'Look at me when I'm talking to you!', or by using other methods of signalling authority, such as skilfully controlling the dialogue, similarly withholding eye gaze, or appearing not to notice the challenge.

Voice

The voice is another key element in preventing and managing behaviour difficulties. Many individuals project the impression of a lack of confidence in themselves as authority figures by speaking too rapidly or breathlessly, allowing the pitch of their voice to rise when anxious, speaking in a flat, monotone way with little rhythm or cadence and by stammering or struggling to find appropriate words to explain themselves. A common failing resides in the false belief that raising one's voice (by shouting, rather than voice projection) necessarily suggests authority. Although cultural differences vary in the extent to which shouting at children is deemed acceptable (e.g. American teachers are often horrified by the raised voices they hear in British classrooms), the occasionally effective use of this measure by skilled teachers may serve as an unhelpful model for those who are struggling to demonstrate their authority. What many fail to recognise is that a lowered voice carries a greater suggestion of intent, self-control and authority.

Body language

The third key area concerns the awareness and use of body language (Neill 1991). Anxious teachers tend to adopt rigid, tense postures. They may cross their arms or legs across their body defensively and may feel challenged by a young person's overly relaxed, non-responsive posture (e.g. leaning back in a chair with arms behind head). Relaxed postures reflect status differentials and are a means by which teacher authority may be tested. Similarly, teachers who lack confidence may not circle the classroom environment in a sufficiently casual or extensive manner to suggest that the classroom is their 'territory'. Standing rigidly at the front of the classroom for prolonged periods, staring at the class as a unit in an unfocused manner and adopting defensive mannerisms such as crossing one's arms or rubbing one's face are all behaviours which dramatically increase the likelihood of indiscipline. Gestures as aids to communication appear to be particularly valuable for children and can serve as an important means of facilitating learning (Hostetter 2011).

Control over communication

At the verbal level it is essential to recognise that authority is usually vested in the individual who is in control of the content and flow of the dialogue. Children may test out adults in authority by posing questions (the answers to which they may have little interest in), making requests, ignoring statements or questions, pausing before replying, and generally seeking control over the communication. Less experienced members of staff may be overly responsive to the child – answering all questions, seeking to maintain a relationship by acquiescing to the child's wishes to as great an extent as possible and proceeding to speak without first gaining the child's full attention. To persevere in such behaviours is to signal to the child that one lacks experience and/or sufficient strength to manage the complexities of classroom life.

Brian, a newly qualified teacher with a class of 8-year-olds, was experiencing considerable difficulties in managing classroom behaviour, despite the fact that he was popular with the class and no one child was displaying severely challenging behaviour. The difficulties he was encountering were largely the result of his own behaviour, as the following event exemplifies.

It was the beginning of the afternoon session and Brian was finishing off his introduction to the class who, seated on the carpet, were breaking off into groups to begin their allotted tasks. The final group, who were going to work in the craft area, were eager to get started, spurred by the knowledge that the area contained a small amount of furry material which was greatly prized by all the children.

Brian's first mistake was to omit to impart some important information about the groups' tasks during the briefing. As the children hurried to the craft table he realised his mistake. His second error was to call further instructions across the room while the children rooted through the materials. As he tried to gain the children's attention (most of whom had their backs to him), he spoke louder with his voice carrying a rather higher pitch. Finally, he was distracted by another child's desire for attention and he left the group to work unassisted for several minutes. Brian's behaviour signalled to the whole class that he did not have control over communication and was unsure as to how this could be gained.

Brian immediately and independently recognised the mistake he had made with respect to the imparting of directions and, as such, was unlikely to repeat this error. He had not, however, appreciated that the tone and pitch of his speech was helping to undermine his authority and was surprised when this was pointed out to him by an observer. Fortunately, he was willing to accept help and agreed to the use of audio recordings of him speaking in the classroom. By modelling voice projection and intonation and analysing the tapes, Brian's adviser helped him to become more skilled in the use of his voice, particularly when he found himself in stressful situations.

Advising and supporting teachers with classroom management problems is problematic for many reasons: often a conceptual framework for understanding behaviour is lacking, opportunities for colleagues to work with the teacher are limited, and resistance to being observed or accepting proffered advice is strong. Skilled professional behaviour often operates at a tacit level and many highly able teachers find it difficult to articulate what it is exactly that they do to maintain classroom discipline (Sternberg and Horvath 1995; Elliott et al. 2011). The common response of many experienced teachers when asked about their practice, 'It's just experience, actually!', is of little help to the novice teacher beset by difficulties. A further problem that results from this is that when teachers seek help from more senior colleagues, the focus of the discussion may all too readily turn to those aspects of practice that are more easily described: pedagogic aspects of teaching and learning such as lesson planning, delivery, pace and task, rather than the more subtle and complex interpersonal aspects of classroom relations.

Although general advice about good practice can be helpful, it is often only detailed observation of practice that can highlight professional shortcomings; unfortunately, constraints upon staffing rarely render such support possible.

An ability to control one's classroom is a key skill which lies at the heart of the teacher's professional identity. Thus for many teachers, in particular those who are relatively experienced, the suggestion that misbehaviour in their classroom stems in part from less than ideal management is highly threatening and a source of shame. In such cases, there may be strong pressure to attribute responsibility to the children rather than to oneself. For this reason, struggling teachers may be loath to be observed, and any advice concerning classroom management may be perceived as a threat to their professional dignity and thus met by defensiveness, resistance and an inability to accept personal responsibility. Despite these difficulties, helping the struggling teacher to develop interpersonal and management skills is generally the single most important means of reducing the prevalence and intensity of disruptive incidents (Elliott 2010).

A number of training manuals or packages have been produced to aid teachers in developing skills for preventing challenging behaviour (e.g. Chisholm et al. 1986; Rogers 2011). While the delineation of such skills can offer the new or trainee teacher a valuable conceptual framework to consider his or her developing knowledge, as has been noted above, for the more experienced teacher, the ability to manage behaviour is a core professional skill which it is often considered shameful to lack. For this reason, some teachers may approach professional development sessions in a defensive manner and feel constrained in their ability to discuss their particular difficulties, strengths and weaknesses. If such a dialogue does not take place, professional development in this area becomes little more than a series of mechanistic prescriptions that are unlikely to become accommodated within the teacher's existing behavioural repertoire.

As a belief grows that all children should be included in mainstream schools, irrespective of the difficulties they encounter, teachers are increasingly finding themselves charged with the education of children with complex emotional and behavioural difficulties. While accepting the general principle of inclusive education, many teachers continue to struggle with the most challenging students (Goodman and Burton 2010). In such circumstances, it is all the more important that the nature and role of teachers' management skills are emphasised and appropriate training is provided. Even the most skilled teachers may find their performance deteriorating when they are under stress, and, in the case of the highly challenging child, they are less likely to utilise positive strategies when they lack confidence in their ability to effect behavioural improvement (Poulou and Norwich 2002).

The shift towards inclusion has also resulted in the greater presence of teaching assistants (TAs) and learning support assistants (LSAs) working alongside the teacher in mainstream settings. While we know a great deal about teacher skills in relation to children's learning and behaviour, our knowledge of the practice, skills and effectiveness of TA/LSAs, and how teachers and TA/LSAs can work most effectively in combination, is still rudimentary. Recently, a large-scale study in the UK has led to suggestions that TAs can have a negative influence upon student learning (Webster *et al.* 2011). In relation to behaviour management, an analysis from the same research group (Rubie-Davies *et al.* 2010) has suggested that teachers observed in classrooms were more proactive and tended to take more responsibility for the behaviour of the whole class group than TAs who were more reactive, and usually dealt solely with the behaviour of individual or small groups of students. Whereas teachers would sometimes reprimand students who were the responsibility of the TA, the reverse scenario was exceedingly rare. Such findings have resulted in greater awareness that increasing the number of adults in classrooms will not automatically result in improved behaviour and learning.

Intervention at the whole-school level

Research in the 1960s and 1970s appeared to suggest that schools, as individual units, made little impact upon student behaviour or attainment. Large-scale surveys in the United States (Coleman *et al.* 1966; Jencks *et al.* 1972) and in Britain (Plowden Report 1967) placed far more emphasis upon family influences. Subsequently, however, the seminal work of Power *et al.* (1967) led to a succession of studies (e.g. Reynolds *et al.* 1976; Rutter *et al.* 1979; Mortimore *et al.* 1988) which provided strong support for the suggestion that schools as social institutions had a significant and differing effect upon the behaviour and attainment of children.

These findings, together with a general emphasis upon whole-school planning and development, have resulted in most schools attempting to develop whole-school behaviour policies. Such policies emphasise the importance of shared visions, values and understandings, consistency of expectations, response and management, the structured use of rewards and, to a lesser extent, sanctions for children's behaviour. Increasingly, the notion of high quality school leadership has been highlighted as key to the creation and maintenance of schools with effective behaviour policies and practices (Reid 2008).

Other whole-school initiatives draw upon rather more narrow behavioural principles in the belief that these will result in a climate in which teachers act consistently to reinforce desirable behaviour and eliminate disruptive and unco-operative behaviour. An early programme of this kind for primary schools, BATPACK (Wheldall and Merrett 1985) was commended by the Elton Report, although this has been overtaken in popularity by a highly structured, yet relatively straightforward American programme, Assertive Discipline (Canter and Canter 1992). Although perceived by some as failing to respect children's and parents' rights (Robinson and Maines 1994), the approach is popular with many teachers who welcome a structured programme in which classroom rules are made clear and relate in contingent fashion to specified rewards and sanctions.

The Assertive Discipline programme is the result of Lee Canter's perception that many teachers with classroom management difficulties are either lacking in asser-tiveness or are hostile in their dealings with children. It emphasises the importance of making classroom rules and procedures clear and explicit and communicating a strong resolve to back up their instructions with actions where necessary. Where children do not observe the rules, the programme offers a series of punishments, the severity of which usually depends upon the number of times the rules are broken. Sanctions usually range from a warning from the classteacher at the first instance to referral to the headteacher for multiple occurrences.

Despite its widespread popularity (Marzano 2009) there has been little struc-tured evaluation of the impact of Assertive Discipline upon schools. In addition, there has been a degree of controversy centring upon the ethics of the techniques advocated (Maines and Robinson 1995; Robinson and Maines 1994; Swinson and Melling 1995). In some cases, such concerns have led schools to adopt many of the techniques involved but avoid the use of the term 'assertive' in describing them. A further difficulty is that while teacher management skills are emphasised in the training manuals, these may be subsequently overlooked in the desire to implement punitive structures for those who misbehave. Thus the programme may become little more than a highly structured system of providing in-class sanctions and referrals to senior management. Rather than using interpersonal skills to prevent or deflect problem situations, the teacher may feel tempted to highlight the 'problem' and seek to invoke punitive consequences in order to demonstrate his or her authority. Thus any attempt to introduce whole-school behaviour programmes should ensure that the day-to-day, preventive skills of the classroom teacher, rather than the school's formal disciplinary procedures, are emphasised.

While the adoption of a whole-school approach is invaluable for increasing the positive climate of school, and should, over time, inevitably reduce the frequency and intensity of disruption, it is unlikely that establishing and operating a whole-school policy on behaviour is sufficient as a solution to problems currently posed by a particularly difficult child. In such circumstances, an examination of inter-personal dealings at school and in the home, exploration of the potential of behav-ioural approaches, and a detailed analysis of the suitability of the educational tasks that are being presented are likely to be more promising in the short term.

Summary: what sort of intervention strategy is appropriate?

In 2006 an influential working group reported to the UK Government on practices that can lead to positive behaviour and discipline (Steer Report 2006). This identified ten aspects of school practice that 'when effective, contribute to the quality of pupil behaviour' (p. 3). These were as follows:

1   A consistent approach to behaviour management, teaching and learning. All members of staff should follow an agreed set of practices in cases where discipline is problematic. High visibility of senior staff around the school was held to be an important means of helping to achieve this end;
2   Effective school leadership that acts to support colleagues, serves as a role model and demonstrates high expectations of behaviour;
3   Good classroom management, learning and teaching. Here, the authors addressed curriculum content, lesson planning and delivery, feedback to students on progress, and the deployment of appropriate classroom routines (see also Bohn *et al.* 2004). A number of commonly agreed management and behaviour strategies were identified such as 'all pupils being greeted at the door, brought into the classroom, stood behind their chairs, formally welcomed, asked to sit and the teacher explaining the purpose of the lesson' (p. 16);
4   The use of systems to reward good work and behaviour, with sanctions available where appropriate;
5   Utilisation of opportunities to teach students how to manage strong emotions, resolve conflict, work cooperatively and to be respectful and considerate to others;
6   Sound provision of staff development and support;
7   Student pastoral support systems with access to specialist support agencies;
8   Positive and regular liaison with parents and other agencies;
9   Smooth transition between different phases of schooling;
10 An organised and attractive school environment that is conducive to personal and social well-being and which minimises opportunities for disruption or anti-social behaviour.

It is interesting to note that these elements variously concern each of the three levels of analysis identified in this chapter. In the main, however, they address whole-school factors drawn from the school effectiveness literature and, in addition, the role of support services. While there are some references to teacher dynamics, these are somewhat superficial and offer little real insight into what characterises skilled interpersonal teacher behaviour (Elliott 2010). Perhaps the primary reason for this is because of the challenges involved in specifying and articulating such complex knowledge.

Ultimately, it is important to retain sensitivity to all three levels by considering the impact of individual child factors, the interactional pattern and skills of teachers' classroom management, and the influence of the school as a social

IN SELECTING AN APPROPRIATE COURSE OF ACTION,
SCHOOLS SHOULD EMPHASISE . . .

Behavioural approach	↔	Skills of classroom management	↔	Whole-school approach

WHERE THERE IS . . .

An isolated but severe problem		General, low-level disruption (mainly classroom based)		General sense of absence of disciplined atmosphere

Figure 8.3 Intervention strategies

institution. The intervention strategy that is adopted will depend upon individual circumstances, particularly the extent to which the problem situation is specific or general (see Figure 8.3). It is important to note that Figure 8.3 refers to an underlying *emphasis* rather than to the employment of discrete strategies. A coherent and structured whole-school approach should reduce the likelihood and frequency of severe behavioural difficulties. Where these do exist, however, improving teachers' classroom management skills and ensuring a high quality of curriculum delivery are more likely to produce a solution in the short term. Where a school is experiencing difficulty with a particular child, especially where this is not specific to one teacher, a behavioural intervention may be the most productive solution. Ideally, however, intervention should operate at all three levels and, indeed, classroom management and behavioural approaches are often considered as part of a broader whole-school approach.

References

Alexander, R. (2000). *Culture and Pedagogy: International Comparisons in Primary Education.* Oxford: Blackwell.

Balli, S.J. (2011). Pre-service teachers' episodic memories of classroom management. *Teaching and Teacher Education* 27: 245–51.

Bohn, C.M., Roehrig, A.D. and Pressley, M. (2004). The first days of school in the classrooms of two more effective and four less effective primary-grades teachers. *The Elementary School Journal* 104: 269–87.

Canter, L. and Canter, M. (1992). *Assertive Discipline.* Santa Monica, CA: Lee Canter Associates.

Chisholm, B., Kearney, D., Knight, G. *et al.* (1986). *Preventive Approaches to Disruption.* London: Macmillan.

Coleman, J.S., Campbell, E., Hobson, C. *et al.* (1966). *Equality of Educational Opportunity.* Washington, DC: US Government Printing Office.

Colley, H. (2003). Engagement mentoring for 'disaffected' youth: A new model of mentoring for social inclusion. *British Educational Research Journal* 29: 521–42.

Cooper, P. (2011). Teacher strategies for effective intervention with students presenting social, emotional and behavioural difficulties: An international review. *European Journal of Special Needs Education* 26(1): 71–86.

Cothran, D.J., Kulinna, P.H. and Garrahy, D.A. (2003). 'This is kind of giving a secret away . . .': Students' perspectives on effective class management. *Teaching and Teacher Education* 19: 435–44.

Cowie, H. and Pecherek, A. (1994). *Counselling: Approaches and Issues in Education.* London: David Fulton.

Elliott, J.G. (2009). Western influences upon post-Soviet Education. In M. Fleer, M. Hedegaard and J. Tudge (eds). *The World Yearbook of Education 2009: Childhood Studies and the Impact of Globalization: Policies and Practices at Global and Local Levels.* New York: Routledge.

Elliott, J.G. (2010). The nature of teacher authority and teacher expertise. *Support for Learning,* 24(4): 197–203.

Elliott, J.G, Stemler, S.E., Grigorenko, E.L. *et al.* (2011). The socially skilled teacher and the development of tacit knowledge. *British Educational Research Journal* 37(1): 83–103.

Elliott, J. and Tudge, J. (2007). The impact of the West on post-Soviet Russian education: Change and resistance to change, *Comparative Education* 43: 93–112.

Elton Report (1989). *Discipline in School.* London: HMSO.

Feldon, D.E. (2007). Cognitive load and classroom teaching: The double-edged sword of automaticity. *Educational Psychologist* 42(3): 123–37.

Furlong, J. (1985). *The Deviant Pupil: Sociological Perspectives.* Milton Keynes: Open University Press.

Goodman, R.L. and Burton, D.M. (2010). The inclusion of students with BESD in mainstream schools: Teachers' experiences of and recommendations for creating a successful inclusive environment. *Emotional and Behavioural Difficulties* 15(3): 223–37.

Hostetter, A.B. (2011). When do gestures communicate? A meta-analysis. *Psychological Bulletin* 137(2): 297–315.

Houts, R.M., Caspi, A., Pianta, R.C. *et al.* (2010). The challenging pupil in the classroom: The effect of the child on the teacher. *Psychological Science* 21(12): 1802–10.

Inglehart, R. and Welzel, C. (2005) *Modernization, Cultural Change and Democracy: The Human Development Sequence.* Cambridge: Cambridge University Press.

Jencks, C., Smith, M., Acland, H. *et al.* (1972). *Inequality: A Reassessment of the Effect of Family and Schooling in America.* New York: Basic Books.

Jones, K., Doveston, M. and Rose, R. (2009). The motivations of mentors: Promoting relationships, supporting pupils, engaging with communities. *Pastoral Care in Education* 27(1): 41–51.

Kounin, J.S. (1970). *Discipline and Group Management in Classrooms.* New York: Holt, Rinehart & Winston.

Langham, M. and Parker, V. (1989). *Counselling Skills for Teachers.* Lancaster: Framework Press.

Maines, B. and Robinson, G. (1995). Assertive discipline: No wheels on your wagon – a reply to Swinson and Melling. *Educational Psychology in Practice* 11(3): 9–11.

Marzano, R.J. (2009). *Classroom Management that Works.* Upper Saddle River, NJ: Pearson Education.

Miller, A., Ferguson, E. and Moore, E. (2002). Parents' and pupils' causal attributions for difficult classroom behaviour. *British Journal of Educational Psychology* 72: 27–40.

Mortimore, P., Sammons, P., Stoll, L. *et al.* (1988). *School Matters: The Junior Years.* Wells: Open Books.

Napper, R. and Keane, D. What's in a name? Mapping the territory of coaches, mentors and others who facilitate learning. *Organisations and People* 11(4): 34–41.

Neill, S. (1991). *Classroom Nonverbal Interaction*. London: Routledge.

Pace, J. (2003). Revisiting classroom authority: Theory and ideology meet practice. *Teachers College Record* 105: 1559–85.

Pace, J.L. and Hemming, A. (2007) Understanding authority in classrooms: A review of theory, ideology and research. *Review of Educational Research* 77: 4–27.

Pearson, G. (1983). *Hooligan: A History of Respectable Fears*. London: Macmillan.

Plowden Report (1967). *Children and their Primary Schools*. London: HMSO.

Poulou, M. and Norwich, B. (2002). Cognitive, emotional and behavioural responses to students with emotional and behavioural difficulties: A model of decision-making. *British Educational Research Journal* 28: 111–38.

Power, M.J., Alderson, M.R., Phillipson, C.M. *et al.* (1967). Delinquent schools. *New Society* 10: 542–3.

Reid, K. (2008). Behaviour and attendance: The national picture – a synopsis. *Educational Review* 60(4): 333–44.

Reynolds, D., Jones, D. and St Leger, S. (1976). Schools do make a difference. *New Society* 37: 321.

Robertson, J. (1990). *Effective Classroom Control*. London: Hodder & Stoughton.

Robinson, G. and Maines, B. (1994). Jumping on a dated wagon. *Educational Psychology in Practice* 9(4): 195–200.

Rogers, W. (2011). *Classroom Behaviour: A Practical Guide to Effective Teaching, Behaviour Management and Colleague Support, Third edition*. London: Sage.

Rose, R. and Jones, K. (2007). The efficacy of a volunteer mentoring scheme in supporting young people at risk. *Emotional and Behavioural Difficulties*, 12(1): 3–14.

Rubie-Davies, C.M., Blatchford, P., Webster, R. *et al.* (2010). Enhancing learning? A comparison of teacher and teaching assistant interactions with pupils, *School Effectiveness and School Improvement*, 21(4): 429–49.

Rutter, M., Maughan, B., Mortimore, P. *et al.* (1979). *Fifteen Thousand Hours*. London: Open Books.

Steer Report (2006). *Learning Behaviour: Principles and Practice – What Works in Schools*. London: Department for Education and Skills.

Sternberg, R.J. and Horvath, J. (1995) A prototype view of expert teaching. *Educational Researcher* 24(6): 9–17.

Swinson, J. and Melling, R. (1995). Assertive discipline: Four wheels on this wagon – a reply to Robinson and Maines. *Educational Psychology in Practice* 11(3): 3–8.

Swinson, J., Woof, C. and Melling, R. (2003). Including emotional and behavioural difficulties pupils in a mainstream comprehensive: A study of the behaviour of pupils and classes. *Educational Psychology in Practice* 19: 65–75.

Webster, R., Blatchford, P., Bassett, P. *et al.* (2010). The wider pedagogical role of teaching assistants. *School Leadership and Management* 31(1): 3–20.

Wheldall, K. and Merrett, F. (1985). *The Behavioural Approach to Teaching Package (BATPACK)*. Birmingham: Positive Products.

Chapter 9

Drug and solvent abuse

Introduction

The use of drugs to create a sense of well-being has been a feature of many cultures throughout the centuries. Within our own culture the use of alcohol and tobacco has been quite acceptable for many years, although health concerns around the use of tobacco are now greatly reducing its acceptability. For almost as long, the use of illicit drugs has been an accepted part of life for the literary elite, as Thomas De Quincy's *Confessions of an English Opium-Eater* testifies. However, in the past forty years the use of illicit drugs such as heroin, cocaine and cannabis has shown a dramatic increase and has become endemic in certain parts of Western culture. For instance, in the UK 30% of 15 year olds reported misusing drugs in 2009 (Health and Social Care Information Centre 2011), and in Canada 13% reported trying substances such as glue, hallucinogens and amphetamines (Hammond *et al.* 2011). There are real risks that misuse of drugs leads to criminal behaviour, with one survey showing that young people who had misused drugs in the past year were over twice as likely to have committed an offence compared with those who reported not having used drugs (Information Centre 2006). In addition, although drug misuse has traditionally been seen as a male behaviour, in recent years the rate of misuse amongst women has increased dramatically (Greenfield *et al.* 2010).

Reasons for drug usage

Adolescence is a time of transition when young people are seeking to establish their own identities. This is partly achieved by experimentation and by challenging adult concepts and expectations. There are, of course, many ways to do this, two of which are under-age drinking and experimenting with drugs. This phase of development is one where the young person feels a need to place great reliance upon friends, and if the friendship group views drug experimentation as an element of their pastimes, then this can exert a powerful influence upon steering a young person to drug usage.

A great deal of work has been carried out in an effort to try to predict who might become a significant drug user. Consistently, such work shows that although drug users often have personality problems, such as being considered immature, there is no specific personality type that predicts future drug addiction. More than three decades of research have however firmly established that genes and environmental factors contribute about equally to the risk of disorders such as alcoholism. However the environment component is quite diverse, with peer drug use, the availability of drugs and elements of family interaction, including parental discipline and family cohesion, being significant risk factors (Frischer *et al.* 2005). It is therefore important to look at all aspects of the young person's life and functioning in order to understand the origins of the problem, and the factors that are helping to maintain it.

Although there can be many reasons for someone to begin taking drugs, a key distinction which needs to be made is between drugs that are being used to cope with the stress of a severe psychiatric illness and their use to be part of a particular youth culture. The former type of user is usually a solitary individual, and often demonstrates many other problems and difficulties. Indeed, results from one review found that in users under the age of 15 years 90% had had at least one mental health problem in the past year, a rate five times higher than their non-abusing peers, with the commonest problems being conduct disorder (74.2%), ADHD (63.6%) and depression.

Mechanisms of addiction

As already mentioned, the origins of abuse are very individual but it has been recognised for some time that such problems can run in families, which has prompted considerable interest in whether addiction problems may actually be inherited. For instance, family, twin and adoption studies reveal a heritability of alcoholism of over 50%, with relatives of alcoholics having a four times greater risk of alcohol dependence (Gunzerath *et al.* 2011). A similar inheritance pattern exists with other forms of addiction, and it is relevant also to note that being adopted does not greatly reduce this risk, again emphasizing the genetic component (Prescott *et al.* 2006).

A considerable research focus has been on how the misuse of drugs is maintained, with the most popular being an assertion that it stimulates the reward system. There have also been great strides in our understanding of the neurobiology of dependence (Volkow and Li 2005), with the brain chemical dopamine being shown to play a significant role. Amphetamine and cocaine, for example, exert their effects by increasing dopamine in the synapse, and so creating a significant change in mood.

As discussed in Chapter 1, there has been an intense interest in the role of epigenetics in many aspects of illness and behaviour, and this is also true of drug misuse. Repeated exposure to numerous drugs of abuse alters gene expression profiles throughout the reward circuitry of the brain. For instance, repeated exposure to cocaine not only changes the way that brain cells function when it is taken, but chronic exposure alters the genetic expression, resulting in a stable and persistent change to the brain's chemistry. These epigenetic mechanisms are increasingly being seen as the explanation why drug misuse has such a long-lasting and potentially permanent hold on its victims (Maze and Nestler 2011).

When is drug use a problem?

For some drugs, such as alcohol and tobacco, usage is so common that it cannot be considered an abnormal activity. In addition, discovering that a teenager has been trying cigarettes or drinking alcohol should not provoke an overreaction. Isolated episodes should be treated as such. Recognising that usage is now becoming regular obviously increases adult concern, and encouraging the young person to seek counselling from local youth projects or drug treatment teams is helpful. The ways that parents, teachers and other concerned adults can help are described towards the end of this chapter.

The pattern of usage can be described as addiction when it is causing problems to the young person's health, or alters social or psychological functioning. At this stage advice from the nearest community addiction team can be invaluable, but it is very rare that real help can be given to drug users until they are willing to receive it. Sadly the commonest scenario is that the young person will only seek help as a last resort. In the early 1990s persistent addicts usually began significant drug taking around 19, but the trend is for usage to increasingly start at a younger age (Gilvarry 2000).

When a young person is addicted to drugs the addiction is not only maintained because of the sense of physical craving, but often by a sense of psychological dependence. In this the addict believes that he or she cannot cope without the drug, and anticipates significant problems if the drug is stopped. It is this anticipation which powerfully contributes to feeling the need to continue. Difficulties within the family, such as seeing marital violence or feeling that parents no longer care about you, can be very potent sources of distress which the young person can only relieve by becoming intoxicated (Braucht *et al.* 1973).

Susan was 9 when her father died in a car crash. In the year before his death there had been concern within the police and social services that he was sexually abusing Susan, but sufficient proof was not found. From the age of 12 Susan began missing school, and she was frequently in trouble with the police for stealing. No matter what the time of day, or night, she was usually to be found sitting in the local park with a group of older boys, in an intoxicated state. On several occasions she needed to be taken to the local hospital because she had taken a cocktail of pills and alcohol which had rendered her incoherent.

Susan's mother acknowledged that she was not able to control her daughter's behaviour, and four weeks after her 14th birthday she was received into the care of the local authority. Initially, she went to live with a local foster family, but she continued to stay out until very late at night, and was usually returned in an intoxicated state either by her friends or the police.

After three months Susan was moved to a children's home that offered closer supervision than the foster family could manage. The first few days were quiet, but Susan gradually became more moody, and would fly into violent rages when thwarted or challenged in any way. She began absconding from the home, and would often be missing for days at a time. When found, she was unkempt and would openly recount stories of criminal activity, drug usage and sexual activity which sometimes included prostitution.

Susan was referred to the local adolescent psychiatry service, and in the sessions there Susan would describe the vivid dreams she had when she tried to sleep. These were always scenes from her early abuse – her bedroom, a sense of being trapped, and feelings of pain and self-disgust. She described how during the day she would sometimes see a flash image of herself in which the front of her nightdress was covered in blood. Susan would avoid looking in a mirror because she said her body disgusted her and explained that the only way she could escape these feelings and images was to 'numb herself' with pills. Susan was, however, adamant that she did not want any psychiatric treatment because she was not a 'nutter'.

After four months in the children's home Susan was arrested for breaking into a chemist's shop. She was remanded to secure accommodation and within two days of arriving began to show the symptoms of withdrawal from sedatives. She successfully completed a withdrawal programme within the secure setting, and after several weeks she began to talk to staff on the unit about her recollections of her abuse.

Susan's story illustrates several of the problems that professionals face when confronted with someone who is routinely abusing drugs. The pattern of self-destruction in this case was being fuelled by recollections of early abuse which were too painful for Susan to deal with. Her method of 'escape' was to be almost permanently intoxicated. Although professional intervention could assist her to deal with these issues, she did not want to cooperate with it, leaving the adults around her feeling powerless to help. Similarly, her drug usage could not be dealt with without her cooperation, and it was only when her general behaviour became totally unruly that formal legal action could be taken. It is sadly true that for most cases of persistent drug usage the situation has to sink to a considerable depth before those concerned for the young person are permitted to offer real help.

An issue that is of growing significance is the impact of maternal drug misuse upon the foetus. Perhaps the best-known of these is the foetal alcohol syndrome which is characterized by three main features: prenatal or postnatal growth deficiency, a characteristic pattern of facial features, and changes to the brain and its functioning. The facial characteristics, namely short fissures at the corners of the eyes, a thin upper lip and a flattened groove above the lip, are only observed in individuals with severe exposure (Bertrand *et al.* 2005), but the cognitive difficulties can emerge with lower exposure. The feature of particular concern in this regard is the impact upon executive functioning – the part of the brain that deals with planning and judgement (Kodituwakku 2009).

In addition to the direct chemical effects, drug misuse reduces the parent's ability to offer the correct family environment, and so family life for these children is typically less stable, with poor consistency of care and a reduced level of emotional support.

Recognising that a child's difficulties may be exacerbated by parental substance misuse is becoming an increasingly important task in the child care field because parental drug use also increases the risk of the child abusing drugs when in their teens. For instance, of children who had parents that were opiate-dependent, almost half go on to misuse drugs themselves (Whitty and O'Connor 2007), although a strong family bond appears to reduce this risk. Some parents try to conceal their substance misuse from their children, but this is rarely successful, with most children becoming aware of their parents' substance misuse much earlier than their parents realize (Barnard and Barlow 2003).

Drugs of abuse

Alcohol

The vast majority of senior secondary schoolchildren admit to under-age drinking. Indeed, in a survey in Scotland and Wales it was found that over half of 15-year-olds had been drunk twice in the previous year (King et al. 1996). In Canada, approximately 21% of young people in grades 7–9 have reported drinking at least once a month in the past year (Hammond et al. 2011). In some this can be a pattern of quite heavy alcohol consumption, but the problems of dependence tend not to occur until adulthood. Excessive consumption can lead to deterioration in day-to-day functioning or in general health, and it is important to realise that young people who use many different drugs will also frequently use alcohol.

Effects

Research has suggested that small amounts of alcohol may be helpful to health by reducing the potential for heart disease (Doll et al. 1994). However, chronic abuse of alcohol is clearly not healthy. As with most drugs of abuse, one of the first signs of addiction is that of tolerance. This is where the young person finds that there is a need to drink increasing amounts in order to achieve the same effect of intoxication. Tolerance occurs because the body, and in particular the liver, becomes more adept at dealing with the alcohol and so minimises its effect more rapidly as time goes on. It is also worth noting that women appear to metabolise alcohol less well than men, and so smaller amounts, at least in the initial stages of chronic abuse, are capable of producing equivalent levels of intoxication (Frezza et al. 1990).

Features of withdrawal

The body's increased capacity to cope with alcohol gradually leads to a steady state in which the normal functioning of the body's systems requires a persistent level of alcohol. When this state has been achieved the young person is said to be showing physiological dependence. At this point, if there is a sudden withdrawal of the alcohol, the young person gradually becomes restless, agitated and tremulous. In severe cases the adolescent may become confused, disorientated and have vivid hallucinations. This severe withdrawal picture (known as delirium tremens) is uncommon in adolescents, but if it should occur, it needs immediate medical treatment.

Initial intervention and responses to acute intoxication

Most adolescents will have episodes when they become significantly intoxicated. The first priority in such situations is to ensure their safety. Because they are liable to vomit, they should not be allowed to lie on their backs, but kept on their sides. With intoxication comes confusion, so a warm soothing tone should be used to keep reassuring them where they are, and that they are safe. Dehydration always follows excess, and is the main cause of the hangover. The drinking of small quantities of water should be encouraged on a frequent basis, and vigilance maintained so that any vomiting does not obstruct the breathing.

If the adolescent is too young to drink, then action needs to be taken. Long lectures or too intense a display of disappointment should be avoided, for this may be counterproductive. It is also important to avoid letting anger colour the intervention. Rather, it should be assumed that such events will happen and the sanction for such behaviour planned in advance. The next day the planned sanction should then be imposed with the minimum of comment. It is the imposition of a sanction that has an impact, not its severity. The cool, brisk intervention is far more effective than long speeches and lengthy punishments. If the episodes begin to form a regular pattern, then a formal behavioural programme may help.

If the drinking is clearly to excess, and is beginning to cause ill-health or problems with maintaining a daily routine, then the situation has reached the abuse stage. The management of alcohol abuse demonstrates many of the approaches that are used to deal with any drug addiction. First, it is important to recognise that the young person must be willing to cooperate with any treatment regime if it is to stand any chance of success. Practitioners are very reluctant to detain people in hospital against their will, and this is reserved for someone who is acutely intoxicated and out of touch with reality. They would also need to be at risk of harm, or harming others, and will be kept in hospital only while this risk persists.

Detoxification

If the young person is willing to cooperate with treatment, the first stage of the process is to look for any physical illness that may be increasing the difficulties. Most regimes routinely give courses of vitamins because young people who have been drinking excessively for any period of time usually have had a very poor diet. The second stage is gradually to reduce the amount of alcohol within the young person's system. This detoxification can cause the adolescent to become very ill, and so it is usual to give regular medication, usually a benzodiazepine (chlordiazepoxide or diazepam), which helps to reduce these effects. Once the effects of stopping the alcohol have been overcome the medication can be gradually withdrawn and the detoxification programme is complete.

Psychological support

If stopping the drinking is to have any chance of success, it is important that at an early stage the issues which started the drinking, and are maintaining it, are explored and addressed. This can take a variety of forms, from brief, focused work which only looks at stopping drinking, to more detailed exploration of life history to understand the origins of the drinking. For most young people detoxification is not necessary, and it is the psychological management which is the central requirement.

In some young people there are clearly social and psychological problems behind the drinking, and dealing with them can be quite a lengthy process. Many programmes involve the use of groups which allow the members to feel they are not alone in trying to deal with their difficulties, and some organisations such as Alcoholics Anonymous offer a very intensive programme of self-analysis and mutual encouragement.

Over the years there have been various attempts to use behavioural techniques to control drinking habits. The most well-established of these is the use of drugs such as disulfram and acamprosate. With this type of drug in the bloodstream any alcohol creates strong feelings of nausea and physical discomfort, including throbbing headache and palpitations, and the intention is to create a sense of aversion to the thought of any further drinking. The decision to use such an approach is now seen as a last resort, especially in the young. In general, this type of intervention shows a degree of success, but the improvement tends to fade over time, with improvements in more general behaviour being the more likely to persist (Tripodi et al. 2010).

Sedatives

Effects

As the name implies, this group of drugs tends to reduce brain activity and clinically they are often used to reduce anxiety or induce sleep. They are also capable of reducing muscle activity and so are sometimes used to help with muscle strains and other such injuries. Although barbiturates were the initial drugs of abuse in this group, the benzodiazepines are now more commonly used.

Young people who abuse sedatives often use other types of drugs as well, especially alcohol. Episodes of violent behaviour are sometimes seen in regular abusers, but generally the picture is one of intoxication similar to alcohol.

Features of withdrawal

The drugs within this group cause physical dependence and so if a regular user is deprived of the drug there can be a withdrawal syndrome which is similar to the one seen with chronic alcoholism. In mild cases the addict becomes restless and anxious, and has great difficulty sleeping. In more severe cases the young person may go on to have seizures, become delirious, develop a high body temperature (hyperthermia) and a very rapid heartbeat (tachycardia). Such reactions can be life threatening and so when present immediate medical attention is necessary. While waiting for medical attention, the person should be kept calm, and someone who understands first aid and resuscitation must remain with them.

Withdrawal from barbiturates usually resolves in about eight to ten days but the longer-acting benzodiazepines cause problems for much longer. Some people still show the effects of withdrawal many months after stopping the drug.

Detoxification

When it is suspected that someone has a sedative addiction it is important to form a clear picture of how much of the drug they have been taking. A regular heavy user will need assistance to detoxify. The first stage in such a process is to transfer from the sedative to a benzodiazepine such as diazepam. This is given to minimise the withdrawal effects of the abused drugs. After stabilisation the dose of diazepam can gradually be reduced. Sometimes antidepressants which have sedative qualities may be used, especially if the patient has clear disturbances of mood.

Psychological support

Even after a successful detoxification programme young people often continue to experience difficulties with sleep, anxiety, depression, headaches and muscle aches, a pattern known as the abstinence syndrome. The chronic presence of such symptoms is a very common reason for the young person to revert to being a drug user, and so the psychological support described above is an important element in any attempt to stop sedative addiction.

Stimulants

Effects

As the name implies, this group of drugs increases certain aspects of thinking and sensation which has led to the use of names such as 'uppers' and 'speed' being used to describe them. Methamphetamine (crystal, meth, ice) creates a rapid feeling of well-being, vigour and physical power. This is described as the 'rush'. Four to six hours later these feelings of increased well-being give way to a sense of unhappiness, anxiety and depression which is known as the 'crash'. This can sometimes be quite profound and suicidal gestures are not uncommon. The tremendous sense of health decreases each time the drug is used. This increasing tolerance to the drug means that larger and larger doses need to be taken in order to create a similar effect. It can produce so intense a change of thinking that the sense of well-being is replaced by a complete disorganisation of thoughts and psychotic symptoms emerge (Marshall and Werb 2010). One of the best-known drugs within this group is cocaine. This comes from the leaves of the coca plant which originally grew in the Andes of South America. It was used by the Incas for some time before becoming a regular treatment in Western medicine for such diverse problems as hysteria and asthma. Although Coca-Cola derived its name from the fact that it contained cocaine, this was actually replaced in 1903 by caffeine and, indeed, in the early part of the century cocaine was a little-used drug, only being popular with artists and people of a bohemian lifestyle.

In the 1960s the drug experienced a renewed popularity and rapidly gained the reputation of being 'glamorous', with the commonest methods of use being by injection or inhaling the powdered form. In the 1970s it was found that the potency of taking cocaine could be increased if it was inhaled while being heated with a solvent. This became known as 'freebasing'. A further refinement to the process was developed in the 1980s, when drug suppliers began to heat cocaine and solvents at higher temperatures, which removes the hydrochloride part of the chemical structure. This process also allows impurities to settle to the bottom, leaving brown crystals. It is these crystals which are heated and inhaled, and because of the distinctive crackling sound that they make when they are heated, this form of cocaine has become known as 'crack'. This form of cocaine gives a very intense sense of well-being which lasts only for a brief time and is inevitably followed by a very profound 'crash'. The intensity of both the positive rush and the after-effects makes this a highly addictive drug, though there is evidence that smoking the drug is less addictive than injecting it (Gossop et al. 1994).

Cocaine creates a sense of well-being, with the young person often talking excessively and perhaps becoming quite agitated. The crash produces sleeplessness, depression and an increasing craving for more cocaine. The effects can remain evident for several weeks afterwards, with the user showing marked lethargy, apathy and depression. Regular cocaine usage also carries with it significant physical problems. It can cause irregular heartbeats, heart attacks and seizures. Crack, in particular, can damage lungs and cause marked breathing difficulties.

Large doses of cocaine can cause people to start having paranoid ideas and sometimes they will have psychotic episodes, with visual and tactile hallucinations, which can last for several days. These are often associated with episodes of violent and antisocial behaviour.

Features of withdrawal

The features of withdrawal may begin quite insidiously, with the young person having no idea why he/she is feeling tired, irritable and lethargic, but usually it is characterised by a more dramatic sense of agitation and depression which begins some hours after the last dose. This is followed by an inability to sleep, despite an increasing sense of fatigue, and a gradual reduction in the sense of craving for more cocaine. This initial withdrawal phase ends with the young person feeling totally exhausted, but with an increased appetite, and sleep patterns which are returning to normal. After this initial phase there may be further periods of feeling miserable and lethargic, which then gives way to feeling more settled and comfortable.

Psychological support

The immediate support for someone in an intoxicated state has been described above. It is always worthwhile to try to determine what the intoxicating agent may be, but always within the context of maintaining a tranquil atmosphere. Treating cocaine addicts rarely requires an alternative drug to be prescribed, and most treatments depend upon using psychological methods. It appears that cognitive behavioural therapy and contingency management have the best impact upon stimulant misuse and its associated dependence (Rawson *et al.* 2002). Unfortunately, relapse rates are very common with this drug, which is why its use is such a cause for concern.

Opiate drugs

Opiate drugs such as heroin have been prescribed by the medical profession for centuries, and at the turn of the century opium dens were features of most large cities. When abused, heroin can quickly become the dominant focus of the young person's life – addiction is easily established, with many users becoming criminals to finance the habit. There are other opiates, the abuse of which is increasing in some countries, such as Canada (Hammond *et al.* 2011).

Features of withdrawal

The opiates can be smoked, injected under the skin ('skin popping') or injected into a vein ('mainlining'). Tolerance to the drug develops quite quickly, and since the young person feels quite unwell as the effect of the drug wears off, addiction to it is rapidly established. If addicts attempt to withdraw they experience severe abstinence symptoms, which begin to appear about eight to twelve hours after the last dose. There is an intense craving to re-use the drug and this is associated with nausea, diarrhoea, a running nose, goosebumps and severe pain within the bones and joints. The young person also begins to sweat profusely, the pupils are constricted and extreme lethargy is apparent, with repetitive yawning. As well as these physical symptoms, the addict will appear to be markedly anxious, restless and depressed. Even when these profound problems have been overcome, the young person can, for several months, feel depressed and anxious and have marked difficulty in sleeping.

Psychological support

In an acutely intoxicated situation the general advice of protection and tranquil atmosphere apply. The health risks associated with overdose require extra vigilance for breathing problems, which in extreme cases may need resuscitation measures to be started.

If an addict is seeking help to overcome a drug habit, the first step is often to substitute the drug with a synthetic opiate such as methadone, or buprenorphine. If the young person is also abusing other drugs, then these have to be reduced before any effort is made to reduce the dose of synthetic substitute. For some abusers, establishing them on a regular replacement programme is the most that can be achieved, with efforts to keep them safe by arrangements such as needle exchange programmes (Dolan *et al.* 2003). The remainder of the programme is focused on offering psychological insight and support with the slow, and at times faltering, process of helping the user rebuild a life.

Hallucinogens

Perhaps the best-known drug within this group is lysergic acid diethylamide (LSD). This drug became very popular in the 1960s and its popularity has continued to rise steadily since then, with 4% of the population reporting having tried it in 1985 compared to 10% in 1992 (Institute for the Study of Drug Dependence 1993). More recently 5–4–4-methyl-amphetamine (MDMA) has become popular among the young. This drug is better known as 'ecstasy'. Also within the group is phencyclidine (PSP), which is often known as 'angel dust'.

Effects

Hallucinogenic drugs tend not to be drugs of habitual use, but are rather used intermittently to enhance social activities, such as rave dancing. Tolerance rapidly develops and so the young person has to take increasing doses to produce the same effect. These drugs alter perception – visual images will flow together and objects will appear to melt. Thoughts assume an unusual clarity and there is often an apparent distortion of time which can make things appear to move very quickly, or very slowly. When intoxicated with the drug there is usually a feeling of euphoria, but users can sometimes feel very panicky, or become paranoid. Switching between such moods can occur abruptly and the distortion of time can make it appear that the bad feelings are lasting for ever. In fact the effects of MDMA and PSP will last for up to eight hours in most cases, although the effects of LSD can last up to twenty-four hours.

When the mood changes are those of panic and fearfulness it is said that the young person is having a 'bad trip'. Such feelings are often associated with breathlessness, and many young people report fearing that they are losing their sanity during such episodes. Although these feelings tend to fade after some hours, they can recur some weeks or months after the drug was last taken. Such re-experiences are known as 'flashbacks' and although usually mild and brief, they can, on occasion, be the source of fear and concern.

Psychological support

If PCP is taken in high doses, it is likely to provoke quite marked violent behaviour, often with psychotic symptoms. In such situations the young person is often poorly coordinated, their blood pressure is quite high, and the heart is often erratic in its beat. In such severe toxicity cases the young person needs to be admitted to hospital to minimise the physical effects. For most young people, however, offering a calming influence until the effect of the drug subsides is usually sufficient. It is also helpful to reassure them of their safety, and that the effects of the drug will pass.

If the young person is experiencing flashbacks then a similar supportive stance is appropriate. The effects are not a sign that they are going crazy, but in the midst of the experience this might be difficult for them to accept.

Inhalants

Solvents, glues, lighter fuel and the propellants within aerosols have all had a vogue with young people as drugs of abuse, but this usage appears to be reducing (Hammond *et al.* 2011). Young people normally experiment with such drugs within groups and continued use is often part of a social routine. The dangers of this type of abuse partially arise from their inflammable nature, and also from the associated risks of choking and suffocation.

Effects

Drugs of this group create an immediate sense of light-headedness, and this is usually associated with a floating sensation. There is a clouding of thinking and the young person may appear quite drowsy, usually with an associated lightening of mood. Commonly, the organic solvents are put in a plastic bag and inhaled to intensify the effect, and, of course, such a mechanism increases the risk that accidental suffocation will occur. The use of aerosol propellants can also be quite dangerous if the spray is a noxious chemical such as fly spray, and some young people will spray through a cloth to try to strain out these other chemicals. For instance lighter fuel, when sprayed on to the back of the throat, irritates the throat lining, causing it to swell, and this can cause severe breathing problems.

A young person intoxicated with solvents appears drunk, with slurring of speech and a slowing of thought processes. The eyes may be red from the irritant nature of the fumes being inhaled, and some users develop inflamed skin round the nose and mouth, also as a result of this irritation.

Psychological support

Even in those who are usually cheerful and biddable, intoxication can prompt a sense of panic, and during this acute phase the aim should be to offer a calm and non-threatening environment in which the effects can wear off. It is important to monitor breathing and pulse to detect any complications that are arising, but usually the effects will simply pass. The decision as to whether medical assistance is needed is determined by whether physical complications, such as breathing problems, are starting to appear. It is unusual for hospital admission to be needed.

There is little evidence to suggest that young people who regularly use solvents experience withdrawal, and so the major thrust of assistance is trying to understand the origins of the use while looking for signs of underlying psychiatric illness. The approach families should take needs to strike a balance between offering support and maintaining a clear rule system which consistently emphasises disapproval of inhalant use. Inhalant use is usually a social activity, and so many young people have no motivation to stop until they outgrow their peer group.

Robert was a 15-year-old boy who had begun sniffing glue when he was 13. His friends within the neighbourhood had introduced him to its use, and most evenings they would gather in a remote corner of a small wood which was next to the estate where they all lived. Glue had become popular because it was easier to steal than alcohol, and there had been a gradual progression from glue to solvents of various kinds.

Robert and his friends began to miss those lessons at school that they did not enjoy, preferring to spend the time in the local shopping centre. Robert's group became very adept at stealing from shops, and would plan what they could do to liven up their evenings – on occasion they would bring off-road motorcycles to ride in the wood, or steal a car and drive it at great speed through the estate.

The search for greater excitement led Robert and his friends into more daring thefts, after which the group would gather in their corner of the wood and inhale solvents to enhance their feelings of elation. At 15, Robert and four of his friends appeared in court on several charges of breaking and entering, and two further court appearances eventually resulted in Robert being given a custodial sentence.

Robert's history illustrates the commonest theme to be found among solvent users. A mixture of peer-group pressure, the search for excitement and accepting delinquent activity as the norm are the elements which tend to maintain solvent use. The lack of motivation to stop means that concerned adults have no real opportunity to intervene. Occasionally the solvent use is a solitary activity to block out psychological or emotional problems, and such users do sometimes recognise that help with these underlying problems is a better solution than solvent usage.

Cannabis

Cannabis is a common drug of experimentation among adolescents and is derived from the cannabis sativa plant. This drug is grown throughout the world and has been used by many cultures over the centuries. It occurs in two forms – a mixture of the dried stems, seeds and leaves which is known as marijuana, and the far more potent resin which is derived from the flowering tops of the plants and is known as hashish. Both forms can be taken orally or smoked, and the strength of the active ingredient in cannabis (delta-9-tetrahydrocannabinol – THC) appears to be increasing over time (Potter et al. 2008).

In the early 1990s in the UK, 3–5% of senior schoolchildren reported having tried cannabis (Health Education Authority 1992), and this increased significantly thereafter, though it is now showing a gradual reduction (Health and Social Care Information Centre 2011). This is an international trend with, for instance, 9% of adolescents in South Africa reporting they have used cannabis (Peltzer et al. 2010), and in Canada about one-half of Grade 10 students had used cannabis at least once in their lifetime (up from one-third in 1990) (Elgar et al. 2011).

However, a quite worrying trend is that the average age that young people begin to use cannabis is getting younger (Potter *et al.* 2008). Given its frequent use there have been concerns about its impact upon the foetus, and intrauterine exposure to cannabis has been shown to be associated with an increased risk for aggressive behaviour and attention problems as early as 18 months of age in girls, but not boys (Marroun *et al.* 2011).

The effects of cannabis begin within a few minutes and last for an hour or two. Visual and physical sensations are often enhanced, and there is some distortion in the perception of time. At the same time the heart rate may often increase, and fine tremors are not uncommon. The user may feel hungry, and usually the drug increases relaxation, though on occasions it can prompt the young person to become agitated and feel anxious. In someone who uses the drug quite regularly there can be a pattern of mild withdrawal with irritability and restlessness, and there can also be features of psychological dependence if there is very heavy usage.

There is a movement which argues that cannabis is no more dangerous than tobacco and is in such common use that it should be legalised. In addition it does appear to have beneficial effects on some physical disorders such as fibromyalgia (Fiz *et al.* 2011), and in palliative care (Carter *et al.* 2011). The symptoms of post-traumatic stress disorder also appear to respond positively to cannabis use (Cougle *et al.* 2011). There is a statistical association between cannabis use and significant mental health problems such as psychosis, though it appears that this risk emerges if the young person began using cannabis at age 14 or younger (Schimmelmann *et al.* 2011). However chronic exposure to cannabis is associated with dose-related impairments in attention, working memory, verbal learning and memory functions (Solowij and Battisti 2008). Use of cannabis also increases the likelihood of physical disorders such as respiratory and cardiovascular disease (Hall and Degenhardt 2009), and changes to the brain structure have also been found, which have probably occurred as a result of brain ischaemia and cerebrovascular changes (Büttner 2011).

There have been various approaches to help young people stop taking cannabis. Brief motivational approaches alone have produced mixed results in samples of young adult marijuana users (Martin and Copeland 2008), which may be due to the fact that the success of the approach appears dependent upon the degree of practitioner commitment to carry out the motivational interviewing with the appropriate energy and enthusiasm (McCambridge *et al.* 2011). Adding elements of CBT may give such approaches more cost-effectiveness (Olmstead *et al.* 2007). To date no specific medication has been found that effectively treats cannabis addiction, but there are some new medications emerging that hold some promise (Hart 2005). However, treatment of any coexisting mental health problem with the appropriate medication may well help in reducing cannabis use.

Given the very high frequency with which cannabis is used in the young there have been several attempts to develop school-based programmes which target cannabis use. In general, these have shown a positive reduction, especially if they are not led by teachers and have an interactive format. They are also more effective when targeting older pupils (Porath-Waller *et al.* 2010).

Anabolic steroids

There has in recent years been an increasing concern that anabolic steroids are being used by athletes and bodybuilders to increase their performances. In such cases it is quite common for two or even three different steroids to be used (Perry *et al.* 1990). While this is not strictly a drug of addiction, some young people can come to believe that they must regularly take the drug to maintain a high performance.

In young people regular use of the drug can cause depression, irritability, hostility, aggression and even psychosis. Many of the longer-term effects are on the sex organs – erectile problems, shrunken testicles, as well as an increase in the risk of heart and liver problems. If these drugs are used by children, growth problems can develop. There is no recognised withdrawal programme, but many of the psychological principles used in helping other types of drug abuser will apply to these young people too.

Newer drugs of abuse

As well as these established drugs of abuse, there is the constant emergence of new chemicals that are found to change mood, and become sought-after as recreational drugs. For example, the anaesthetic ketamine has become a popular drug in some quarters because of its ability to produce vivid dreams or hallucinations, and the way it makes the user feel as though the mind is separated from the body. Another anaesthetic that has become a drug of abuse particularly at parties is GHB (Gammahydroxybutyrate). This causes both hallucinations and a great sense of euphoria, but is particularly dangerous if mixed with alcohol, and there have sadly been several deaths. The continual emergence of new substances means that there cannot be complacency because as these substances become available new risks and dangers to the young people using them emerge.

General recognition and management of an addict

The regular use of drugs has the potential to have a profound effect upon a young person's future life and functioning and, quite naturally, parents and others who come into contact with the young person become very concerned by such behaviour. However, it is important to realise that many young people move away from drug use without any formal treatment.

A clear change of behaviour may be the first indication that a young person is starting to establish a drug habit. The sudden onset of stealing, a marked drop in school performance, changing friendships and alliances, and becoming more irritable and bad tempered can all be features of a young person trying to cope with adolescence, but should also prompt consideration that they may also be abusing drugs. At this stage it is important to voice suspicions in the correct way. Direct confrontation will only provoke denial and prompt the young person to be more secretive. Suspicion should be followed by a period of looking for supporting signs, especially periods of intoxication. If a drug habit is developing it will be increasingly difficult for a young person to hide the drug's effects.

The pattern of response described for alcohol is generally applicable to all drug usage situations. Although detoxification can be an important step in a successful programme, engaging the young person in appropriate psychological support is the fundamental factor in determining whether drug usage can be stopped.

Some young people may lack the motivation to stop drug usage, and in such cases the approach needs to be a careful mix of education and gentle encouragement. For some, the most that can be achieved in the short term is harm minimisation – and developments such as needle exchange programmes and education about which inhalants carry the greatest risk are examples of this approach (Anderson 1990). If the drug use is too disruptive for a household or school to tolerate, then intoxication may mean being barred. This is not a punishment for misbehaviour, it is protection for the home or school from further disruption. This 'tough love' approach places a great strain on caring adults but helps to impress upon a user the terms on which they can rejoin their family or community.

Formal treatment programmes

Professional agencies tend to offer treatment which falls into two categories. The first is treatments which focus upon the young person, and may take the form of counselling, behavioural techniques or group meetings. Contingency management appears to be most useful for single element interventions, such as attending for physical examinations (Perlman et al. 2003), but is not effective in the long term. Relapse-prevention CBT focuses on helping drug users to identify situations or states where they are most vulnerable to drug use, to avoid high-risk situations, and to use a range of cognitive and behavioural strategies to cope more effectively with these situations. It has been shown to have limited effectiveness, especially in the long term, and this is also true for the more standard forms of CBT (National Institute for Health and Clinical Excellence 2007). Self-help groups can be beneficial in helping users to recognise that the problems they face are commonly shared, but young people tend to be reluctant to participate in such meetings. The second approach is to focus upon the family, and the network in which the adolescent lives. Youths with more severe drug use and greater psychiatric comorbidity do appear to benefit more from programmes which take this wider view, for instance multidimensional family therapy (Henderson et al. 2010).

Although three treatment approaches – multidimensional family therapy, functional family therapy, and group CBT – have become established models for substance abuse treatment, a number of other models are probably efficacious, and none of the treatment approaches appears to be clearly superior to any others in terms of treatment effectiveness for adolescent substance abuse (Aldron and Turner 2008). In addition, motivational interviewing is often a helpful approach with the young person (see Chapter 2), though its success does appear to be quite dependent upon the personal qualities and commitment of the practitioner (McCambridge et al. 2011).

The multifaceted nature of many young people's drug problems makes it difficult for a single type of intervention to succeed. Because of this, in recent years

Multisystemic Therapy (Henggeler 1999) has been the focus of considerable research interest. This is an intervention which tries to address the elements within the individual, school, home, peer group and community that may be contributing to the substance misuse. Its focus is maintaining continual engagement with the programme, and the long-term results are not only very hopeful (Henggeler *et al.* 2002), but the overall cost of the programme is less than many other options (Schoenwald *et al.* 1996).

Issues of prevention

The major concerns that exist around drug use have naturally prompted considerable work on programmes of prevention. There is a suggestion that the rate of increase in usage of certain drugs is slowing down (Health and Social Care Information Centre 2011), and reviews of school-based prevention programmes show that the most promising prevention approaches are those that target individuals at the beginning of adolescence, and teach drug resistance skills, as well as seeking to improve the young person's coping mechanisms and social skills (Botvin 2000). The most effective of such programmes offer a wide target database, are interactive in format, and tend to be more effective if they go on for longer and are not facilitated by their teachers (Porath-Waller *et al.* 2010). They can also be effective in reducing the usage of substances such as tobacco and alcohol, but their effects appear to decrease over time, with booster interventions being necessary to maintain and in some instances even enhance prevention effects (Griffin *et al.* 2003).

Sources of further help

www.uk-rehab.com/
www.talktofrank.com/
www.re-solv.org
www.aona.co.uk
www.nida.nih.gov/nidahome.html
www.adfam.org.uk
www.eata.org.uk
www.release.org.uk

References

Anderson, H.R. (1990). Increase in deaths from deliberate inhalation of fuel gases, and pressurised aerosols. *British Medical Journal* 301: 41.

Barnard, M. and Barlow, J. (2003) Discovering parental drug dependence: Silence and disclosure. *Children and Society* 17: 45–56.

Bertrand, J., Floyd, R.L. and Weber, M.K. (2005). Guidelines for identifying and referring persons with fetal alcohol syndrome. *Morbidity and Mortality Weekly Report, Recommendations and Reports* 54: 1–14.

Botvin, G.J. (2000). Social and competence enhancement approaches targeting individual-level etiologic factors. *Addictive Behaviors* 25: 887–97.

Braucht, G.N., Brakarsh, D. and Follingstad D. (1973). Deviant drug use in adolescence: A review of psychosocial correlates. *Psychological Bulletin* 79: 92–106.

Büttner, A. (2011). Review: The neuropathology of drug abuse. *Neuropathology and Applied Neurobiology* 37: 118–34.

Carter, G.T., Flanagan, A.M., Earleywine, M. *et al.* (2011). Cannabis in palliative medicine: Improving care and reducing opioid-related morbidity. *American Journal of Hospice and Palliative Care* 28: 297–303.

Cougle, J.R., Bonn-Miller, M.O., Vujanovic, A.A. *et al.* (2011). Post-traumatic stress disorder and cannabis use in a nationally representative sample. *Psychology of Addictive Behaviors* 25: 554–8.

Dolan, K., Rutter, S., Wodak, A.D. (2003) Prison-based syringe exchange programmes: A review of international research and development. *Addiction* 98: 153–8.

Doll, R., Peto, R. and Hall, E. (1994). Mortality in relation to consumption of alcohol: 13 years' observations on male British doctors. *British Medical Journal* 309: 911–18.

Elgar, F.J., Phillips, N. and Hammond, N. (2011). Trends in alcohol and drug use among Canadian adolescents, 1990–2006. *Canadian Journal of Psychiatry* 56: 243–7.

Fiz, J., Durán, M., Capellà, D. *et al.* (2011). Cannabis use in patients with fibromyalgia: Effect on symptoms relief and health-related quality of life. *PLoS One* 6: e18440.

Frezza, M., di Padova, C., Pozzato, G. (1990). High blood alcohol levels in women: The role of decreased gastric alcohol dehydrogenase activity and first pass metabolism. *New England Journal of Medicine* 322: 95–9.

Frischer, M., Crome, I. and Macleod, J. (2005) *Predictive Factors for Illicit Drug Use Among Young People: A Literature Review.* London: Home Office.

Gossop, M., Griffiths, P. and Powis, B. (1994). Cocaine: Patterns of use, route of administration and severity of dependence. *British Journal of Psychiatry* 164: 660–4.

Greenfield, S.F., Back, S.E., Lawson, K. *et al.* (2010). Substance abuse in women. *Psychiatric Clinics of North America* 33: 339–55.

Griffin, K.W., Botvin, G.J., Nichols, T.R. *et al.* (2003). Effectiveness of a universal drug abuse prevention approach for youth at high risk for substance use initiation. *Preventive Medicine* 36: 1–7.

Gunzerath, L., Hewitt, B.G., Li, T.-K. *et al.* (2011). Alcohol research: Past, present, and future. *Annals of the New York Academy of Science* 1216: 1–23.

Hall, W. and Degenhardt, L. (2009). Adverse health effects of non-medical cannabis use. *Lancet* 374: 1383–91.

Hammond, D., Ahmed, R., Yang, W.S. *et al.* (2011). Illicit substance use among Canadian youth: Trends between 2002 and 2008. *Canadian Journal of Public Health* 102: 7–12.

Hart, C.L. (2005). Increasing treatment options for cannabis dependence: A review of potential pharmacotherapies. *Drug and Alcohol Dependence* 80: 147–59.

Health and Social Care Information Centre (2011). *Statistics on Drug Misuse: England, 2010.* London: Health and Social Care Information Centre.

Health Education Authority (1992). *Tomorrow's Young People: 9–15 Year Olds Look at Alcohol, Drugs, Exercise and Smoking.* London: Health Education Authority.

Henderson, C.E., Dakof, G.A., Greenbaum, P.E. *et al.* (2010). Effectiveness of multi-dimensional family therapy with higher severity substance-abusing adolescents: Report from two randomized controlled trials. *Journal of Consulting and Clinical Psychology* 78: 885–97.

Henggeler, S. (1999). Multisystemic therapy. *Child Psychology and Psychiatry Review* 4: 2–10.

Henggeler, S., Clingempeel, W.G., Brondino, M.J. *et al.* (2002). Four-year follow-up of Multisystemic therapy with substance-abusing and substance-dependent juvenile offenders. *Journal of the American Academy of Child and Adolescent Psychiatry* 41: 868–74.

Information Centre (2006) *Statistics on Young People and Drug Misuse: England, 2006*. London: NHS.

King, A., Wold, B., Tudor-Smith, C. *et al.* (1996). *The Health of Youth: A Cross-National Survey*. European Series No. 69. Geneva: WHO Regional Publications.

Kodituwakku, P. (2009). Neurocognitive profile in children with fetal alcohol spectrum disorders. *Developmental and Disability Research Review* 15: 218–24.

Marroun, H.E., Hudziak, J.J., Tiemeier, H. *et al.* (2011). Intrauterine cannabis exposure leads to more aggressive behavior and attention problems in 18-month-old girls. *Drug and Alcohol Dependence* 118: 470–4.

Marshall, B.D. and Werb, D. (2010). Health outcomes associated with methamphetamine use among young people: A systematic review. *Addiction* 105: 991–1002.

Martin, G. and Copeland, J. (2008).The adolescent cannabis check-up: Randomized trial of a brief intervention for young cannabis users. *Journal of Substance Abuse and Treatment* 34: 407–14.

Maze, I. and Nestler, E.J. (2011). The epigenetic landscape of addiction. *Annals of the New York Academy of Science* 1216: 99–113.

McCambridge, J., Day, M., Thomas, B.A. *et al.* (2011). Fidelity to motivational interviewing and subsequent cannabis cessation among adolescents. *Addictive Behaviors* 36: 749–54.

National Institute for Health and Clinical Excellence (2007). Drug misuse: Psychosocial interventions. Clinical Guideline No. 51. July 2007. www.nice.org.uk/guidance/index.jsp?action=byIDando=11812. Accessed June 12, 2011.

Olmstead, T.A., Sindelar, J.L., Easton, C.J. *et al.* (2007). The cost-effectiveness of four treatments for marijuana dependence. *Addiction* 102: 1443–53.

Perlman, D.C., Friedmann, P. and Horn, L. (2003) Impact of monetary incentives on adherence to referral for screening chest x-rays after syringe exchange-based tuberculin skin testing. *Journal of Urban Health* 80: 428–37.

Perry, P.J., Andersen, K.H. and Yates, W.R. (1990). Illicit anabolic steroid use in athletes: A case series analysis. *American Journal of Sports Medicine* 18: 422–8.

Porath-Waller, A.J., Beasley, E. and Beirness, D.J. (2010). A meta-analytic review of school-based prevention for cannabis use. *Health Education and Behavior* 37: 709–23.

Potter, D.J., Clark, P. and Brown, M.B. (2008). Potency of delta 9-THC and other cannabinoids in cannabis in England in 2005: Implications for psychoactivity and pharmacology. *Journal of Forensic Science* 53: 90–4.

Prescott, C.A., Madden, P.A.F. and Stallings, C. (2006) Challenges in genetic studies of the etiology of substance use and substance use disorders. *Behavioral Genetics* 36: 473–82.

Rawson, R.A., Gonzales, R. and Brethen, P. (2002). Treatment of methamphetamine use disorders: An update. *Journal of Substance Abuse Treatment* 23: 145–50.

Schimmelmann, B.G., Conus, P., Cotton, S.M. *et al.* (2011). Cannabis use disorder and age at onset of psychosis: A study in first-episode patients. *Schizophrenia Research* 129: 52–6.

Schoenwald, S., Ward, D., Henggeler, S. *et al.* (1996). MST treatment of substance abusing or dependent adolescent offenders: Costs of reducing incarceration, inpatient, and residential placement. *Journal of Child and Family Studies* 5: 431–44.

Solowij, N. and Battisti, R. (2008). The chronic effects of cannabis on memory in humans: A review. *Current Drug Abuse Reviews* 1: 81–98.

Tripodi, S.J., Bender, K., Litschge, C. *et al.* (2010). Interventions for reducing adolescent alcohol abuse: A meta-analytic review. *Archives of Pediatric and Adolescent Medicine* 164: 85–91.

Volkow, N. and Li, T.K. (2005) The neuroscience of addiction. *Nature Neuroscience* 8: 1429–30.

Waldron, H.B. and Turner, C.W. (2008). Evidence-based psychosocial treatments for adolescent substance abuse. *Journal of Clinical Child and Adolescent Psychology* 37: 238–61.

Whitty, M. and O'Connor, J. (2007) Opiate dependence and pregnancy: 20-year follow-up study. *Psychiatric Bulletin* 31: 450–3.

Chapter 10

Depression

Introduction

Over recent years, there has been an intense interest in the concept of depression in childhood. The issue is particularly complex because sadness and tears are common parts of all children's lives and so cannot form any true basis for a diagnosis of a depressive illness. Moreover, the term itself has become so much part of common usage that it has begun to lose value as a description of a particular illness process. In addition, it is important not to lose sight of other emotional reactions in children and adolescents that can at first sight appear similar to depression but are a normal age variant. An excellent example of this is the mood lability which is common in the early teenage years, and presents as rapid changes of mood which are sometimes quite marked. It is occasionally difficult to distinguish this type of marked mood swing from the illness process where profound depression alternates with a very elated and over-cheerful period (known as bipolar illness – see Chapter 7), but the distinction is important since the ways to respond to these two types of mood variation are substantially different.

Reaching a diagnosis

To confirm that a depressive syndrome is present, the young person must not only appear miserable and unhappy, but demonstrate a negative style of thinking and present a daily routine which illustrates a loss of interest and concentration. For some clinicians, there must be clear anhedonia – which means that the young person has lost all enjoyment of life and now portrays a picture dominated by gloom and despondency.

Julie, a 14-year-old girl, presented with a six-week history of not attending school. When asked about this, she explained that for some months she found it difficult to concentrate at school and was concerned that all of her friends had turned against her, and that the teachers no longer liked her. Her mother said that Julie was previously a happy and cheerful girl, but over recent months she had become quiet and withdrawn, and would quickly become tearful and

> distressed at any difficulty or problem. She no longer went out with her friends, preferring to spend most of her time in her bedroom watching television. She had stopped eating and, although she constantly felt tired, was finding it difficult to settle to sleep and was waking consistently at 4.00 a.m. Throughout the interview, Julie emitted a sense of sadness and misery and, when asked directly, confirmed that she saw no future for herself, and had thought about suicide, although she insisted she would not kill herself since she did not want to cause additional distress to her family.

It is only in recent years that it has been established that the definition of depressive disorder which is used in adults is also appropriate to use when trying to assess children. Previously, there had been a view that depression did not occur until adult life, or that if it did present in children, it was in a 'masked' form. This theory suggested that a variety of difficulties within childhood, for example soiling and wetting, were the manifestations of depression in a child (Frommer 1968). This theory drew its support, in part, from the fact that conditions such as bedwetting improved when treated with antidepressants.

Prevalence

Depressive disorder affects 1–6% of adolescents each year, and early onset heralds a more severe and persistent illness in adult life (Thapar *et al.* 2010). Of course, when considering prevalence, it is important to bear in mind the distinction between the presence of depressive symptoms and the more profound depressive disorder. For example, a community-based study in Cambridge found 21% of the girls reported having symptoms of depression in the previous year, but when a syndrome definition was used the rate was 6% (Cooper and Goodyer 1993). Overall 5–10% of adolescents will have a major depressive illness during their teenage years (Fleming and Offord 1990), with the majority of these starting after puberty, especially in girls (Kessler *et al.* 2001). Having depression in adolescence carries with it a significantly increased risk of suicide (Gould *et al.* 2003).

Impact of the disorder

As already described, depressed young people are persistently miserable, gloomy and unhappy. They may feel so bad that the effort to express such negative emotions is too much, and they then become inert and withdrawn. There is often an associated slowing of speech and movement which can sometimes be mistaken by the uninformed as disinterest. Not surprisingly, such behaviours cause these young people to have impaired peer and family relationships, and there is usually a deterioration in school performance (Puig-Antich *et al.* 1993). In some cases these features, rather than the depressive symptoms themselves, may be more evident to the casual observer (Kent *et al.* 1995). Depression also has a wider impact, having long-term negative consequences on adult physical health and functioning.

The nature of the disorder can have a significant impact on trying to find out details of history from the young person. The withdrawal and general slowing up of thought processes mean that they are unlikely to volunteer information, and any answers they do give are likely to be slowly given. Many questions will be met with 'don't know', but since this is almost a universal adolescent reply, it is not very helpful diagnostically.

Causes of depression

There is a great deal of scientific endeavour focused upon trying to understand what causes depression. Although the vast majority of this work is focused on the illness in adults, some parallel work is being undertaken in children. Perhaps predictably the lines of enquiry have been those followed for adults – genetic, brain chemistry, the role of historical themes and significant life events. None of these has so far been proven to be the total explanation for the onset of depression, and at present it seems to be a mixture of the factors that ultimately leads to the onset of the illness. Children, perhaps even more than adults, are sensitive to atmospheres, and perhaps this is relatively more influential in children as a consequence (Kendler et al. 1992).

Overall it does appear, based on the evidence from twin studies, that depressive symptoms in young people are inheritable to a degree, with genetic factors becoming more important from childhood to adolescence (Rice et al. 2002). It is clear that a parent having depression poses a risk to their children because the child is three times more likely to develop a depressive illness, with at least 50% affected by about the age of 20, and the depression beginning earlier than their peers (Williamson et al. 2004).

One of the most enduring theories in the causation of depression is the amine hypothesis (Deakin and Crow 1986). This suggests that depression arises because there is a problem with a particular family of chemical transmitters, the monoamines. If these are depleted, then depression results. The evidence for this comes from the fact that if drugs are given which are known to reduce monoamines, then depression occurs, and, conversely, many of the drugs used to ease depression are known to increase these brain chemicals. However the cause of depression is far from being a simple deficiency of central monoamines. The drugs which alter amine levels (monoamine oxidase inhibitors and serotonin specific reuptake inhibitors) do produce immediate increases in monoamine transmission, but the positive changes to mood take weeks to appear. Conversely, reducing monoamines in healthy volunteers produces virtually no deterioration in mood (Ruhe et al. 2007).

It is now thought that the increases in the amount of synaptic monoamines that the medications bring about produce actual physical changes to the brain, and that it is these changes in the cells of the brain that bring about the improved mood (Pittenger and Duman 2008). The degree of these changes is dependent upon genetic issues, and it is clear that people with different genetic make-up respond to antidepressants to different degrees (Holsboer 2008). Several other brain chemicals show a degree of association with depression and are prompting significant research interest – for instance growth factors (called neurotrophic factors) that regulate plasticity within the brain, a brain transmitter called glutamate, and cytokines, chemicals which carry messages between cells (Krishnan and Nestler 2008).

What is very clear is that there is no single mechanism that is the cause of depression. Consider, for instance, cortisol. Studies suggest that high levels of cortisol are almost exclusively a feature of very severe depressive episodes, and chemicals that alter this (called glucocorticoid antagonists) show some therapeutic efficacy (Schatzberg and Lindley 2008). By contrast, depression found in chronic fatigue syndrome and post-traumatic stress disorder is associated with low cortisol (Gold and Chrousos 2002).

Given that these brain chemical changes can be long-lasting, epigenetics has been invoked to explain several aspects of depression. In essence, epigenetic changes offer a mechanism by which environmental experiences can modify gene function in the absence of DNA sequence changes (see Chapter 1). For instance, differences have been noted in the brain network responsible for managing stress (through the control of cortisol) in people who have had different early life experiences. Significant differences were found between the brain networks of those who committed suicide and had been abused during childhood compared to the brain networks of those who were not abused, and those of a group that had died in a car accident (McGowan et al. 2009). The implications of this are that poor early life experience may significantly increase the risk of depression, altering the young person's ability to cope with stressful events. Such epigenetic mechanisms have also been suggested to be important in explaining the high discordance rates between monozygotic twins, the chronic relapsing nature of the illness, and the strikingly higher prevalence of depression in women.

Alongside the interest in chemical causes, there has been a vast amount of work done looking at how environmental issues, stress, life events and other such changes in a particular person's circumstances might affect the onset of depressive illness. The fact that for each successive generation the prevalence of depression is increasing, and the age of onset is decreasing (Klerman and Weissman 1989), has tended to reinforce the belief that life issues are also playing a significant part in the causation of depression, perhaps through the epigenetic mechanisms described above.

There is clear evidence that family factors play a role in the development, maintenance and course of youth depression, with abusive family relationships predicting depression, while less severe relationship problems do not (Weich et al. 2009). This tends to confirm the idea that genetic vulnerability and provoking events are both needed to prompt the emergence of depression (Eley et al. 2004). The events may include poverty, exposure to violence, social isolation, family breakup, and a parent losing their job.

More recently there has been greatly increased interest in the diagnosis and treatment of bipolar disorders in children and adolescents. Bipolar disorders are recurrent disturbances in mood that include periods both of depression and mania. Classic bipolar disorders, with manic episodes lasting for at least several days, often start in adolescence, but have traditionally been considered very uncommon in earlier childhood. In recent years the similarity of the symptoms with severe ADHD (see Chapter 7) has raised the question of whether it could start at a younger age. Distinguishing the two disorders is possible with neuro-cognitive assessments (Leibenluft et al. 2007), but the diagnosis in young children remains controversial (Youngstrom et al. 2008).

The depressive symptoms of bipolar disorder show no real difference from those already described, but it is important to distinguish the two because the evidence suggests that both pharmacotherapy and psychotherapy are more effective if instituted early in the course of bipolar illness, and that with multiple episodes and disease progression there is a noticeable decline in treatment response (Berk et al. 2010).

Self-harm and parasuicide

Over recent years there has been a growing concern about the increasing frequency of young people who harm themselves, and one of the most under-recognised mechanisms is that of cutting. These young people often cut their bodies in places that are not easily seen, and the severity of the cuts can vary very widely. The actual frequency of the behaviour is quite hard to determine because young people who cut themselves are rarely assessed by healthcare professionals. In a review of the literature, the Mental Health Foundation (2006) found about 10% of young people were significant cutters, and in a study we carried out (Hall et al. 2010), 23% of senior school pupils reported cutting themselves at some time.

The literature on deliberate self-harm is quite substantial, with the origin of the behaviour often being seen as an attempt to bring relief from a stressful, or distressing, situation. There are generally two types of cutting behaviour presenting to clinics (Dimmock et al. 2007) and reported in community surveys (Hall and Place 2010). There are those young people who are emotionally troubled, with no effective way of coping, and young people for whom cutting is part of the youth culture to which they belong. Usually parents are unaware of the behaviour, and most studies suggest it is more common in girls (Laye-Gindhu and Schonert-Reichl 2005). In the vast majority of cases, these young people are not seeking to die (Madge et al. 2008), and the picture appears similar in many countries around the word (Scoliers et al. 2009).

Intervention focuses upon easing any provoking issues, and helping the young person find better ways of coping with life's stresses. These tend to be only modestly successful, and it is perhaps the development of preventative strategies that offers the best opportunity to reduce this behaviour (Hall et al. 2009).

There is a clear difference between this behaviour and the actions prompted, albeit often very briefly, by the intention to die (usually termed parasuicide). Twin and adoption studies have shown that both completed and attempted suicide tends to run in families. Thus, suicide attempt rates are elevated in the families of suicide completers and suicide rates are elevated in family members of attempters (Brent and Melhem 2008).

Perhaps not surprisingly, thoughts about committing suicide are strongly associated with suicidal attempts, and if there is coexisting depression the risk increases.

Of those presenting to hospital, children under 12 are more likely to have a family history of depression than adolescents. Furthermore, these children are more likely to report being bullied as a factor in their attempt, while adolescents tend to have a history of self-harming behaviour (Sarkar *et al.* 2010). It is also interesting to note that heavy binge drinking increases the risk of suicidal behaviour among younger adolescents, and is actually a greater risk than being depressed (Aseltine *et al.* 2009). A history of maltreatment and social factors such as parental separation, divorce and family discord, as well as child abuse, bullying, and copying peers or events that appear in the media, are all associated with suicidal behaviour (De Leo and Heller 2009).

It must also not be forgotten that adolescence is a time when thoughts of suicide are not uncommon, with perhaps 9% of young people having such ideas from time to time (Thompson *et al.* 2011). The fact that vulnerable young people can find sites on the internet that encourage suicide (Recupero *et al.* 2008) increases their risk. Adolescents who have made previous suicide attempts are particularly at risk, and unfortunately, despite progress in the identification of risk factors for attempted and completed suicide, there are no interventions that have been shown to reliably decrease the risk of further episodes in these young people (Bridge *et al.* 2006).

Associations with other disorders

Where more than one disorder appears to be present at the same time there is said to be comorbidity, and with regards to depression there is a strong comorbidity with anxiety. When severe, anxiety is quite a disabling symptom. Anxiety is an important emotion since it helps protect us from potentially dangerous situations, and we all experience a degree of anxiety from time to time, such as when taking tests, because the bodily changes it brings help us perform and focus better. A diagnosis of anxiety disorder merely indicates that the young person is experiencing anxiety that has stopped being helpful and is now causing significant distress and preventing routine day-to-day functioning. As many as 75% of depressed young people will show anxiety features (Merikangas and Angst 1994). In the more marked forms, the anxiety tends to precede the onset of the depressive illness (Brady and Kendall 1992). However, there is no evidence to suggest that this is a particular type of illness; rather is it that having two such difficulties occurring together multiplies the impact upon the sufferer's life.

Another common comorbidity is oppositional behaviour and conduct disorder. Why there should be a link with conduct problems is not understood, but it is probably significant that the overall outcome for young people with conduct problems does not seem to be influenced by whether they have depression or not (Harrington *et al.* 1991). When they occur together the young person usually shows more serious levels of maladjustment, especially relating to school success and substance dependence, than would be expected with each disorder alone (Marmorstein and Iacono 2003).

Intervention

As one might imagine, a young person presenting with a depressive illness often has other difficulties and problems associated with it, and it is important that these are assessed and dealt with appropriately. In many cases the correct resolution of wider family difficulties, and addressing issues such as poor peer relationships, can have a major beneficial effect upon the young person's mood. It is therefore important to recognise all the elements which may be contributing to the low mood, and to ensure that each element is given due weight in the intervention plan.

The treatment of depressive illness in adults has been exhaustively researched, and several approaches have been delineated. Although somewhat dependent upon the philosophy of the service offering treatment, and the views of the individual, developing a positive therapeutic relationship with the young person and their family is crucial for a successful outcome.

Medication

In significant depressive illness in adults, medication has a part to play in the treatment programme (Paykel and Priest 1992). The first successful group of antidepressants were the tricyclic antidepressants. Before being superseded by drugs with fewer side-effects they were the main medication used in depression, proving effective in treating the disorder in about 80% of cases. Nowadays these are not used for depression, though imipramine continues to find a small role in easing bedwetting, and as a potential alternative treatment in managing ADHD.

All antidepressants show a distinct response profile. There is usually little benefit evident in the first two weeks, but then the physical and motor features which are associated with depression, such as changes to appetite and sleep, and being slow in movements, begin to improve. The patients usually do not actually feel any better themselves at this stage, but observers see the improvements. It is usually six to eight weeks before the full impact of the drug is felt upon mood.

The discovery that serotonin influences depression produced a new family of drugs which have quickly become the treatment of choice in adult depression. These are known as selective serotonin reuptake inhibitors (SSRIs). The most commonly used drug in this family is fluoxetine (Prozac), and it is the first antidepressant that it is almost fashionable to admit to be taking. Although these drugs are far less toxic than the older tricyclics, they do have side-effects of their own, most notably gastrointestinal problems such as nausea and vomiting, which are dose-related.

There has been a period of great concern about giving antidepressants to young people because some have reported having suicidal ideas while taking them. As described above, such feelings are not rare in adolescents, and it is also worth noting that early in treatment the low mood is not improved, but feeling motivated to act on the low mood can be. These concerns led to a considerable reduction in their use, but studies since then have increasingly confirmed that, while caution is needed, the benefits of their use are greater than the risk of suicidal ideation and suicide attempts (Dudley *et al.* 2010). The current advice is that a cautious and well-monitored use of antidepressant medications should be the first-line treatment option in adolescents with moderate to severe depression (Masi *et al.* 2010).

With regards to the illnesses that may be present with the depression, the medication that treats depression can often have a modestly beneficial effect upon anxiety symptoms. Cognitive behaviour therapy can also help with such symptoms as well as reducing behavioural problems (see below). When there is drug misuse, effectively treating the depression is associated with a reduction in the misuse, but more intensive psychological interventions, rather than brief interventions, may be required to bring about lasting improvement. The most helpful in this regard are motivational interviewing and drug misuse focused cognitive-behavioural therapy (Baker *et al.* 2010).

Psychological approaches

Almost since the beginning of modern psychiatry there have been efforts to help people overcome psychological difficulties by using techniques which work with mental processes directly. These have taken many forms, but generally focus upon:

- changing behaviour directly through behavioural programmes;
- changing the thinking processes which are influencing the mood and behaviour – this is known as cognitive therapy;
- exploring the young person's inner world by looking at history, belief systems and issues such as loss – this is the basis of most psychotherapies.

These approaches are discussed in detail elsewhere (Chapter 2), and although the focus will be somewhat different for a depressed child, the principles are very similar. For instance, behavioural programmes aim to reduce behaviours which are maintaining the problem, and reduce them, or introduce new behaviours which are incompatible with being depressed. In practice, behavioural programmes are not used in isolation, but as part of a wider psychological approach using cognitive therapy.

In recent years the use of cognitive therapy for people with depression has become recognised as a helpful approach (Vostanis and Harrington 1994). This type of therapy is based on the assumption that behaviour and moods are produced as a result of what the person is thinking, and so changing the thinking can change the behaviour. Since its original focus was dealing with depressive illness, it is perhaps not surprising that its value in treating young people has been explored.

In practice, this type of intervention depends upon understanding the processes which are governing a particular person's thinking. Although there are several elements to the thinking process, two of the key ones from a therapeutic point of view are cognitive processes and cognitive products. Cognitive processes are the procedures which the brain uses to perceive and interpret experiences. The cognitive products are the thoughts which result from the interpretation and its interaction with experience, opinions, and so on. If the young person has distortions in the cognitive processes then it becomes very easy to develop a distorted view of the world, and the depressing thoughts that stem from this act as strong reinforcement that the original view was a correct one. For example, if a young person believes he or she is useless at schoolwork, every low mark or comment by a teacher helps to confirm for the young person that this is a true summary of the situation. This view has been supported by the finding that such negative cognitions (such as self-criticism) are stable and often precede the emergence of depressive symptoms (Nolen-Hoeksema *et al.* 1992).

These cognitive processes can give rise to problems such as depression in two different ways. The first is that there is a necessary skill or area of understanding which the young person still has to grasp fully. An example of this might be the young person feeling they need to develop a way of controlling temper outbursts, or learning to cope with a hurtful remark without taking it to heart. The second type of problem is that the thinking becomes distorted in some way – for instance, seeing a group of people talking always makes the young person believe that they are being discussed in a derogatory way.

The basic approach in cognitive therapy is always one of collaboration, with therapist and patient working as a team. For depressed young people this is often hard to establish, since they feel worthless and without a future. Engaging them in the therapy process usually means that initially they have to be led, and that enthusiasm for help needs to be nurtured and encouraged rather than being the prerequisite to commencing, which it is in other types of therapy.

To be of any help it is necessary to gain an understanding of the thoughts that are fuelling the depressive feelings. Typically, this process has three stages. First, it is important to confirm that the young person understands the concepts of emotion – happiness, sadness, and so on. Much of the work requires an accurate reporting of feelings and emotions, and so it is vital that these are fully recognised and labelled correctly. Using the knowledge, the young person begins to self-monitor, recording feelings and moods – when they occur and what they are associated with. This allows the young person and therapist together to identify the behavioural sequences which are associated with the problem. In this way the elements that require changing are clarified. This is the starting point for looking at the thought processes. If thought triggers mood which triggers behaviour, then examining the sequences most associated with gloomy moods should help to bring out the originating thoughts.

Having found the thought, then the cognitive restructuring can begin. The overall aim is to help the young person change the underlying cognitive processes which determine the interpretation that is being placed upon events. This is done in as concrete a way as possible, trying all the time to challenge the child's 'beliefs' with evidence that cannot be misinterpreted. Using such techniques helps the young person gradually to replace belief with knowledge, and with that knowledge comes a lessening of symptoms.

Marie was a 15-year-old girl who for the last year had felt increasingly miserable and unhappy. One morning her mother had not been able to rouse her for school, and hospital investigations revealed that she had taken about twenty of the tablets her grandmother was prescribed for her anxiety illness. Although her mother said Marie had been a little more subdued in recent weeks, she was shocked by this event, for the family saw Marie as sensible and very level headed. The parents could not identify any particular stresses in Marie's life which might have prompted the overdose, but accepted that since becoming a teenager she had tended to stay in her room and no longer confided in her mother about her problems or worries.

Marie described a pattern of increasing sadness in which she had lost interest in schoolwork and hobbies. She felt her friends no longer liked her, and the overdose had been prompted because she had finally become convinced that all of the girls in her class despised her. She had reached this conclusion because she had come to realise that whenever the girls were whispering together they were making derogatory remarks about her.

The thought-identification approach drew out this negative attribution and Marie was asked to think of an alternative explanation for the huddle. She decided upon 'so the boys can't hear', and every time she saw the huddle she used a particular sequence which commenced with visualising a road stop sign and repeating 'stop' under her breath. She then took a deep breath and repeated the new explanation to herself. Self-scoring showed that over the subsequent week her concern about these huddles of girls reduced. Similar measures were used to tackle the other specific issues which arose through the course of therapy, and Marie showed a full return to school-work and hobbies, and a new interest in boyfriends, over the next three months. Marie still did not share with her parents, but when therapy ended she was talking intently with her two best friends and was telling them 'everything'!

It is important to realise that there are many variations of the approach that can be adopted, although most contain elements similar to those described.

In young people the evidence suggests that cognitive therapy may not be as positive as first thought. Recent work has shown that cognitive behaviour therapy has a more modest effect than the early studies suggested, especially in more complicated cases (Klein et al. 2007). In moderate to severe depression, adding it to a medication regime does not significantly reduce depressive symptoms or suicidal thinking (Dubicka et al. 2010), and in one of the largest studies to date it was found to be no better than a placebo (Treatment for Adolescents with Depression Study (TADS) Team 2009).

Another intervention which is regularly used to reduce the symptoms of depression is interpersonal psychotherapy. This is a therapy which uses a relationship between patient and therapist as a basis for change, and the focus is very much upon the individual's inner world. The primary aim of such therapy is to give insight into the events and situations that prompted the difficulties, and more importantly into the unresolved issues which are maintaining them. A more detailed discussion of interpersonal psychotherapy can be found in Chapter 2, but when working with a young person who is depressed the therapy is often focused on exploring painful historical events or losses. Although difficult to carry out, there is a growing evidence base that this type of therapy can be effective in treating adolescent depression (Mufson et al. 2004). Finally, the part that various aspects of family functioning plays in the causation and maintenance of depression is increasingly being recognised (Restifo and Bögels 2009) and, as a consequence, work with families is sometimes part of the treatment programme.

As discussed in Chapter 2, diet and exercise are also a focus of interest. In the case of depression, some of these approaches are based on the association between depression and the levels of elements such as magnesium, and fatty acids (Colangelo et al. 2009). The evidence for the value of such approaches is still largely anecdotal, and although omega-3 fatty acids may well be helpful in the early stages of bipolar disorder (McNamara et al. 2010), dietary management should certainly not be the main approach for any but the mildest of difficulties. With regards to exercise, it seems that aerobic exercise may be helpful in moderating the effects of the depression, but it needs to be strenuous if it is to have any significant effect (Dunn et al. 2005), and there continues to be doubt about its actual value (Mead et al. 2009).

Outcome

In trying to form a view of how young people with depression might fare in adult life it is important to distinguish those who only have a moderate form of depression from those with severe depression or bipolar illness. As was described earlier, there is probably a genetic loading in the severe disorder groups which makes the development of longer-term problems more likely.

The research evidence suggests that early detection and intervention is effective in ameliorating the poor psychosocial outcome that often accompanies depressive illness, and although having an episode of depression in childhood does make it more likely that there will be episodes of depression in adult life, if there is only one episode throughout the teens and twenties, then the outlook is good (Rao et al. 1995). There are factors that can offer reassurance that this may be the only episode – for instance high self-esteem, good coping skills, school achievement, outside interests and positive relationships with family and friends. It is also clear that continuation of treatment is necessary in all patients after the acute phase of the illness, and for some patients long-term maintenance is required if relapse is to be prevented (Birmaher et al. 1998).

The outlook for the severely ill group may be less positive, for it has been estimated that the risk of a repeat episode of depression in this group is about 60% (Harrington et al. 1990), with as many as 80% of adults with bipolar illness beginning their illness before puberty (Geller et al. 1994). An adult with a confirmed major depressive illness experiences, on average, between five and six recurrences during his or her lifetime (Zis and Goodwin 1979), and they usually take about nine months to resolve.

No matter which type of illness it is, there can be more subtle long-term problems, for although treatment may reduce the immediate depressive symptoms, this is not always followed by improvement in other areas, such as social functioning. If the young person has a second episode of depression in adolescence, then there is a far greater likelihood of disruption to interpersonal relationships and a persistent sense of dissatisfaction with life (Rao *et al.* 1995). Also, as adults, they are more likely to present with overdoses and other suicidal gestures than is the general population (Kovacs *et al.* 1993).

Preventative strategies

With the knowledge that exists about predicting the frequency of future problems in at-risk groups, it is natural to ask what is being done to try to prevent this heavy psychological toll on these young people. Some work in adults has looked at whether the continued prescription of antidepressants is able to prevent relapse, and the results suggest long-term treatment does reduce the likelihood of relapse but does not abolish the likelihood of some symptoms returning (Paykel 1993).

The main efforts in prevention have been focused upon fostering elements that appear protective against further relapse. These include a positive emotional atmosphere at home, and a perceived sense of family support for the child, elements that are more important in protecting against mental illness than merely having the appearance of an average family make-up (Garrison *et al.* 1997). Indeed, the reverse is the case, that family discord increases the risk of depressive illness (Nomura *et al.* 2002), as does living with a parent who has a depressive illness (Beardslee *et al.* 1998).

Such findings also point to methods by which at-risk children might be made more resilient to the risks to which they are exposed (Place *et al.* 2002). These are elements such as developing outside interests; strengthening positive relationships with family and friends; developing good coping skills; correcting any educational deficits so that the young person can experience school achievement. These interventions will also strengthen self-esteem and so reduce the likelihood of further problems. However, the evidence is that prevention strategies are only likely to be effective when given to high-risk groups of adolescents rather than to the whole population (Stice *et al.* 2009).

Conclusion

Depressive illness is a debilitating, and often recurrent problem, which exerts influences far beyond the immediate ways that it affects the patient. It often seems to begin in adolescence, and although our understanding of it in this age group is increasing there is still much to learn about how it influences the young person's adult life. The treatment is principally by medication and cognitive therapy, and although work still continues to try to find more powerful ways to intervene, it remains a challenging condition in diagnosis, in treatment, and in prevention.

Sources of further help

www.teen-depression.info
www.depressionalliance.org/
www.nimh.nih.gov/health/topics/depression/depression-in-children-and-adolescents.
    shtml
www.youthinmind.com/
www.depressioninteenagers.co.uk

References

Aseltine, R.H., Schilling, E.A., James, A. *et al.* (2009). Age variability in the association between heavy episodic drinking and adolescent suicide attempts: Findings from a large-scale, school-based screening program. *Journal of the American Academy of Child and Adolescent Psychiatry* 48: 262–70.

Baker, A.L., Hides, L. and Lubman, D.I. (2010). Treatment of cannabis use among people with psychotic or depressive disorders: A systematic review. *Journal of Clinical Psychiatry* 71: 247–54.

Beardslee, W.R., Versage, E.M. and Gladstone, T.R.G. (1998). Children of affectively ill parents: A review of the past 10 years. *Journal of the American Academy of Child and Adolescent Psychiatry* 37: 1134–41.

Berk, M., Hallam, K., Malhi, G.S. *et al.* (2010). Evidence and implications for early intervention in bipolar disorder. *Journal of Mental Health* 19: 113–26.

Birmaher, B., Brent, D.A. and Benson, R.S. (1998). Summary of the practice parameters for the assessment and treatment of children and adolescents with depressive disorders. *Journal of the American Academy of Child and Adolescent Psychiatry* 37: 1234–8.

Brady, E.U. and Kendall, P.C. (1992). Comorbidity of anxiety and depression in children and adolescents. *Psychological Bulletin* 111: 244–55.

Brent, D.A. and Melhem, N. (2008). Familial transmission of suicidal behavior. *Psychiatric Clinics of North America* 31: 157–77.

Bridge, J.A., Goldstein, T.R. and Brent, D.A. (2006). Adolescent suicide and suicidal behavior. *Journal of Child Psychology and Psychiatry* 47: 372–94.

Colangelo, L.A., He, K., Whooley, M.A. *et al.* (2009). Long-chain omega-3 polyunsaturated fatty acids are inversely associated with depressive symptoms in women. *Nutrition* 25: 1011–19.

Cooper, P. and Goodyer, I. (1993). A community study of depression in adolescent girls: I. Estimates of symptom and syndrome prevalence. *British Journal of Psychiatry* 163: 369–74.

Deakin, J.F.W. and Crow, T.J. (1986). Monoamines, rewards and punishments: The anatomy and physiology of the affective disorders. In J.F.W. Deakin (ed.) *The Biology of Depression*. London: Royal College of Psychiatrists.

De Leo, D. and Heller, T. (2008). Social modeling in the transmission of suicidality. *Crisis* 29: 11–19.

Dimmock, M., Grieves, S. and Place, M. (2007). Young people who cut themselves: A growing challenge for educational settings. *British Journal of Special Education* 35: 42–8.

Dubicka, B., Elvins, R., Roberts, C. *et al.* (2010). Combined treatment with cognitive-behavioural therapy in adolescent depression: Meta-analysis. *British Journal of Psychiatry* 197: 433–40.

Dudley, M., Goldney, R. and Hadzi-Pavlovic, D. (2010). Are adolescents dying by suicide taking SSRI antidepressants? A review of observational studies. *Australasian Psychiatry* 18: 242–5.

Dunn, A.L., Trivedi, M.H., Kampert, J.B. *et al.* (2005). Exercise treatment for depression: Efficacy and dose response. *American Journal of Preventive Medicine* 28: 1–8.

Eley, T.C., Sugden, K., Corsico, A. *et al.* (2004). Gene-environment interaction analysis of serotonin system markers with adolescent depression. *Molecular Psychiatry* 9: 908–15.

Fleming, J. and Offord, D. (1990). Epidemiology of childhood depressive disorders: A critical review. *Journal of the American Academy of Child and Adolescent Psychiatry* 29: 571–80.

Frommer, E. (1968). Depressive illness in children. *British Journal of Psychiatry*, Spec. Pub. 2: 117–36.

Garrison, C.Z., Waller, J.L., Cuffe, S.P. *et al.* (1997). Incidence of major depressive disorder and dysthymia in young adolescents. *Journal of the American Academy of Child and Adolescent Psychiatry* 36: 458–65.

Gold, P.W. and Chrousos, G.P. (2002) Organization of the stress system and its dysregulation in melancholic and atypical depression: High vs low CRH/NE states. *Molecular Psychiatry* 7: 254–75.

Gould, M.S., Greenberg, T., Velting, D.M. *et al.* (2003). Youth suicide risk and preventative interventions: A review of the past 10 years. *Journal of the American Academy of Child and Adolescent Psychiatry* 42: 386–405.

Hall, B. and Place, M. (2010). Cutting to cope: A modern adolescent phenomenon. *Child; Care, Health and Development* 36: 623–9.

Hall, B., Haddow, S. and Place, M. (2009). VAST: A tool for recognising vulnerable children in the classroom and developing a care pathway of intervention. *International Journal of Education* 1(1): E10.

Hall, B., Elliott, J. and Place M. (2010). Self-harm through cutting: Evidence from a sample of schools in the North of England. *Pastoral Care in Education* 28: 33–43.

Harrington, R.C., Fudge, H., Rutter, M. *et al.* (1990). Adult outcomes of childhood and adolescent depression: I. Psychiatric status. *Archives of General Psychiatry* 47: 465–73.

Harrington, R.C., Fudge, H., Rutter, M. *et al.* (1991). Adult outcomes of childhood and adolescent depression: II. Links with antisocial disorders. *Journal of the American Academy of Child and Adolescent Psychiatry* 30: 434–9.

Holsboer, F. (2008). How can we realize the promise of personalized antidepressant medicines? *Nature Reviews in Neuroscience* 9: 638–46.

Kendler, K., Neale, M., Kessler, R. *et al.* (1992). A population-based twin study of major depression in women: The impact of varying definitions of illness. *Archives of General Psychiatry* 49: 257–66.

Kent, L., Vostanis, P. and Feehan, C. (1995). Teacher-reported characteristics of children with depression. *Educational and Child Psychology* 12: 62–70.

Kessler, R.C., Avenevoli, S. and Merikangas, K. (2001). Mood disorders in children and adolescents: An epidemiologic perspective. *Biological Psychiatry* 49: 1002–14.

Klein, J.B., Jacobs, R.H. and Reinecke, M.A. (2007). Cognitive-behavioral therapy for adolescent depression: A meta-analytic investigation of changes in effect-size estimates. *Journal of the American Academy of Child and Adolescent Psychiatry* 46: 1403–13.

Klerman, G.L. and Weissman, M.M. (1989). Increasing rates of depression. *Journal of the American Medical Association* 261: 2229–35.

Kovacs, M., Goldston, D. and Gatonis, C. (1993). Suicidal behaviors and childhood onset depressive disorders: A longitudinal investigation. *Journal of the American Academy of Child and Adolescent Psychiatry* 32: 8–20.

Krishnan, V. and Nestler, E.J. (2008). The molecular neurobiology of depression. *Nature* 455: 894–903.

Laye-Gindhu, A. and Schonert-Reichl, K.A. (2005) Nonsuicidal self-harm among community adolescents: Understanding the 'whats' and 'whys' of self-harm. *Journal of Youth and Adolescence* 34: 447–57.

Leibenluft, E., Rich, B.A., Vinton, D.T. *et al.* (2007). Neural circuitry engaged during unsuccessful motor inhibition in pediatric bipolar disorder. *American Journal of Psychiatry* 164: 52–60.

Madge, N., Hewitt, A., Hawton, K. *et al.* (2008). Deliberate self-harm within an international community sample of young people: Comparative findings from the child and adolescent self-harm in Europe (CASE) study. *Journal of Child Psychology and Psychiatry* 49: 667–77.

Marmorstein, N.R. and Iacono, W.G. (2003). Major depression and conduct disorder in a twin sample: Gender, functioning, and risk for future psychopathology. *Journal of the American Academy of Child Adolescent Psychiatry* 42: 225–33.

Masi, G., Liboni, F. and Brovedani, P. (2010). Pharmacotherapy of major depressive disorder in adolescents. *Expert Opinions in Pharmacotherapy* 11: 375–86.

McGowan, P.O., Sasaki, A., D'Alessio, A.C. *et al.* (2009). Epigenetic regulation of the glucocorticoid receptor in human brain associates with childhood abuse. *Nature Neuroscience* 12: 342–8.

McNamara, R.K., Nandagopal, J.J., Strakowski, S.M. *et al.* (2010). Preventative strategies for early-onset bipolar disorder: Towards a clinical staging model. *CNS Drugs* 24: 983–96.

Mead, G.E., Morley, W., Campbell, P. *et al.* (2009). Exercise for depression. *Cochrane Database of Systematic Reviews*, Issue 3.

Mental Health Foundation (2006) *Truth Hurts: Report of the National Inquiry into Self-Harm among Young People.* London: Mental Health Foundation and Camelot Foundation.

Mufson, L., Dorta, K.P., Wickramaratne, P. *et al.* (2004). A randomized effectiveness trial of interpersonal psychotherapy for depressed adolescents. *Archives of General Psychiatry* 61: 577–84.

Nolen-Hoeksema, S., Girgus, J. and Seligman, M. (1992). Predictors and consequences of childhood depressive symptoms. *Journal of Abnormal Psychology* 101: 405–22.

Nomura, Y., Wickramaratne, P.J., Warner, V. *et al.* (2002). Family discord, parental depression, and psychopathology in offspring: Ten-year follow-up. *Journal of the American Academy of Child and Adolescent Psychiatry* 41: 402–9.

Paykel, E.S. (1993). The place of antidepressants in long-term treatment. In S.A. Montgomery and J.H. Corn (eds) *Psychopharmacology of Depression.* Oxford: Oxford University Press.

Paykel, E.S. and Priest, R.G. (1992). Recognition and management of depression in general practice: Consensus statement. *British Medical Journal* 305: 1198–202.

Pittenger, C. and Duman, R.S.(2008). Stress, depression, and neuroplasticity: A convergence of mechanisms. *Neuropsychopharmacology* 33: 88–109.

Place, M., Reynolds, J., Cousins, A. *et al.* (2002). Developing a resilience package for vulnerable children. *Child and Adolescent Mental Health* 7: 162–7.

Puig-Antich, J., Kaufman, J., Ryan, N. *et al.* (1993). The psychosocial functioning and family environment of depressed patients. *Journal of the American Academy of Child and Adolescent Psychiatry* 32: 244–53.

Rao, U., Ryan, N.D., Birmaher, B. *et al.* (1995). Unipolar depression in adolescents: Clinical outcome in adulthood. *Journal of the American Academy of Child and Adolescent Psychiatry* 34: 566–78.

Recupero, P.R., Harms, S.E. and Noble, J.M. (2008). Googling suicide: Surfing for suicide information on the Internet. *Journal of Clinical Psychiatry* 69: 878–88.

Restifo, K. and Bögels, S. (2009). Family processes in the development of youth depression: Translating the evidence to treatment. *Clinical Psychology Review* 29: 294–316.

Rice, F., Harold, G. and Thapar, A. (2002). Assessing the effects of age, sex and shared environment on the genetic aetiology of depression in childhood and adolescence. *Journal of Child Psychology and Psychiatry* 43: 1039–51.

Ruhe, H.G., Mason, N.S. and Schene, A.H. (2007). Mood is indirectly related to serotonin, norepinephrine and dopamine levels in humans: A meta-analysis of monoamine depletion studies. *Molecular Psychiatry* 12: 331–59.

Sarkar, M., Byrne, P., Power, L. *et al.* (2010). Are suicidal phenomena in children different to suicidal phenomena in adolescents? A six-year review. *Child and Adolescent Mental Health* 15: 197–203.

Schatzberg, A.F. and Lindley, S. (2008) Glucocorticoid antagonists in neuropsychotic disorders. *European Journal of Pharmacology* 583: 358–64.

Scoliers, G., Portzky, G., Madge, N. *et al.* (2009). Reasons for adolescent deliberate self-harm: A cry of pain and/or a cry for help? Findings from the child and adolescent self-harm in Europe (CASE) study. *Social Psychiatry and Psychiatric Epidemiology* 44: 601–7.

Stice, E., Shaw, H., Bohon, C. *et al.* (2009). A meta-analytic review of depression prevention programs for children and adolescents: Factors that predict magnitude of intervention effects. *Journal of Consulting and Clinical Psychology* 77: 486–503.

Thapar, A., Collishaw, S., Potter, R. *et al.* (2010). Managing and preventing depression in adolescents. *British Medical Journal* 340: C209.

Thompson, R., Proctor, L.J., English, D.J. *et al.* (2011). Suicidal ideation in adolescence: Examining the role of recent adverse experiences. *Journal of Adolescence* Apr 8. *Early View.*

Treatment for Adolescents with Depression Study (TADS) Team. (2009). The treatment for adolescents with depression study (TADS): Outcomes over one year of naturalistic follow-up. *American Journal of Psychiatry* 166: 1141–9.

Weich, S., Patterson, J., Shaw, R. *et al.* (2009). Family relationships in childhood and common psychiatric disorders in later life: Systematic review of prospective studies. *British Journal of Psychiatry* 194: 392–8.

Williamson, D.E., Birmaher, B., Axelson, D.A. *et al.* (2004). First episode of depression in children at low and high familial risk for depression. *Journal of the American Academy of Child and Adolescent Psychiatry* 43: 291–7.

Youngstrom, E.A., Birmaher, B. and Findling, R.L. (2008). Pediatric bipolar disorder: Validity, phenomenology, and recommendations for diagnosis. *Bipolar Disorders* 10: 194–214.

Zis, A.P. and Goodwin, F.K. (1979). Major affective disorder as a recurrent illness: A critical review. *Archives of General Psychiatry* 36: 835–9.

Chapter 11

Dyslexia

Introduction

In every country one will find a significant number of children whose performance in reading, writing and spelling is considered to be problematic. Although the origins of such difficulties can be easily explained for some – for example, because of hearing/visual impairment, autism, brain damage – there are many others for whom the cause is less evident. Many of this latter group are considered to have a specific disorder, often known as developmental dyslexia or reading disability.

Many educationalists, objecting to dyslexia's quasi-medical tone, prefer to speak of 'specific learning difficulties'. Unlike the use of the term 'dyslexia', which tends to involve a diagnosis on the basis of various symptoms and signs (British Psychological Society 1999), 'specific learning difficulties' is essentially an exclusionary construct that refers to a situation where the child's level of functioning in reading and writing and associated areas is significantly weaker than one would expect on the basis of his or her general academic or cognitive performance. Rather than being wholly synonymous terms, then, dyslexia may be considered to be one common type of specific learning difficulty. Another term widely employed in the research literature is 'reading disability' which, for many, describes all those who experience difficulty with accurate and fluent reading. However, this term is also understood in differing ways, and many reading researchers do not differentiate between the terms reading disability and dyslexia (Wagner 2008; Pennington and Bishop 2009) and here the terms are often used interchangeably. For researchers who seek to understand the biological or cognitive origins of reading difficulties, fine distinctions between such terms are often of secondary importance. However, problems are more likely to emerge in clinical or educational contexts where a diagnosis of dyslexia is widely believed to offer additional valuable information to assist intervention planning and resource allocation.

The focus of this chapter concerns what is meant by the terms 'dyslexia' and 'reading disability' and the extent to which these terms add to our ability to understand and remedy the problems of children who have difficulties in learning to read. First, however, it is necessary to differentiate between the problems of those who struggle to understand and use the alphabetic principle in order to develop accurate and fluent reading, and other types of difficulties involving reading comprehension or motivation to read. Generally, those who use the terms dyslexia or reading disability (e.g. Torgesen 2005) are concerned with the first of these – decoding – although poor reading motivation and comprehension will often result from such difficulties (Morgan *et al.* 2008). However, as is noted below, some do not consider all who experience decoding difficulties to be dyslexic and others contend that dyslexia concerns far more than difficulties involving accurate reading. The focus of this chapter, however, is upon those with single word decoding difficulties. Single word reading is important here because the reader can only use decoding skills to read each word, rather than also drawing upon the syntactic and semantic cues that are typically available when reading passages of text.

The British Psychological Society (BPS) Working Party Report (1999) on dyslexia offered a 'working definition':

> Dyslexia is evident when accurate and fluent word reading and/or spelling develops very incompletely or with great difficulty. This focuses on literacy learning at the 'word' level and implies that the problem is severe and persistent despite appropriate learning opportunities. It provides the basis for a staged process of assessment through teaching.
>
> (BPS 1999: 64)

Relatively general definitions of this sort have resulted in criticism from otherwise opposing camps. Some have argued that such definitions are too inclusive as, on this basis, all children with decoding problems could be considered to be dyslexic (Regan and Woods 2000). Norwich (2009) makes a similar point, adding that this would also include those with severe problems of intellectual functioning. Others (e.g. Herrington and Hunter-Carsch 2001) criticise the definition for providing no underlying causal elements which might be employed to differentiate dyslexics from other poor readers. In contrast, the definition has also been criticised (e.g. Cooke 2001) for excluding those who may be adequate readers but still considered to be dyslexic on the basis of other difficulties (e.g. planning, organisation, dealing with form filling, and mathematical or musical notation).

A more detailed definition is provided by the Orton Dyslexia Society. Here dyslexia is seen as

> one of several distinct learning disabilities. It is a specific language-based disorder of constitutional origin characterized by difficulties in single word decoding, usually reflecting insufficient phonological processing abilities. These difficulties in single word decoding are often unexpected in relation to age and other cognitive and academic abilities; they are not the result of generalized developmental disability or sensory impairment. Dyslexia is manifested by variable difficulty with different forms of language, often including, in addition to problems reading, a conspicuous problem with acquiring proficiency in writing and spelling.
>
> (Lyon 1995: 9)

Such a definition of dyslexia reflects the influence of a growing, and increasingly sophisticated, research base which appears to point strongly towards language processing as the basis for the problems observed. However, dyslexia remains a highly controversial condition, with some denying its very existence and others arguing that arriving at a diagnosis is problematic, both conceptually and also in relation to its value for practitioners (Elliott and Gibbs 2008).

The perceived value of a dyslexia diagnosis

There have been many accounts in the popular press of children who have struggled through their education, often under great stress, who, it is claimed, were subsequently discovered to be dyslexic. This finding, it is sometimes alleged, proved to be a turning point in their lives as they could now benefit from remedial teaching geared for dyslexics and begin to make the gains which one would anticipate, given their intellectual abilities. For other individuals, however, a failure to diagnose the condition, it has sometimes been claimed, resulted in a ruined education and limited options in adult life. For some, litigation is now a justifiable consequence. The following quotation, taken from a newspaper article, is representative of many:

> A 22-year-old woman was condemned to 'temporary menial tasks' because her former schools did not realise she was dyslexic, the High Court heard yesterday. Pamela Phelps claims that she is of average intelligence but because her learning difficulty was not discovered until two months before she left school, she never learned to read and write properly . . . It was not the disorder that prevented her from being able to read. She had originally been 'lumped in' with children of low intelligence when she needed special tuition. Tests were carried out on her at infant, junior and comprehensive schools. At the age of 10 she was found to be four years behind in reading and writing skills but the reason was never identified.
>
> (*Guardian*, 27 July 1997: 5)

The above account suggests that if a diagnosis of dyslexia had been arrived at earlier, appropriate treatment would have resolved her difficulties. In July 2000, Ms Phelps' case was upheld and she was awarded substantial damages (see *The Times* Law Report of 28 July 2000 for details). However, it should be noted that her primary school had not failed to recognise that she had reading difficulties – this was the reason for her referral to an educational psychologist. When transferring to secondary school she had a reading age equivalent of 7 years and 3 months. Any secondary school in such a situation should ensure that help is given to remedy such difficulties as, without specialist teaching, problems of this severity are highly unlikely to be overcome (Brooks 2002). However, the high visibility of the case was not because a child with reading difficulties failed to be given help but, rather, because dyslexia was not formally diagnosed. Such a diagnosis, it was suggested, would have resulted in more appropriate forms of intervention being provided. The key questions here are: What are the key criteria for arriving at a diagnosis?; to what extent does such a diagnosis point us to appropriate forms of intervention?; and, finally, should additional resources or special arrangements be made available for diagnosed dyslexics?

Diagnosing dyslexia

While advocates argue that there is no such thing as a typical dyslexic, there are a number of underlying signs and symptoms which are often associated with the condition. These may include:

- speech and language difficulties (particularly as a young child);
- poor short-term verbal memory;
- difficulties in ordering and sequencing;
- clumsiness;
- lack of consistent hand preference;
- frequent use of letter reversals (b for d, p for q);
- poor verbal fluency.

Such difficulties, however, are also frequently found in people without reading difficulties and in poor readers who are not considered to be dyslexic. Furthermore, it is a point of some debate whether such symptoms are causes, consequences or merely correlates of reading failure. Thus, as is so often the case with the types of problem discussed in this book, the existence of certain signs and symptoms does not necessarily assist the practitioner in making a diagnosis.

There are many reasons why a child may experience difficulties in learning to read. Heaton and Winterton (1996) suggest that key factors are:

- low intelligence;
- inadequate schooling in the form of poor teaching or inappropriate content;
- socio-economic disadvantage;
- physical disability (e.g. hearing or visual difficulties);
- 'visible' neurological impairment which goes beyond reading and writing;
- emotional and behavioural factors which might affect attention, concentration and responsiveness to teacher direction, thus jeopardising the child's ability to learn;
- dyslexia.

One of the major difficulties of such analyses is that dyslexia may simply be identified on the basis of the absence of the first six factors (Lyon 1995). Difficulties abound here, particularly with respect to the relationship of intelligence to dyslexia (see discussion below), and the fact that those with reading difficulties are also more likely to experience emotional and behavioural difficulties (Morgan *et al.* 2008). The role of socio-economic factors as a potential excluding criterion is similarly problematic for, as Rutter (1978) points out, consideration of social factors may rule out the possibility of a diagnosis of dyslexia in those from disadvantaged backgrounds. It is partly for this reason that dyslexia has sometimes been criticised as a 'middle-class syndrome'.

Given the lack of current consensus about what constitutes dyslexia, and whether it differs from more general reading disability, it is hardly surprising that prevalence estimates vary substantially. For those researchers who consider the terms dyslexia and reading disability to be synonymous, estimates tend to be greater than for those who see dyslexics as a subset of a broader reading disabled population. A further complication is that reading abilities are now widely considered to lie along a continuum with no clear-cut distinction between normal and disabled readers. As a result, prevalence rates vary greatly according to where the cut-off point has been applied. Shaywitz (2005) provides a figure of 17.5%, although estimates can be a great as 20%. In contrast, Hulme and Snowling (2009) offer a more conservative estimate of 4–8%. Fletcher et al. (2007) suggest a prevalence rate of between 6% and 17%, depending upon the definitions and cut-off points selected.

There is also some disagreement about gender ratios for reading difficulties. Generally, it is considered that there is a higher prevalence of males, although estimated ratios of 3:1 or 4:1 (e.g. Goswami 2009) are most likely excessive. This proportion is likely to be inflated by the greater tendency of teachers to refer boys to clinical services as they are more likely than girls to present with other comorbid behavioural difficulties (Shaywitz 2005; Pennington 2009). In general, it is now widely considered that the true ratio of males to females with reading difficulties is in the range 1.3:1 to 1.5:1 (Fletcher et al. 2007).

Dyslexia is perceived as a problem in developed countries around the world (Brunswick et al. 2010) although rates of reading difficulty are particularly high in English-speaking countries, primarily because of the highly irregular nature of the English language. In countries where the language is more transparent, such as Italy or Finland, presenting problems typically concern speed of reading (fluency) rather than accuracy.

In the field of learning difficulties, it is important to recognise that definitions are designed both for research purposes and for professional decisions concerning intervention and resource allocation. For advocacy groups, and others seeking to maximise the availability of resources, strict conceptual rigour may not be a primary concern. Even here, agendas may differ. For some, the issue will be to widen the net to cover as many children as possible; for others, the emphasis will be upon retaining available resources by excluding those whose difficulties fall outside of a narrow predetermined range of deficits (Elliott and Grigorenko 2012).

What causes dyslexia/reading disability?

Factors underpinning any learning difficulty can be considered at a variety of levels: the biological, the cognitive and the behavioural (Frith 1997).

Biological factors

No single cause of dyslexia/reading disability has been discovered, and it is now widely agreed that multiple factors are at play (Pennington 2009). Much research has focused on biomedical accounts which emphasise brain structure and genetic influences. Early research into the workings of the brain focused upon structural factors and often involved post-mortem studies. More recently *in vivo* techniques such as magnetic resonance imaging, voxel-based morphometry and diffusion tensor imaging have enabled more sophisticated examination of what structures in the brain are engaged in the task of reading. These approaches have pointed to a number of structural abnormalities in those with reading disabilities (see Leonard *et al.* 2001).

Another line of research concerns the use of various imaging techniques to examine brain functioning. In contrast to studies of brain structure, functional imaging reveals *in vivo* changes in the brain that are caused by various experimental manipulations (e.g. when asking the participant to undertake a cognitive task of some kind). There are many types of functional imaging of which functional magnetic resonance imaging (fMRI) is probably the best known. While there are significant differences in the approaches and samples used by various research groups, there are clear indications of a deficient functional profile for those with a reading disability.

Despite the wealth of information that neuroscience has provided about the structure and function of the 'reading brain', our understandings continue to be rudimentary and much further work will be necessary before insights can be applied in any meaningful way to inform practice in educational contexts (Elliott and Grigorenko 2012). At the current time, neuroscience is unable to provide individual assessments of poor readers or point to particular forms of intervention for those with reading difficulties. Practitioners, therefore, should be circumspect about any over-simple analyses and claims for intervention based upon brain studies.

The common finding that dyslexia runs in families has resulted in a familiar genes versus environment debate. While it is quite possible that the quality of a child's literacy experiences will be significantly affected by living with one or more parents who have encountered difficulties in learning to read, the existence of a genetic component in reading ability (and disability) is now clearly established (Grigorenko and Naples 2009; Scerri and Schulte-Körne 2010). Although heritability estimates vary according to the particular language involved and the samples and measures employed, it is generally assumed that an accurate figure lies within the range 40–60% (Grigorenko 2004), indicating an important genetic influence. However, moving from statistical estimates to the identification of particular genetic mechanisms, and specific genes underpinning these, has proven more difficult. At the present time, there are six genes that are under close examination with several other possible candidates having been suggested. It should be noted, however, that research linking genes to mechanisms is still at a rudimentary stage and it is not yet possible to offer a sound hypothetical model.

While genes are unlikely to cause reading difficulties in any direct sense, they serve to increase the likelihood that an individual will be affected. Thus it would appear that genetic susceptibility for some individuals will be minimised or maximised by subsequent life experiences. The investigation of environmental factors has resulted in the identification of a number of 'risk or protective' factors for reading difficulties. Among these are socio-economic status (Nicholson 1997), family traditions and values concerning education and literacy (Kamhi and Laing 2001), exposure to printed material (Cunningham and Stanovich 1997), and protected time for reading (Carter et al. 2009). While these factors are not considered to play a causal role, when they are low, they may be considered to be risk factors, and protective factors when high.

Detailed discussion of the role of biological factors – neuroscience and genetics – in reading disability can be found in Elliott and Grigorenko (2012).

Cognitive processes in dyslexia/reading disability

Although early accounts of reading disability, provided largely by medical practitioners, assumed that the core problems were primarily visual, research undertaken during the past forty years has increasingly emphasised its linguistic origins (Vellutino et al. 2004). At the current time, the dominant account is the phonological deficit hypothesis (Stanovich and Siegel 1994) in which the three most commonly identified elements are phonological awareness, verbal short-term/working memory, and rapid retrieval of phonological information stored in long-term memory, as exemplified by rapid naming tasks (Wagner and Torgesen 1987).

Phonological awareness

Phonological decoding is an important process for reading unfamiliar words and involves a process of mapping speech sounds on to patterns of letters. Children with reading disability tend to experience difficulties in accurately representing speech sounds, and this results in difficulties of phonological awareness, alphabetic knowledge, mapping together sounds and letters, and orthographic awareness (Vellutino et al. 2004). Phonological awareness, the ability to detect and manipulate different sounds in spoken language, can operate both at the level of phonemes (the smallest units of sound which enable us to distinguish one word from another) and that of syllables. According to current theorising, the beginning reader needs to be able to perceive phonemes in syllables and words and then be able to manipulate these in order to be able to make a connection between speech and writing and to employ an alphabetic system to read and spell (Adams 1990).

The emphasis upon phonological awareness was stimulated by research findings (Bradley and Bryant 1983; Lundberg 1994) indicating that young pre-readers who showed difficulties in perceiving rhyme and alliteration and segmenting words into their constituent sounds were more likely to demonstrate reading difficulties later in life. Subsequently, it has been shown that phonological awareness and letter-sound knowledge are key predictors of early reading development (National Early Literacy Panel 2008).

Interest in the role of phonological factors in reading has been spurred by intervention studies such as that of Lundberg *et al.* (1988) which showed that pre-school children who receive phonological awareness training through listening and rhyming games made greater gains in reading and spelling than comparable control groups. Since this time, a great number of phonologically based interventions have been shown to be helpful for young children at risk of reading failure (e.g. Scanlon *et al.* 2005, 2008), although gains may not always persist unless structured interventions continue in the subsequent school years (Slavin *et al.* 2011).

It is important to recognise, however, that while deficiencies in phonological awareness appear to be the most significant factors in studies of children with reading difficulties, there remain a significant proportion of poor readers who do not demonstrate such problems (White *et al.* 2006) and we are still a long way from being clear about their precise nature and role. Despite more than thirty years of research into the phonological deficit, 'we still don't know what it is' (Ramus and Szenkovits 2009: 165).

Short-term/working memory difficulties

Memory difficulties have long been considered as playing a role in reading disability. While there has been some interest in the role of long-term memory processes (Menghini *et al.* 2010), most research has focused upon short-term or working memory, both of which involve holding information for brief periods of time. Whereas short-term memory solely involves brief storage (e.g. holding a telephone number in one's mind while searching for a pen and paper), working memory involves both storage and processing (e.g. mentally undertaking a complex mathematical calculation). While evidence for a relationship between short-term verbal memory and reading disability has proven variable, with some finding such a link (Wagner and Torgesen 1987) and others failing to do so (Savage *et al.* 2007), evidence involving working memory has proven stronger (Alloway *et al.* 2009). Complicating this picture somewhat is the distinction between verbal and visual working memory, in which the former appears to be most problematic for poor readers (Johnson *et al.* 2010).

While memory problems are a feature of many with reading disability, it should be noted that a significant proportion of poor readers show no memory-related difficulties and this appears to be a less powerful predictor than phonological awareness (Savage *et al.* 2007). However, working memory appears to play a particularly important role in reading comprehension (Swanson *et al.* 2006) rather than the process of decoding which lies at the heart of reading disability.

Rapid naming

An interesting finding from experimental studies was that those with reading disability tended to encounter greater difficulty than their normal reader peers in rapidly naming familiar items such as letters, colours or everyday objects, placed before them. This finding led to the creation of the double deficit model (Wolf and

Bowers 1999) which located those with reading difficulties into three groups: those with normal naming speed but with phonological difficulties, those with a rapid naming deficit but sound phonological skills, and those with weaknesses in both phonological and naming abilities. According to Wolf and her colleagues (2000), it is this third group that will encounter greatest difficulty in learning to read. This position is controversial, however, and some have challenged the suggestion that, for the English language, there is a significant group of poor readers with rapid naming problems but intact phonological skills (Vukovic and Siegel 2006).

While the presence of rapid naming difficulties in many poor readers is incontrovertible there is some disagreement about the meaning of this phenomenon and the viability of the double deficit hypothesis (Vellutino *et al.* 2004). It should also be noted that rapid naming difficulties are more closely associated with reading fluency than single word decoding (Manis *et al.* 2000) and so this problem may be particularly influential for transparent languages where, unlike single word decoding, the major problem is not decoding accuracy but, rather, slow, laborious reading (Torppa *et al.* 2010).

Low-level auditory and visual processing factors

In recent years, there has been a resurgence of interest in the role of basic auditory and visual processing which may underlie phonological and other proximal reading-related difficulties.

The quality of one's phonological awareness is likely to be affected by any difficulty in being able to reflect upon the sounds in words that are spoken (Corriveau *et al.* 2010). In the light of findings more than three decades ago that children with language impairment appeared to perform poorly on tasks involving acoustic sensitivity, Tallal (1980) sought to ascertain whether this was also true of struggling readers. Here, the theory was that deficits in auditory processing would affect speech perception, which, in turn, would undermine the development of phonological awareness and ultimately, the acquisition of reading skills.

Tallal's findings supporting this hypothesis have been subject to significant criticism although they have served to foster other related lines of enquiry. Perhaps the leading research in this area at the current time is that undertaken by Goswami and her colleagues (Goswami *et al.* 2010; Corriveau *et al.* 2010). These researchers argue that auditory impairments that undermine the perception of speech rhythm and stress may render it difficult for the child to draw upon key speech cues that are important for language learning. However, findings are inconclusive. While poor performance on auditory measures has been found for poor readers, this appears to affect only a minority, and the range reported varies significantly (Boets *et al.* 2007; Griffiths *et al.* 2003). Furthermore, interventions geared to enhancing the auditory processing of children with reading difficulties have failed to demonstrate resultant gains in reading performance (McArthur *et al.* 2008; Pokorni *et al.* 2004). Several researchers have suggested that auditory processing problems are unlikely to be the cause of reading disability; rather, they may act as risk factors that aggravate existing phonological processing difficulties (Boets *et al.* 2007).

Given the nature of the reading process, it is unsurprising that visual processing deficits have long been held to play a causal role. Such a perspective, however, was largely undermined by the work of Vellutino (1987, 1979; Vellutino *et al.* 2004) which demonstrated that deficits in a variety of visual processes (e.g. visual perception and visual sequencing) did not appear to play a causal role. More recently, there have been several new lines of enquiry with some supporting evidence, although conceptual and methodological difficulties continue to render this area of enquiry problematic (Skottun and Skoyles 2008). At the current time, there are insufficient grounds for claims that visual processing problems cause reading disability/dyslexia (American Academy of Pediatrics, 2011).

The development of our understanding of the role of visual factors has not been assisted by journalists' enthusiasm for much-heralded 'miracle cures' which have often promised more than could be delivered and which have not been subsequently validated by well-designed research evaluations. One approach that has received extensive media coverage involves treatments designed to reduce glare from bright lighting or white page backgrounds and limit the strain upon eyes resulting from sustained focusing. Such difficulties have been variously labelled as visual stress (Singleton 2009), Meares-Irlen syndrome (Irlen 1991), or scotopic sensitivity. Irlen (1983), who is largely credited with highlighting the condition and designing treatment approaches, has claimed that between 50% and 75% of children with dyslexic profiles may suffer from such sensitivity.

In response to the widespread publicity which resulted from Irlen's work, Wilkins (2003) designed the Intuitive Colorimeter, a piece of apparatus which can throw light of various shades and strength on to texts, that is now employed by some optometrists. Assessment, with the aid of this machine, it is argued, permits the prescription of coloured lenses individually tailored to the client's specific requirements. He argues that while tinted glasses or overlays can lead to gains in reading speed for reading disabled children, gains do not appear to be significantly greater than for normal readers with visual stress difficulties. Wilkins (2003) has been careful to differentiate between reading disability/dyslexia and visual stress, and researchers are now increasingly understanding these as problems with different symptoms and origins.

Perceptuo-motor difficulties

The frequent observation that many poor readers show signs of mild clumsiness, particularly postural stability and balance problems, has resulted in a degree of research interest. Perhaps the most popular theory stemming from such observations is that involving cerebellar dysfunction. According to this theory's proponents (Nicolson et al. 2001; Stoodley and Stein 2011), cerebellar dysfunction results in a failure to achieve high-level automaticity of a variety of skills that are important for reading acquisition. According to Nicolson and Fawcett (1995), motor difficulties do not directly act as causal factors in reading disability but, rather, reflect underlying cerebellar impairments.

As is the case for many processes underlying reading difficulty, research studies have produced conflicting findings. The majority of studies report that between 35% and 65% of struggling readers demonstrate some level of motor difficulty (Ramus *et al.* 2003; Chaix *et al.* 2007). However, the evidence for a causal relationship is generally considered to be weak (Rochelle and Talcott 2006), and many studies in this area have been criticised for being of varied quality (Savage 2004).

The role of intelligence in the diagnosis of dyslexia

At the heart of the dyslexia debate lies the thorny issue of intelligence. In work with those with reading difficulties, the frequent parental comment, 'I know he can't read but he's not daft!' typically reflects the concern and frustration often felt by those who perceive the stigmatising impact of their child's difficulties in learning to read. In our society, illiteracy is often perceived as shameful, and the humiliation involved can be a painful experience that may be carried and sustained throughout adulthood (McNulty 2003). It is no wonder, then, that parents are often happy for their child to receive a quasi-medical diagnosis of dyslexia. In the minds of many, such a diagnosis helps to separate intellectual from literacy weakness and offers a picture of the dyslexic as someone who, while perfectly 'normal', has a particular difficulty which hinders their development in a highly specific area of functioning. In addition, as is the case in medicine, it is hoped that a diagnosis will help to indicate an effective method of intervention.

For many, then, the dyslexic is typically frustrated and thwarted by being unable to read and write at a level commensurate with his or her intellectual functioning. Thus, it is unsurprising that perhaps a widely used criterion employed in diagnosis has involved searching for a discrepancy between IQ and measured reading ability (Presland 1991). The most common method of ascertaining this is by predicting an individual's expected reading score on the basis of his or her IQ score. Where the difference between predicted and actual scores is great, it has been widely argued that a specific difficulty is present (McNab 1994).

Despite IQ's continuing resonance with many practitioners, multiple findings from research studies have clearly shown that decoding ability is largely independent of intellectual functioning (e.g. Fletcher *et al.* 1994; Stanovich and Stanovich 1997). While poor readers with low IQ scores may, by virtue of their more limited reasoning skills, be less able to use meaning, inference and syntactic knowledge to help them to make sense of text, they tend to experience no greater or lesser problems than their 'dyslexic' peers when they try to read individual words – the crucial area for dyslexia (Stanovich 1991). In addition, IQ appears not to offer meaningful information about how well the poor reader will respond to intervention (Stuebing *et al.* 2009). Such findings, then, have seriously called into question the suggestion that poor readers can be differentiated on the basis of discrepancies between intellectual functioning and reading ability. In the light of these findings, a key piece of special education legislation in the United States, the

Individuals with Disabilities Education Improvement Act 2004 (IDEA), now states that an IQ discrepancy is not necessary for a diagnosis of learning disability, as was formerly the case.

As noted above, one reason why dyslexia is a sought-after diagnosis is that there is a very real danger that reading difficulty will be equated with limited academic ability. When this is the case, some children may encounter low teacher, peer and, possibly, parental expectations and, as a result, intellectual challenge may be reduced. Because of the widespread perception that the dyslexic is often highly intelligent, it is sometimes considered that being assigned such a label will raise teacher expectations. In turn, it is hoped that this will result in the provision of a stimulating and demanding education which will stretch rather than demotivate the child. An example of the power of expectations is provided in the case study of Aidan, below.

Aidan, aged 13, was the younger of two brothers, both of whom had a long-standing history of reading difficulty. He attended a local comprehensive school, which, while enjoying a sound record of public examination success, employed a rigid system of streaming, based upon end-of-term examinations.

Assessment of Aidan's reading demonstrated a significant mismatch between his reading accuracy and reading comprehension (as measured by a standardised reading test). Aidan's reading accuracy was consistent with that of an average 9-year-old while his comprehension was superior by approximately two and a half years. Aidan's performance on a standardised spelling test was at an age equivalence of 8 years and 4 months.

Intellectual assessment, using the Wechsler Intelligence Scales for Children (Revised), indicated that Aidan was functioning within the top 5% of the population. He performed well on spatial tasks (such as recreating patterns using wooden blocks and ordering pictures to tell a story) and excelled on a number of verbal measures involving general knowledge, comprehension and reasoning. His only significant weakness involved a short-term memory task where he was required to repeat a string of numbers spoken aloud.

It was clear that Aidan could compensate for his poor decoding skills by employing his high intellect to assist him to make sense of text. In a manner similar to that when one is attempting to master a foreign language, he would use his understanding of the grammatical structures of language, and inferential skills, to guess words difficult to recognise and thus draw meaning from the text.

Reliance upon internal examinations for streaming decisions had resulted in Aidan being placed in the lowest stream. In discussion with him, it became clear that this was proving highly problematic. Aidan complained that his classmates often teased him for displaying enthusiasm in class and for the fact that his orientation to school life and peer relationships often seemed to mark him out as different. A further frustration stemmed from what was, for him, an unstimulating and unchallenging curriculum. Although Aidan experienced difficulty in achieving high grades in his examinations, this was largely a reflection of his underdeveloped literacy skills rather than an inability to understand the ideas and concepts which were presented to him. His teachers confirmed the fact that he was quick to grasp ideas and had a sound analytic ability yet, surprisingly, the possibility of inappropriate placement had not appeared to register with them.

In a series of meetings with school staff, the educational psychologist highlighted Aidan's superior intellectual ability, his frustration with the content of many of his lessons and his unhappiness in being placed within a class of somewhat disaffected, unmotivated youngsters. After prolonged debate, the teachers accepted the recommendation that Aidan should be placed in a higher stream. Furthermore, it was agreed that his written performance in end-of-term examinations should not be seen as adequately representing his learning. Aidan's teachers were asked to ensure that his schoolwork was intellectually challenging and not impeded by his difficulties in reading. This, of course, made significant demands upon his teachers who, in large part, were enthusiastic and diligent in tailoring aspects of their lesson delivery to meet his needs.

As note-taking was an important element of schoolwork, Aidan was subsequently encouraged to record notes using audiotapes. This necessitated the employment of a highly structured filing system in order to ensure ready access to these materials. Aidan's capacity for organisation, coupled with a high level of motivation and support from volunteer sixth-formers, ensured that this proved highly effective. Direct intervention aimed at helping him to develop reading and spelling skills continued outside of classroom hours. Some months later his teachers reported that Aidan was far more cheerful and, despite ongoing difficulties with reading and spelling, was making excellent progress in his learning.

The key issue here is not that intelligence proved to be an important factor in diagnosing dyslexia. Nor can it be considered that by demonstrating his above-average intelligence, the appropriate 'treatment' was indicated. What intellectual assessment did help to highlight was that Aidan's ability to grasp and work with difficult ideas and concepts was being obscured by an inappropriate system of assessment placing too great a reliance upon written scripts. Confirmation of Aidan's abilities by the educational psychologist resulted in a changed classroom environment and higher teacher expectations, which, while not a 'cure' for his literacy difficulties, at least ensured that intellectual challenge was maintained.

The above case study serves as a good illustration of the benefits to an individual of a thorough assessment of strengths and weaknesses, rather than the use of a diagnostic label. Not only did Aidan receive a more appropriate education, recognition of his intellectual abilities may have helped him to cope with the threats to his self-esteem caused by his placement and treatment by his peers. There is much evidence (e.g. Edwards 1994) that the dyslexic child may be treated harshly, feel humiliated, be discriminated against or undervalued, experience a range of highly negative emotions, and, as a result, develop a diminished sense of self. However, we should question whether such experiences are any less demeaning or harmful for those poor readers who are not labelled dyslexic. Indeed, does the case for sensitivity and special treatment for the dyslexic leave other poor readers feeling even more stigmatised as a result? It is possible that what may benefit some will prove costly to others. This is not to say that the unfortunate experiences of some dyslexics should be discounted, rather that schools need to provide sensitive and supportive environments for all children who encounter learning difficulties.

Intervention approaches

As has been noted, it has often proven difficult to differentiate between dyslexic and other poor readers. If causes and symptoms cannot be clearly identified for such a subgroup, does a diagnosis of dyslexia assist in formulating a clear intervention strategy?

It is widely accepted that poor readers require teaching approaches which focus upon the ability to decode words using a knowledge of letter sounds, singly and in combination. One of the teaching techniques most associated with dyslexic children is multisensory learning. This highly structured approach involves the child learning the names, sounds and shapes of letters by accessing a number of sensory channels – hearing, touch, vision and movement. Such work is conducted individually or in small groups either in school or, typically, in a specialist centre for dyslexic children. A variety of multisensory programmes exist, some of the most common being based upon the Fernald Approach (Fernald 1943) and the Orton-Gillingham Method (Orton 1967). Despite its popularity with dyslexia specialists, much of the endorsement cited by advocates has arisen from case study material (e.g. Riccio et al. 2010), and high-quality research evidence for the multisensory component of structured approaches to reading intervention is sparse (Everatt and Reid 2009) and not overly convincing (Pennington et al. 2007).

Much debate has focused upon whether the teaching of reading should focus upon the explicit instruction of decoding skills involving knowledge of letters and letter combinations or through 'whole-language' approaches in which phonic knowledge is acquired explicitly, or implicitly, through everyday reading and writing activities. It is important here to recognise that the naturalistic, whole-language (sometimes misleadingly called the 'real books') approach to instruction, sometimes undertaken in isolation, has been found to be ill-suited for those who experience complex reading difficulties (see Elliott and Grigorenko 2012, for a detailed review of the 'reading wars' between proponents of these two contrasting approaches). Children with reading disability do not generally need significantly different forms of reading instruction. Like all beginning readers, they require inputs on print-related concepts, phonological awareness, phonics, an emphasis upon reading smoothly and fluently, vocabulary, comprehension, spelling and writing, which are differentially weighted according to their own particular strengths and weaknesses and which will maximise their interest and motivation (Wharton-Macdonald 2011). However, unlike their more skilled peers, those with reading difficulties will also require interventions that are more individualised, more structured, more explicit, more systematic and more intense, in ways by which nothing is left to chance (Torgesen 2004).

The importance of identifying and intervening with those at risk of reading difficulties at as young an age as possible is now widely accepted (Scanlon et al. 2005). Many countries now operate variants of a response to intervention (RTI) model in which children receive additional, highly structured support in small groups or, individually, in cases of severe difficulty, as soon as signs of poor academic progress are noted. Such an approach has been contrasted with a traditional 'wait to fail' model, whereby intervention only occurs after a lengthy period of observation and assessment. RTI has proven particularly popular in the United States although its emphasis upon academic skills, rather than underlying cognitive processes, has resulted in fierce criticism in some quarters (Reynolds and Shaywitz 2009). In response to such criticisms, proponents argue that there is little evidence that cognitive profiling is of sufficient value for informing individualised reading interventions to justify the high costs involved (Fletcher and Vaughn 2009). In similar vein, Vellutino et al. conclude that 'intelligence tests have little utility for diagnosing specific reading disability' (2004: 29) and recommend that practitioners should

> shift the focus of their clinical activities away from emphasis on psychometric assessment to detect cognitive and biological causes of a child's reading difficulties for purposes of categorical labelling in favour of assessment that would eventuate in educational and remedial activities tailored to the child's individual needs.
>
> (Vellutino et al. 2004: 31)

There is little evidence that, within the general pool of children with reading disability, there exists a subset of dyslexics who require alternative, specialised forms of intervention (Stanovich 1991; Vellutino et al. 2000). Indeed, it is generally considered that the highly structured, phonics-based approach that is widely advocated for those diagnosed as dyslexics is equally appropriate for all poor readers (Rice and Brooks 2004), as are other rather broader intervention programmes (Hatcher and Hulme 1999; Shaywitz et al. 1992).

The desire to discover ways of treating dyslexia other than through educational interventions has persisted over the past century and there continue to be many claims for the utility of various alternative or complementary therapies including visual and auditory training, biofeedback, dietary supplements, and perceptual-motor training. However, evidence offered to support such programmes tends to place over-reliance upon personal testimonials, anecdotes, case-studies and in-house investigations (Hyatt et al. 2009). When subjected to the rigours of scientific evidence-based scrutiny, there is little evidence that these approaches are effective in overcoming complex reading difficulties (Snowling 2010). In relation to visual programmes, for example, a joint technical report produced by the American Academy of Pediatrics concludes that

> scientific evidence does not support the efficacy of eye exercises, behavioral/ perceptual vision therapy, training glasses, or special tinted filters or lenses in improving the long-term educational performance in these complex pediatric neurocognitive conditions.
>
> (American Academy of Pediatrics 2011: e849)

The case study of Aidan has indicated the importance of recognising that reading difficulties may mask true levels of intellectual functioning. Having understood this principle, teachers may be more likely to reflect upon the content and mode of their educational delivery in order to ensure that the able child with reading difficulties is appropriately challenged. Recognition of the need to assist the child in such a fashion, however, does not mean that his or her needs for additional resources are greater than those of other poor readers whose cognitive abilities are weaker. Indeed, one might go so far as to argue that ongoing adult support, guidance and regulation may be more necessary in the case of those with more global difficulties.

Outcomes

While, if tackled early with specialised and structured teaching, many children with reading difficulties can be helped to progress to functioning within normal levels (Torgesen 2005), there continues to be a significant proportion who fail to make adequate progress, with problems persisting throughout the school years and remaining a problem in adulthood (Rutter et al. 2006). Some young children, when provided with highly structured, high-quality intervention, will make initial gains but drop back when they reach the age of 8 or 9, when the nature of reading demands increases substantially (Vellutino et al. 2008). In the United States, it has been estimated that these 'treatment resisters' account for between 2% and 6% of the school population (Vaughn and Roberts 2007). In adolescence, the situation becomes even more complex as the precise nature of students' reading difficulties will become more varied. Some will continue to struggle at the letter–sound level, others will only encounter problems with relatively complex multisyllabic words. Some may no longer encounter problems in decoding words but find it difficult to read fluently. As a result of many years of arduous and laborious reading, many students may be left with a limited vocabulary and poor concept knowledge, struggle to comprehend passages of text, and lack motivation to read (Biancarosa and Snow 2006). Unfortunately, systematic, well-funded research projects geared to helping those with the greatest difficulties continue to yield disappointing results (Scammacca et al. 2007; Vaughn et al. 2010) and, other than calling for even more intense and individualised interventions, there seems to be little knowledge as to how this problem may be overcome.

Sadly, many poor readers will take the burden of associated emotional insecurity and low self-esteem into their adult lives (McNulty 2003). Given this picture, it is hardly surprising that there is some (albeit limited) evidence that those with reading disability tend to stop their education at an earlier age and have less success in employment (Spreen 1987). We are, however, familiar with accounts of famous people – such as Churchill and Leonardo da Vinci – who, despite reading and spelling difficulties, achieved greatness. From such individuals, perhaps, we should recognise the fact that reading difficulties are not necessarily barriers to success. In addition to tackling reading difficulties directly, therefore, parents, teachers and others should ensure that assistance focuses upon the use of technological aids, the development of organisational strategies and, perhaps most importantly, the enhancement of the child's perceived competence and sense of self-esteem.

The way forward?

Rutter (1998) has criticised the dyslexia literature on the grounds that attempts have been made to define the term before it has been made clear what exactly is being investigated. There continue to be significant differences in understandings of terms such as dyslexia and reading disability both across and within academic disciplines and professional groupings. Perhaps the most appropriate way forward at the present time is to use the terms 'dyslexia' or 'reading disability' to describe the problem of all those who struggle to decode single words (Elliott and Grigorenko 2012). Such an approach would seem to avoid the need to differentiate poor readers into groupings that have questionable validity or have little value for informing intervention.

While our understandings of the biological bases of reading difficulty have advanced significantly, these continue to offer little to those who seek to assist in the education of those with such problems. Cognitive science has also identified a number of processes that appear to be important for understanding reading disability, yet it appears that none of these can fully account for the problems of all poor readers and there continues to be much debate and inconsistency in respect of research findings. To date, most work in this area has had only limited relevance for the planning of individually tailored intervention programmes.

The literature is replete with a large variety of intervention techniques with varying support from high-quality, rigorous research evaluations. Some of these directly address specific language-based deficits, some utilise a variety of alternative or complementary therapies, some draw upon new technologies to tackle or circumvent literacy difficulties, and others reflect existing good practices in the teaching of reading (e.g. paired or shared reading). We now have much information about the best ways to intervene with those at risk of reading disability from an early age – through the operation of intense, explicit, structured instruction centring upon the development of early reading skills. We have also learned much about how best to intervene with older struggling readers although, despite the availability of highly intensive and systematic programmes that cater for individual differences, we continue to struggle to help a small proportion with the most severe difficulties to develop adequate reading skills.

The insights we have gained from rigorous intervention studies have typically involved a general pool of struggling readers that has not been selected on the basis of some dyslexic cognitive profile. It seems likely that, despite the contradictions and inconsistencies of professional opinion, decisions about the nature of intervention should continue to focus upon the general needs of those with reading difficulties, with some adjustment according to individual circumstances, rather than any division into dyslexic/poor reader camps. Similarly, at the current time, there would appear to be insufficient moral or empirical grounds for allocating additional resources, or high-stakes testing accommodations, to those who are labelled dyslexic while leaving other poor readers – those, perhaps, deemed by some to have limited potential – to struggle unaided.

Sources of further help

http://www.interdys.org/
http://www.bda-dyslexia.org.uk
http://www.dyslexiaaction.org.uk/
http://www.fcrr.org/

References

Adams, M.J. (1990). *Beginning to Read: Thinking and Learning about Print*. Cambridge, MA: MIT Press.

Alloway, T.P., Gathercole, S.E., Kirkwood, H.J. *et al.* (2009). The cognitive and behavioral characteristics of children with low working memory. *Child Development* 80: 606–21.

American Academy of Pediatrics (2011). Joint technical report: Learning disabilities, dyslexia and vision. *Pediatrics* 127(3): e818–56.

Biancarosa, G. and Snow, C.E. (2006). *Reading Next: A Vision for Action and Research in Middle and High School Literacy. A Report to the Carnegie Corporation of New York, Second Edition*. Washington, DC: Alliance for Excellent Education.

Boets, B., Wouters, J., van Wieringen, A. *et al.* (2007). Auditory processing, speech perception and phonological ability in preschool children at high-risk of dyslexia: A longitudinal study of the auditory temporal processing theory. *Neuropsychologia* 45: 1608–20.

Bradley, L. and Bryant, P.E. (1983). Categorising sounds and learning to read: A causal connection. *Nature* 301: 419–21.

British Psychological Society (1999). *Dyslexia, Literacy and Psychological Assessment: Report by a Working Party of the Division of Educational and Child Psychology of the British Psychological Society*. Leicester: British Psychological Society.

Brooks, G. (2002). *What Works for Children with Literacy Difficulties? The Effectiveness of Intervention Schemes*. Department for Education and Skills Research Report 380. London: DfES.

Brunswick, N., McDougall, S. and de Mornay Davies, P. (eds) (2010). *Reading and Dyslexia in Different Orthographies*. New York: Psychology Press.

Carter, D.R., Chard, D.J. and Pool, J.L. (2009). A family strengths approach to early language and literacy development. *Early Childhood Education Journal* 36: 519–26.

Chaix, Y., Albaret, J., Brassard, C. *et al.* (2007). Motor impairment in dyslexia: The influence of attention disorders. *European Journal of Paediatric Neurology* 11: 368–74.

Cooke, A. (2001). Critical response to 'Dyslexia, Literacy and Psychological Assessment, (Report by a Working Party of the Division of Educational and Child Psychology of the British Psychological Society)': A view from the chalk face. *Dyslexia* 7(1): 47–52.

Corriveau, K.H., Goswami, U. and Thomson, J.M. (2010). Auditory processing and early literacy skills in a preschool and kindergarten population. *Journal of Learning Disabilities* 43(4): 369–82.

Edwards, J. (1994). *The Scars of Dyslexia*. London: Cassell.

Elliott, C.D., Murray, D.J. and Pearson, L. (1983). *British Ability Scales*. Windsor: NFER-Nelson.

Elliott, J.G. and Gibbs, S. (2008). Does dyslexia exist? *Journal of Philosophy of Education* 42(3/4), 475–91.

Elliott, J.G. and Grigorenko, E.L. (2012). *The Dyslexia Debate*. New York: Cambridge University Press.

Everatt, J. and Reid, G. (2009). Dyslexia: An overview of recent research. In G. Reid (ed.) *The Routledge Companion to Dyslexia* (pp. 3–21). New York: Routledge.

Fernald, G. (1943). *Remedial Techniques in the Basic School Subjects*. New York: McGraw-Hill.

Fletcher, J.M., Lyon, G.R., Fuchs, L.S. *et al.* (2007). *Learning Disabilities: From Identification to Intervention*. New York: Guilford Press.

Fletcher, J.M., Shaywitz, S.E., Shankweiler, D. *et al.* (1994). Cognitive profiles of reading disability: Comparisons of discrepancy and low achievement definitions. *Journal of Educational Psychology* 86: 6–23.

Fletcher, J.M. and Vaughn, S. (2009). Response to intervention: Preventing and remediating academic difficulties. *Child Development Perspectives* 3(1): 30–7.

Frith, U. (1997). Brain, mind and behaviour in dyslexia. In C. Hulme and M.J. Snowling (eds) *Dyslexia: Biology, Cognition, and Intervention* (pp. 1–19). London: Whurr.

Goswami, U. (2009). Memorandum submitted by Professor Usha Goswami. In House of Commons, Science and Technology Committee, *Evidence Check 1: Early Literacy Interventions* (pp. Ev83–5). London: Stationery Office.

Goswami, U. (2010). Neuroscience in education. In C.L. Cooper, J. Field, U. Goswami *et al.* (eds) *Mental Capital and Mental Wellbeing* (pp. 55–62). Oxford: Blackwell.

Goswami, U., Gerson, D. and Astruc, L. (2010). Amplitude envelope perception, phonology and prosodic sensitivity in children with developmental dyslexia. *Reading and Writing* 23: 995–1019.

Griffiths, Y.M., Hill, N.I., Bailey, P.J. *et al.* (2003). Auditory temporal order discrimination and backward recognition masking in adults with dyslexia. *Journal of Speech, Language, and Hearing Research* 46: 1352–66.

Grigorenko, E.L. (2004). Genetic bases of developmental dyslexia: A capsule review of heritability estimates. *Enfance* 3: 273–87.

Grigorenko, E.L. and Naples, A.J. (2009). The devil is in the details: Decoding the genetics of reading. In P. McCardle and K. Pugh (eds) *Helping Children Learn to Read: Current Issues and New Directions in the Integration of Cognition, Neurobiology and Genetics of Reading and Dyslexia* (pp. 133–48). New York: Psychological Press.

Hatcher, P.J. and Hulme, C. (1999). Phonemes, rhymes and intelligence as predictors of children's responsiveness to remedial reading instruction: Evidence from a longitudinal intervention study. *Journal of Experimental Child Psychology* 72(2): 130–53.

Heaton, P. and Winterton, P. (1996). *Dealing with Dyslexia*, Second edition. London: Whurr.

Herrington, M. and M. Hunter-Carsch. 2001. A social interactive model of specific learning difficulties. In M. Hunter-Carsch (ed.) *Dyslexia: A Psycho-Social Perspective* (pp. 107–33). London: Whurr.

Hulme, C. and Snowling, M.J. (2009). *Developmental Disorders of Language Learning and Cognition*. Oxford: Wiley-Blackwell.

Hyatt, K.J., Stephenson, J. and Carter, M. (2009). A review of three controversial educational practices: Perceptual motor programs, sensory integration, and tinted lenses. *Education and Treatment of Children* 32(2): 313–42.

Irlen, H. (1983). Successful treatment of learning disabilities. Paper presented at the 91st Annual Convention of the American Psychological Association, Anaheim, CA.

Irlen, H. (1991). *Reading by the Colours*. New York: Avery.

Johnson, E.S, Humphrey, M., Mellard, D.F. *et al.* (2010). Cognitive processing deficits and students with specific learning disabilities: A selective meta-analysis of the literature. *Learning Disability Quarterly* 33(1): 3–18.

Kamhi, A.G. and Laing, S.P. (2001). The path to reading success or failure: A choice for the new millennium. In J.L. Harris, A.G. Kamhi and K.E. Pollock (eds) *Literacy in African American Communities* (pp. 127–45). Mahwah, NJ: Lawrence Erlbaum.

Leonard, C.M., Eckert, M.A., Lombardino, L.J. *et al.* (2001). Anatomical risk factors for phonological dyslexia. *Cerebral Cortex* 11: 148–57.

Lundberg, I. (1994). Reading difficulties can be predicted and prevented: A Scandinavian perspective on phonological awareness and reading. In C. Hulme and M. Snowling (eds) *Reading Development and Dyslexia*. London: Whurr.

Lundberg, I., Frost, J. and Petersen, O.P. (1988). Effects of an extensive programme for stimulating phonological awareness in pre-school children. *Reading Research Quarterly* 33: 263–84.

Lyon, G.R. (1995). Towards a definition of dyslexia. *Annals of Dyslexia* 45: 3–27.

Manis, F.R., Doi, L.M. and Bhadha, B. (2000). Naming speed, phonological awareness, and orthographic knowledge in second graders. *Journal of Learning Disabilities* 33: 325–33.

McArthur, G.M., Ellis, D. Atkinson, C.M. *et al.* (2008). Auditory processing deficits in children with reading and language impairments: Can they (and should they) be treated? *Cognition* 107(3): 946–77.

McNab, I. (1994). *Specific Learning Difficulties: How Severe is Severe?* (BAS Information Booklet). Windsor: NFER-Nelson.

McNulty, M.A. (2003). Dyslexia and the life course. *Journal of Learning Disabilities* 36: 363–81.

Menghini, D., Carlesimo, G.A., Marotta, L. *et al.* (2010). Developmental dyslexia and explicit long-term memory. *Dyslexia* 16: 213–25.

Morgan, P.L., Fuchs, D., Compton, D.L. *et al.* (2008). Does early reading failure decrease children's reading motivation? *Journal of Learning Disabilities* 41(5): 387–404.

National Early Literacy Panel (2008). *Developing Early Literacy: Report of the National Early Literacy Panel*. Washington, DC: National Institute for Literacy. Available at http://www.nifl.gov/earlychildhood/NELP/NELPreport.html.

Nicholson, T. (1997). Social class and reading achievement: Sociology meets psychology. *New Zealand Journal of Educational Studies* 32: 105–8.

Nicolson, R.I. and Fawcett, A.J. (1995). Dyslexia is more than a phonological disability. *Dyslexia* 1: 19–36.

Nicolson, R.I., Fawcett, A.J. and Dean, P. (2001). Developmental dyslexia: The cerebellar deficit hypothesis. *Trends in Neurosciences* 24: 508–12.

Norwich, B. (2009). How compatible is the recognition of dyslexia with inclusive education? In G. Reid (ed.) *The Routledge Companion to Dyslexia* (pp. 177–92). New York: Routledge.

Orton, J.L. (1967). The Orton-Gillingham Approach. In J. Mooney (ed.) *The Disabled Reader.* Baltimore, MD: Johns Hopkins University Press.

Pennington, B.F. (2009). *Diagnosing Learning Disorders: A Neuropsychological Framework,* Second edition. New York: Guilford Press.

Pennington, B.F and Bishop, D.V.M. (2009). Relations among speech, language and reading disorders. *Annual Review of Psychology* 40: 663–81.

Plomin, R. and Rutter, M. (1998). Child development, molecular genetics, and what to do with genes once they are found. *Child Development* 69: 1223–42.

Pokorni, J.L., Worthington, C.K. and Jamison, P.J. (2004). Phonological awareness intervention: Comparison of Fast ForWord, Earobics, and LiPS. *Journal of Educational Research* 97: 147–57.

Presland, J. (1991). Explaining away dyslexia. *Educational Psychology in Practice* 6(4): 215–21.

Ramus, F., Pidgeon, E. and Frith, U. (2003). The relationship between motor control and phonology in dyslexic children. *Journal of Child Psychology and Psychiatry* 44: 712–22.

Ramus, F. and Szenkovits, G. (2009). Understanding the nature of the phonological deficit. In K. Pugh and P. McCardle (eds) *How Children Learn to Read* (pp. 153–70) New York: Psychology Press.

Regan, T. and Woods, K. (2000). Teachers' understandings of dyslexia: Implications for educational psychology practice. *Educational Psychology in Practice* 16: 333–47.

Reynolds, C.R. and Shaywitz, S.E. (2009). Response to intervention: Ready or not? Or, from wait-to-fail to watch-them-fail. *School Psychology Quarterly* 24(2): 130–45.

Riccio, C.A., Sullivan, J.R. and Cohen, M.J. (2010). *Neuropsychological Assessment and Intervention for Childhood and Adolescent Disorders.* New Jersey: John Wiley.

Rice, M. and Brooks, G. (2004) *Developmental Dyslexia in Adults: A Research Review.* London: NRDC.

Rochelle, K.S. and Talcott, J.B. (2006). Impaired balance in developmental dyslexia? A meta-analysis of the contending evidence. *Journal of Child Psychology and Psychiatry* 47(11): 1159–66.

Rutter, M. (1978). Prevalence and types of dyslexia. In A. Benton and D. Pearl (eds) *Dyslexia: An Appraisal of Current Knowledge* (pp. 5–28). New York: Oxford University Press.

Rutter, M. (1998). Dyslexia: Approaches to validation. *Journal of Child Psychology and Psychiatry Review* 3(1): 24–5.

Rutter, M.., Kim-Cohen, J. and Maughan, B. (2006). Continuities and discontinuities in psychopathology between childhood and adult life. *Journal of Child Psychology and Psychiatry* 47(3/4): 276–95.

Savage, R.S. (2004). Motor skills, automaticity and developmental dyslexia: A review of the research literature. *Reading and Writing: An Interdisciplinary Journal* 17: 301–24.

Savage, R.S., Lavers, N. and Pillay, V. (2007). Working memory and reading difficulties: What we know and what we don't know about the relationship. *Educational Psychology Review* 19: 185–221.

Scammacca, N., Roberts, G., Vaughn, S. *et al.* (2007). *Reading Interventions for Adolescent Struggling Readers: A Meta-Analysis with Implications for Practice.* Portsmouth, NH: RMC Research Corporation Center on Instruction.

Scanlon, D.M., Gelzheiser, L.M., Vellutino, F.R. *et al.* (2008). Reducing the incidence of early reading difficulties: Professional development for classroom teachers versus direct interventions for children. *Learning and Individual Differences* 18: 346–59.

Scanlon, D.M., Vellutino, F.R., Small, S.G. *et al.* (2005). Severe reading difficulties: Can they be prevented? A comparison of prevention and intervention approaches. *Exceptionality* 13: 209–27.

Scerri, T. and Schulte-Körne, G. (2010). Genetics of developmental dyslexia. *European Child and Adolescent Psychiatry* 19: 179–97.

Shaywitz, B.A., Fletcher, J., Holahan, J. *et al.* (1992). Discrepancy compared to low achievement definitions of reading disability: Results from the Connecticut Longitudinal Study. *Journal of Learning Disabilities* 25: 639–48.

Shaywitz, S.E. (2005). *Overcoming Dyslexia*. New York: Alfred Knopf.

Singleton, C. (2009). Visual stress and dyslexia. In G. Reid (ed.) *The Routledge Companion to Dyslexia* (pp. 43–57). London: Routledge.

Skottun, B.C. and Skoyles, J.R. (2008). Dyslexia and rapid visual processing: A commentary. *Journal of Clinical and Experimental Neuropsychology* 30(6): 666–73.

Slavin, R.E., Lake, C., Davis, S. *et al.* (2011). Effective programs for struggling readers: A best-evidence synthesis. *Educational Research Review* 6(1): 1–26.

Snowling, M.J. (2010) Dyslexia. In C.L. Cooper, J. Field, U. Goswami *et al.* (eds), *Mental Capital and Mental Wellbeing* (pp. 775–83). Oxford: Blackwell.

Spreen, O. (1987). *Learning Disabled Children Growing Up: A Follow-Up into Adulthood*. Lisse, Netherlands: Swets & Zeitlinger.

Stanovich, K.E. (1991). Discrepancy definitions of reading disability: Has intelligence led us astray? *Reading Research Quarterly* 26: 7–29.

Stanovich, K.E. and Siegel, L.S. (1994). The phenotypic performance profile of reading-disabled children: A regression-based test of the phonological-core variable-difference model. *Journal of Educational Psychology* 86: 24–53.

Stanovich, K.E. and Stanovich, P. J. (1997). Further thoughts on aptitude/achievement discrepancy. *Educational Psychology in Practice* 13(1): 3–8.

Stoodley, C.J. and Stein, J.F. (2011) The cerebellum and dyslexia, *Cortex* 47(1): 101–16.

Stuebing, K.K., Barth, A.E., Molfese, P.J. *et al.* (2009). IQ is not strongly related to response to reading instruction: A meta-analytic interpretation. *Exceptional Children* 76(1): 31–51.

Swanson, H.L., Howard, C.B. and Sáez, L. (2006). Do different components of working memory underlie different subgroups of reading disabilities? *Journal of Learning Disabilities* 39(3): 252–69.

Tallal, P. (1980). Auditory temporal perception, phonics, and reading disabilities in children. *Brain and Language* 9: 182–98.

Torgesen, J.K. (2004). Lessons learned from research on interventions for students who have difficulty learning to read. In P. McCardle and V. Chhabra (eds) *The Voice of Evidence in Reading Research* (pp. 355–82). Baltimore, MD: Brookes.

Torgesen, J.K. (2005). Recent discoveries on remedial interventions for children with dyslexia. In M.J. Snowling and C. Hulme (eds) *The Science of Reading: A Handbook* (pp. 521–37). Oxford: Blackwell.

Torppa, M., Lyytinen, P., Erskine, J. *et al.* (2010). Language development, literacy skills, and predictive connections to reading in Finnish children with and without familial risk for dyslexia. *Journal of Learning Disabilities* 43(4): 308–21.

Vaughn, S. and Roberts, G. (2007). Secondary interventions in reading: Providing additional instruction for students at risk. *Teaching Exceptional Children* 39(5): 40–6.

Vaughn, S., Denton, C.A. and Fletcher, J.M. (2010). Why intensive interventions are necessary for students with severe reading difficulties. *Psychology in the Schools* 47(5): 432–44.

Vellutino, F.R. (1979). *Dyslexia: Theory and Research*. Cambridge, MA: MIT Press.

Vellutino, F.R. (1987). Dyslexia. *Scientific American*, 1 March: 34–41.

Vellutino, F.R., Scanlon, D.M. and Lyon, G.R. (2000). Differentiating between difficult-to-remediate and readily remediated poor readers: More evidence against the IQ-achievement discrepancy definition for reading disability. *Journal of Learning Disabilities* 3: 223–38.

Vellutino, F.R., Fletcher, J.M., Snowling, M.J. *et al.* (2004). Specific reading disability (dyslexia): What have we learned in the past four decades? *Journal of Child Psychology and Psychiatry* 45: 2–40.

Vellutino, F.R., Scanlon, D.M., Zhang, H. *et al.* (2008). Using response to kindergarten and first grade intervention to identify children at-risk for long-term reading difficulties. *Reading and Writing* 21: 437–80.

Vukovic, R.K. and Siegel, L.S. (2006). The double-deficit hypothesis: A comprehensive analysis of the evidence. *Journal of Learning Disabilities* 39(1): 25–47.

Wagner, R.K. (2008). Rediscovering dyslexia: New approaches for identification and classification. In G. Reid, A. Fawcett, F. Manis and L. Siegel (eds). *The Sage Handbook of Dyslexia* (pp. 174–91). London: Sage.

Wagner, R.K. and Torgesen, J.K. (1987). The nature of phonological processing and its causal role in the acquisition of reading skills. *Psychological Bulletin* 101: 192–212.

Wharton-McDonald, R. (2011). Expert classroom instruction for students with reading disabilities: Explicit, intense, targeted . . . and flexible. In A. McGill-Franzen and R.L. Allington (eds) *Handbook of Reading Disability Research*. New York: Routledge.

White, S., Milne, E., Rosen, S. *et al.* (2006). The role of sensorimotor impairments in dyslexia: A multiple case study of dyslexic children. *Developmental Science* 9(3): 237–69.

Wilkins, A. (2003). *Reading Through Colour*. London: Wiley.

Wolf, M. and Bowers, P.G. (1999). The double-deficit hypothesis for the developmental dyslexias. *Journal of Educational Psychology* 91: 415–38.

Wolf, M., Bowers, P.G. and Biddle, K. (2000). Naming-speed processes, timing, and reading: A conceptual review. *Journal of Learning Disabilities* 33: 387–407.

Chapter 12

Developmental coordination disorder (dyspraxia)

Introduction

The clumsy individual is a longstanding and traditional figure of fun, although this often masks the distressing and incapacitating nature of such problems. While clinical accounts of motor difficulties featured in the scientific literature throughout the twentieth century, it is only relatively recently that detailed consideration has been given to the particular needs of this population. Burgeoning interest in this field has led to a proliferation of terms to describe this condition, which has not always resulted in conceptual clarity. Terms employed include: developmental dyspraxia, minimal brain dysfunction, perceptuomotor dysfunction, sensory integrative dysfunction, apraxia, physical awkwardness, developmental coordination disorder and the clumsy child syndrome. For many lay people, 'dyspraxia' is the more recognisable term. Derived from Greek, *dys* is a prefix meaning 'bad'. 'Praxis' relates to 'the learned ability to plan and carry out sequences of controlled movements in order to achieve an objective' (Ripley *et al.* 1999: 1). This emphasis upon planning highlights a strong cognitive element that impacts upon motor skills and co-ordinated movements.

Despite the hold the term dyspraxia has among the lay public and, in the UK, its widespread use by health and education professionals (Peters *et al.* 2001), 'developmental coordination disorder' (DCD) has been chosen by most international specialists as the preferred term (Polatajko *et al.* 1995a) and this is borne out by scrutiny of the terms used in the research literature (Magalhães *et al.* 2006).

According to the American Psychiatry Association's Diagnostic and Statistical Manual (DSM-IV) (APA 1994), four criteria are listed for DCD:

1 There is a significant impairment in the development of motor coordination.
2 The condition interferes with the academic progress of the child or with day-to-day activities.
3 The condition is not due to a general medical condition such as cerebral palsy or muscular dystrophy.
4 The condition is not primarily due to mental retardation.

It should be noted, however, that for some specialists, DCD and dyspraxia do not describe exactly the same condition. While the term DCD is now used in the majority of scientific publications, it remains, 'a fuzzy term without a precise definition' that describes 'a broad band of mild motor problems that researchers and practitioners are still struggling to refine' (Cermak *et al.* 2002: 22). DCD, it is argued (e.g. Kaplan *et al.* 1998), is unlikely to be a discrete condition, and almost certainly describes a heterogeneous grouping of difficulties. Attempts to derive subtypes, however, have resulted in only minimal success (Dewey 2002).

DCD's conceptual relationship with dyspraxia is similarly uncertain. Kimball (2002: 210) considers it 'debatable' whether the two terms are synonymous, and some consider that dyspraxia may describe a subgroup of children who have more severe motor planning problems. Steinman *et al.* (2010) have a rather different understanding and consider the term developmental dyspraxia to describe a sub-group of clumsy children whose problems are deemed to be neurological in origin and primarily concern skilled learned movements (or gestures), rather than more general problems of basic motor, perceptuomotor, linguistic or general cognitive functioning. Kirby and Drew (2003) differentiate between dyspraxia and DCD by contending that the former places greater emphasis upon planning. For these authors, DCD relates more closely to coordination and execution. Whereas the dyspraxic 'does not know what to do and how to move . . . the child with DCD has difficulties with coordination and execution' (2003: 6). Dewey and Kaplan (1994) offer another perspective and distinguish between three main groups of children with DCD: those with problems of balance, coordination and carrying out everyday motor activities, those who experience difficulty in planning and subsequently undertaking a series of motor actions (the group who are seen by many as being dyspraxic), and those who have problems in both of the above. Yet again, others differentiate between planning/sequencing and motor execution in relation to dyspraxia. In cases of ideomotor dyspraxia, the individual is seen as experiencing difficulty in performing even simple motor tasks when requested. This is less of a problem in the case of ideational dyspraxia where it is undertaking a sequence of multistep motor tasks rather than executing simple movements that is seen as parti-cularly problematic. While it is helpful to differentiate between cognition and action components of motor difficulties, it should be noted that current conceptualisations and labels do not consistently reflect this distinction (Missiuna and Polatajko 1995).

Prevalence

Irrespective as to whether psychiatric classification systems or standardised mea-sures of motor skill are employed, there is no clear, widely agreed quantifiable means of determining DCD or dyspraxia. For this reason, a consensus about preva-lence rates is not easily reached and different degrees of severity and forms of difficulty are often employed. Lewis (2003), for example, notes that studies using one of the most popular standardised assessment tools of motor performance have utilised a range of cut-off points for identifying children with DCD, ranging from the fifth to the twentieth centile.

Estimates for the primary school population range between 5% and 15% (Wilson 2005) although the two major classification systems, DSM-IV and the

World Health Organization's classification system (ICD-10) (1992), both provide estimates of approximately 5–6 % for children. A more conservative figure was provided by a large population-based study of children aged 7–8 years. Employing strict criteria, the study reported a prevalence rate of 1.8% although it was also noted that on the basis of broader cut-offs, the probable rate was 5% (Lingam *et al.* 2009). The proportion of children who actually receive a formal diagnosis from a medical professional is actually far smaller, in part because of a lack of professional knowledge of the condition (Missiuna *et al.* 2008). Males are more likely to be affected (Zoia *et al.* 2006), although the ratio of boys to girls in clinical samples (e.g. Miller *et al.* 2001) tends to be higher; this most likely reflecting the greater salience of boys with such problems. The condition becomes less prevalent in adulthood although difficulties often persist (Cantell *et al.* 1994).

Symptoms

If one itemised the various symptoms of DCD and dyspraxia described in the literature, the resulting list would be very long. However, not all children with DCD display exactly the same motor problems and there is little consensus as to the specific deficits that should underpin a diagnosis (Wilson 2005). Some children will have very specific difficulties while others may have a more generalised impairment (Polatajko and Cantin 2006). A high proportion of, but not all, children with DCD reach motor milestones (e.g. crawling, walking, speaking) at a later than average age. Others tend to show difficulties only with respect to the acquisition of more complex motor skills.

In addition to general difficulties of gross and fine motor coordination, common symptoms include: poor organisational skills, poor sense of direction, poor short-term memory, sensitivity to touch (including intolerance of having nails cut or hair and teeth brushed), and difficulty in establishing hand dominance. In addition, such children often exhibit emotional and behavioural difficulties such as obsessive or phobic behaviour, poor social maturity and skills, and a tendency to impatience.

The nature and impact of symptoms vary according to the child's age although in many cases a meaningful difficulty is often not identified until the child starts school. However, from early infancy, the child with DCD is more likely to exhibit attentional, feeding and sleeping difficulties. As noted above, independent crawling and walking may be delayed. During the primary school years, managing the difficulties that result from their poor gross and fine motor actions, and coping with the threat to their sense of self that results from this, are often key tasks. In adolescence, problems stemming from poor peer relations and, as academic and self-regulatory demands increase, a disorganised and unsystematic approach to learning often become increasingly salient.

In addition to a tendency to emotional immaturity, there appears to be a variety of secondary socio-emotional and behavioural problems that may result from the individual's attempts to cope with the shame and humiliation that the less physically adept so often experience in childhood. In the early years of life, play has a strong motoric nature and, as the child moves through the school years, poor performance in sports and other physical pursuits becomes a hindrance to achieving social status, leading to a greater likelihood of exclusion from the peer group (Livesey *et al.* 2011). As described in the case study below, children with DCD can easily become isolated onlookers (Smyth and Anderson 2000; Cairney *et al.* 2005). While emotional and behavioural problems may not emerge until adolescence (Hellgren *et al.* 1994) their social foundations can begin from a relatively early age (Short and Crawford 1984; Schoemaker and Kalverboer 1994). Children with poor motor skills are more likely to become withdrawn, develop a low sense of self-worth, and find themselves the victims of bullying (Piek *et al.* 2006).

Among this group are children who find it difficult to concentrate at school and become the class nuisance, children who are unhappy in school because they are bullied or socially isolated, children who cope with their clumsiness by becoming the class clown and children who withdraw completely from participation and remain unnoticed until it is too late to help them (Henderson and Sugden 1992: 6).

Given the above, it is hardly surprising that many such children have difficulties with academic subjects at school, despite their generally average IQ profile. In particular, studies have repeatedly demonstrated difficulties with written language, spelling and arithmetic (Fletcher-Flinn *et al.* 1997; Dewey and Kaplan 1994; Kadesjo and Gillberg 1999).

Danny's parents recognised early in his infancy that his motor skills were failing to develop in line with those of his peers. Rather than achieving the usual walking milestones, he tended to sit and watch others and liked to be carried. As he matured, he often bumped into inanimate objects, had a poor sense of balance, and encountered difficulty with dressing and tying laces. When seated, he would lock his legs behind the legs of his chair as if to anchor himself into a stable position from which he would not slide. Riding a bike or roller-skating were activities that were beyond his capabilities. Food was regularly spilled when eating, and a plastic table cloth that could be easily wiped clean proved indispensable. Although he received physiotherapy, his parents believe that this achieved little. At school, Danny proved to be an excellent reader and a quick learner although his handwriting was poor. For several years, he was provided with remedial handwriting exercises by occupational therapists and teachers but these only served to make him feel increasingly frustrated and self-conscious. As a young child, he tended to avoid the rough and tumble of the playground, preferring sedentary activities such as playing on the computer or reading. He enjoys film and drama, often creating complex imaginary plots in his head, but avoids singing and dancing. Although he is 14, Danny's parents still feel that they must organise his daily life as he appears to have little sense of time, and continues to react to events, rather than planning ahead. He appears uninterested in his personal appearance, and his mother feels obliged to assist in his daily grooming.

Danny's parents have always been far more concerned about his social than his physical difficulties. Watching him enter the schoolyard as an 8-year-old, his mother noted that he circled the periphery, hoping to be invited over to join his peers. When he commenced secondary school, Danny's earlier experience of relative social isolation as a young child was replaced by the challenges of a more hostile environment and he soon became a victim of bullying. Transfer to another school with stronger teacher regulation has proven beneficial and he has been far happier in this more structured environment. Harassment has now ceased and his mother often invites his schoolmates over to the house. Sadly, reciprocal invitations to their homes are relatively rare.

Comorbidity

Children with motor difficulties often display features of other conditions such as Asperger's syndrome, dyslexia and attention disorders. Indeed, Wilson (2005) claims that for DCD, comorbidity with other disorders is more the norm than the exception. The greater the severity of the coordination difficulties, the more will be the range and severity of other problems. In a study of children with ADHD, Kadesjo and Gillberg (2001) found that 47% had DCD. Kaplan et al. (1998) found that 69% of their ADHD and 63% of their dyslexic samples had DCD. In an examination of DCD clinic samples in Canada, Miller et al. (2001) found that where comorbidities were evident, 41% had reports of attention deficit disorder, 38% demonstrated a learning disability, 3% showed developmental delay, and 18% had other comorbidities. Portwood (1999) reported that approximately half of the clinical cases with which she was working experienced difficulty with language production.

Gaining a clear picture of clinical samples is often compounded by a tendency only to examine for DCD/dyspraxia in cases of severe difficulty (Ramus et al. 2003). Language problems are also often difficult to classify and the dyspraxic child may be seen by some to have semantic pragmatic disorder, a term used to describe difficulty in grasping the meaning of language used in its social context. Thus differential diagnosis may, in part, be determined by whether this is undertaken by a psychologist, psychiatrist, physiotherapist, speech and language therapist or paediatrician (Kirby 1999).

Causes

While the causes of DCD/dyspraxia are unknown, it is generally considered that these involve multiple factors that result in immature or atypical brain development (Kaplan et al. 1998). However, given that identifiable neurological disorders are exclusionary criteria for a diagnosis of DCD, this is a rather grey area (Dewey and Wilson 2001). Certainly research in this field is considerably less advanced than that in other areas such as dyslexia. Thus, while texts such as those of Portwood (1999), Macintyre (2001) and Kirby and Drew (2003) provide simple descriptions of how the brain functions and offer suggestions as to the origins of such conditions, it is important to recognise how little is actually known about the mechanisms involved. As with most developmental disorders, there appears to be some family link that is indicative of a genetic component (Martin *et al.* 2006).

At the cognitive level, a range of processing deficits has been examined. Problems have been found in visual perception (Lord and Hulme 1987), kinaesthetic perception (concerning awareness of limb position and movement (Laszlo *et al.* 1988b), the transfer of information from one sensory modality (e.g. vision, vestibular (inner-ear) functioning, proprioception, touch) to another (Newnham and McKenzie 1993), and the ability to select the most appropriate motor responses (van Dellen and Geuze 1988) and programme these in an effective fashion (Smyth 1991). One line of research (Mandich *et al.* 2002, 2003) has suggested that children with DCD have particular difficulty with inhibitory function; they tend to encounter difficulty ignoring irrelevant information and suppressing the production of unwanted responses. Such responses may concern either motor or cognitive (e.g. attention) functions.

In a wide-ranging review of motor control in children with DCD, Williams (2002: 137) states that, despite the rather limited amount of research available, the following underlying difficulties are often observed:

- significantly slower reaction – movement and times;
- universal difficulty with timing (e.g. rhythmic) control;
- frequent difficulty with force control (i.e. exerting an appropriate amount of pressure);
- over-reliance upon visual information as a means to regulate posture/ balance;
- greater vulnerability to situations where balance is disturbed (perturbation);
- an inability to adapt quickly to changes in movement demands;
- inefficient coordination of muscle-group activation to regulate balance;
- poor intersensory integration, especially concerning visual and proprioceptive information.

Assessment of motor skills

While a degree of conceptual and diagnostic confusion continues to prevail, researchers and clinicians are agreed that early recognition and assessment of children's motor difficulties are essential (Polatajko *et al.* 1995a). Not only can various forms of physical therapy be introduced but, equally important, all those who live and work with the child can be sensitised to the broader difficulties concerned, helped to modify the child's environment, and helped to recognise the need to minimise potential threats to the child's social and emotional well-being.

While a variety of tools are employed, there is still no 'gold standard' of assessment instruments for DCD (Sugden and Chambers 2003: 15). One of the most widely employed standardised measures for children is the Movement Assessment Battery for Children (M-ABC) (Henderson and Sugden 1992), now in revised format as the Movement ABC-2. (Henderson *et al.* 2007). Originally published two decades earlier as the Test of Motor Impairment (TOMI), this measure is concerned with both gross and fine motor skills and assesses manual dexterity, ball skills and balance. The second edition has been designed for use with children aged between 3 and 16 (the earlier version was for children aged 4–12). Despite the popularity of the M-ABC with researchers screening for DCD (Wilson 2005), as in the case for other widely used measures, it has been criticised for lacking a sound theoretical base (Cantell and Kooistra 2002). Other widely employed tests are the Bruininks-Oseretsky Test of Motor Proficiency (BOTMP) (Bruininks 1978) and the Developmental Test of Visual-Motor Integration (VMI) (Beery 1997). The BOTMP is widely used as a diagnostic tool by therapists (Miller *et al.* 2001). The VMI is popular with occupational therapists, although Missiuna and Pollock (1995) have recommended that it should be supplemented by assessment of the child's grasp, and of the time taken to complete the test. It is important to note, however, that the correlation between measures is not always high and the two most popular tests, the M-ABC and the BOTMP, do not consistently identify the same children as having motor impairments (Dewey and Wilson 2001). To overcome this, it is recommended that test results should be combined with observations of specialist clinicians (Crawford *et al.* 2001).

As measures that require individualised assessment of performance on standardised tasks are time-consuming and thus expensive for screening purposes, a variety of checklists has become available for this purpose. Some are designed to be completed by parents – the Developmental Coordination Disorder Questionnaire (DCDQ) (Wilson *et al.* 2000). Others, such as that forming part of the M-ABC2, are designed for therapists to obtain information from teachers and parents.

Schoemaker *et al.* (2003) testify to the M-ABC Checklist's psychometric properties although they found evidence that this measure, covering a broader range of motor skills, did not always confirm diagnoses derived from the M-ABC Test. Although it was anticipated that the Checklist would identify more children with motor problems (Henderson and Sugden 1992), there is some evidence to suggest that, for some age groups, it may identify a significant number of false positives, thus resulting in time-consuming and unnecessary diagnostic follow-up investigations (Schoemaker *et al.* 2003). It also appears that the Checklist may fail to highlight the movement problems of some children that are revealed by the Test (Junaid *et al.* 2000).

Intervention

Intervention for the physical aspects of DCD is usually undertaken by physiotherapists or occupational therapists, although teachers and educational psychologists may have an important role in respect of cognitive difficulties such as planning and organisation which can cause significant problems for schooling.

Intervention programmes may involve one or both of two broad forms (Sugden 2007). A focus can be placed upon addressing underlying processes of motor performance such as those concerning perception, memory, vision and kinaesthetics (sometimes known as 'bottom-up' approaches) or, alternatively, emphasis can be placed upon helping with task-specific problems ('top-down' or functional approaches).

Bottom-up approaches tend to be clustered into sensory integration training, process-orientated treatment or perceptual motor training (Mandich *et al.* 2001). Sensory integration, originally designed for children with learning disabilities, is based upon a belief that providing sensory stimulation will lead to an improvement in brain and motor functioning. Therapy involves full body movements that provide various forms of sensory stimulation – for example, vestibular, proprioception (awareness of one's own body) and tactile awareness. Much of the thinking in this area stems from the work of Ayres who defined sensory integration as

> a neurological process that organizes sensation from one's own body and from the environment, and makes it possible to use the body effectively within the environment. The spatial and temporal aspects of inputs from different sensory modalities are interpreted, associated and unified.
>
> (Ayres 1989: 11)

The evidence in support of bottom-up approaches is generally unpromising (Wilson 2005) and, where gains on test measures have been shown, there is an underlying question as to their generalisability to other situations and contexts (Mandich *et al.* 2001). Davidson and Williams (2000), for example, carried out a ten-week individualised programme of therapy that was followed by a year's activities recommended to the children's parents and teachers. The programme emphasised sensory integration of vestibular functioning, body awareness and touch, and perceptual-motor training of fine and gross motor activities. Although there was small improvement in some areas of functioning at twelve-month follow-up, the authors concluded that the clinical benefit of the intervention could not be demonstrated. Another research group (Laszlo and Bairstow 1985; Laszlo *et al.* 1988a) has produced evidence supporting the efficacy of their kinaesthetic approach; however, their experimental design has been criticised and other studies have failed to show similar gains (e.g. Polatajko *et al.* 1995b; Sims *et al.* 1996a, 1996b).

In a review of processing deficits in DCD, Wilson and McKenzie (1998) noted that while impaired processing of visual information appeared to be significant, no studies had examined whether training to improve visuo-spatial processing would result in improved motor coordination problems. However, a review of the role of visual perception in DCD (Rösblad 2002) concluded that there was little evidence to suggest that this was a major factor.

Top-down approaches appear to offer greater potential. The emphasis of such interventions is upon addressing directly specific difficulties encountered in the child's daily life. Thus the actual tasks that the child would normally encounter are identified and guidance is given on how these can be undertaken. Where necessary, the task is broken down into discrete steps that can be taught in isolation before being subsequently linked together. A second, cognitive, component of such approaches involves teaching the child various problem-solving strategies that are related to the performance of particular motor tasks.

Although it is generally argued that intervention can prove helpful, there is a dearth of well-controlled studies that can help indicate what forms of treatment are most effective with the various types of difficulties encountered. Chu (1998) argued that research of this kind was virtually non-existent although, more recently, researchers have begun to undertake such evaluations. As is the case in many clinical fields, the absence of a control group is a common feature. This is unsurprising given the concerns of many about the ethics of having groups of needy children who receive no intervention (Howard 1998).

Much of the earlier treatment evaluation work focused upon bottom–up approaches, although it would appear that the emphasis is shifting; two meta-analyses of research studies having pointed to the greater efficacy of top–down approaches (Pless and Carlsson 2000; Chen et al. 2003). In their review of six top–down approaches, Chen and colleagues found that these resulted in significant gains in motor skill acquisition and rather weaker indications of transfer of motor skills. However, it was acknowledged that these results have to be treated with caution (described by the authors as 'suggestive' rather than 'confirmatory') as the studies involved relatively small samples and none utilised control groups. Furthermore, all the studies ignored social and communication skills, which, as has been demonstrated in the case study of Danny above, often prove to be the more incapacitating difficulties.

One of the top–down programmes currently receiving significant attention in the literature is the Cognitive Orientation to daily Occupational Performance (CO-OP) (Polatajko et al. 2001a, 2001b). Reflecting a general shift towards the utilisation of cognitive approaches for those with special needs (Figg and Elliott 2003), the CO-OP is an individualised programme involving twelve one-hour training sessions. The programme has three major objectives: skill acquisition, cognitive strategy development, and generalisation and transfer. Initially, children are asked to select three skills that are important to them in daily life. During the intervention phases they are continually asked to analyse their performance and, where difficulties emerge, identify and try out possible means of overcoming these. The cognitive strategy employed, with theoretical and clinical roots in the work of Vygotsky, Feuerstein and Meichenbaum, is similar to many existing approaches in special education (Ashman and Conway 1997). These emphasise a cyclical process involving selecting goals, planning the means to undertake the task, carrying this out, and evaluating its effectiveness.

A repeated difficulty in intervention programmes concerns the problem of generalisation and transfer although, here too, top–down approaches appear to be more promising (Wilson 2005). While children with various forms of special need can often be taught knowledge or skills in a specific context, too often this new learning cannot be demonstrated at other times and in other settings. To help overcome this, CO-OP continually emphasises the application of strategies to everyday situations on the part of both the children and their parents (see Polatajko et al. 2001a, for further details).

Polatajko et al. (2001b) have suggested four particular reasons for the apparent efficacy of their approach:

1 Children select their own tasks which might result in enhanced motivation and greater understanding of goals.
2 The approach utilises verbal self-guidance that can subsequently develop into an internal means of self-regulation.
3 Emphasis is placed upon gaining rapport between therapist and child that facilitates a discovery-based approach to problems and solutions.
4 Children are asked to evaluate their performance. Recognition of their gains may result in a heightened sense of self-efficacy and confidence to tackle other motor difficulties.

In their review of several top-down approaches, Chen *et al.* (2003) found that CO-OP demonstrated the largest gains in skill acquisition. While there was some evidence that it resulted in skill transfer, this was weaker than for skill acquisition. Chen *et al.* suggest that this relatively weaker effect may be explained by the criteria employed, standardised measures, as these shared few characteristics with the children's self-selected tasks and may have appeared less meaningful to them. CO-OP has been described by one leading specialist in learning disorders (Pennington 2009: 233) as 'the one empirically validated best practice for particular motor disorders in childhood'.

Many of the interventions described in the literature are conducted by highly skilled physiotherapists and occupational therapists. Clearly, with prevalence rates so high, it is important that others, in daily contact with the child, are enabled to assist in programmes. Noting a dearth of controlled studies examining the efficacy of such approaches, Sugden and Chambers (2003) carried out a detailed evaluation of a top-down (task-orientated) programme (Henderson and Sugden 1992) in which teachers and parents were asked to provide individualised sessions lasting approximately twenty minutes for three to four sessions a week. The approach involved children performing functional tasks in (preferably) everyday settings and emphasised a problem-solving approach involving the planning, execution and evaluation of action. The teachers and parents involved in the intervention were charged with selecting appropriate skills (e.g. the manipulation of objects) and locating these in relevant settings. A high proportion of the children made, and sustained, gains as measured by the M-ABC and teacher and parent reports. Of course, fixed-term intervention studies undertaken by prestigious university researchers are more likely to result in parental and teacher engagement than everyday clinical recommendation. Such programmes require commitment and time and teachers often encounter difficulties in providing individualised pro-grammes. While some of the activities in the Sugden and Chambers study – for example, correctly gripping writing equipment or cutlery – were ongoing and thus dealt with routinely, both the teacher and parent groups reported that it had often been hard to find time in the daily routine to fit in the extra activities involved. To assist them, some teachers had drawn upon the services of teaching assistants, and several parents had enlisted the help of other family members. A further difficulty, noted by the authors, was that some children appeared to have gained little despite regular intervention. Whether these individuals would have benefited more from specialist intervention was unclear. Clearly, as with most developmental conditions, it is unlikely that children with DCD can be deemed to represent an homogeneous population that will respond similarly to one form of intervention. While teachers and parents may make an important contribution to intervention, it is important to make a distinction between roles. 'To pass responsibility for remediation to the school is to fail to distinguish between therapeutic intervention and educational practice' (Stephenson et al. 1991: 111).

In addition to supporting therapists in delivering therapy, parents and teachers need to focus upon whether there is a need to modify the child's environment. Many of the secondary difficulties that arise are less likely to occur if accommodations are made. Thus teachers are advised to substitute handouts or other note forms for conventional means of student written recording (Johnstone and Garcia 1994). Here, electronic aids may prove valuable, for example, children should be taught to use a keyboard early rather than labour with handwriting as this often continues to be slow and effortful (Missiuna and Pollock 1995).

In 2006, a seminar series on DCD, involving many of the leading researchers in the field, produced a Consensus Statement (Sugden 2006). In relation to intervention, the Statement outlined a number of key principles which should underpin the selection of approaches:

a) Activities should be functional and based on everyday operations. They should be meaningful to the child, their parents, teachers, and other key figures in their lives.
b) The child should have an active role in helping to determine elements of the intervention. This would include the selection and prioritisation of tasks and targets, and monitoring their progress over time.
c) Key adult figures in the child's life, family and professionals, should be encouraged to assist in generalisation and application of skills in everyday life.
d) The contextual life of the family (e.g. time, routines, sibling needs, finance) should be taken into account when planning activities.
e) Interventions should be based on sound theory and supported by evidence of their effectiveness in relevant contexts.

Prognosis

At one time it was considered that clumsiness reflected developmental delay that would be resolved spontaneously by adolescence (Gubbay 1978) although it is now recognised that this is not the case for all, with studies often providing contradictory findings (Cantell and Kooistra 2002). This most likely reflects real differences in prognosis for individual children. In addition, prognosis is affected by the complex interrelationship of overlapping conditions such as attention deficit disorder (Sugden and Wright 1998). What is clear is that, although a number of children outgrow their motor difficulties, for many, problems continue in adulthood and can affect occupational choices (Sugden 2006; Rasmussen and Gillberg 2000). Two studies, each involving ten-year follow-up investigations of children deemed clumsy at ages 5 and 6 (Losse *et al.* 1991; Cantell *et al.* 1994) found continuing evidence of motor difficulties in mid-adolescence. The latter study also noted that, in comparison with controls, they also had lower levels of achievement and aspiration.

Sources of further help

http://www.canchild.ca/en/measures/gmfcs.asp
http://www.dyspraxiafoundation.org.uk/professionals/pr_occupational.php

References

American Psychiatric Association (APA) (1994). *Diagnostic and Statistical Manual of Mental Disorders*, Fourth Edition. Washington, DC: American Psychiatric Association Press.

Ashman, A.F. and Conway, R.N.F. (1997). *An Introduction to Cognitive Education: Theory and Applications*. London: Routledge.

Ayres, A.J. (1989). *Sensory Integration and Praxis Tests*. Los Angeles: Western Psychological Services.

Beery, K.E. (1997). *Developmental Test of Visual–Motor Integration*, Fourth Edition, revised. Los Angeles: Western Psychological Services.

Bruininks, R.H. (1978). *Bruininks-Oseretsky Test of Motor Proficiency Examiners' Manual*. Circle Pines, MI: American Guidance Service.

Cairney, J., Hay, J., Faught, B. *et al.* (2005). DCD, self-efficacy towards physical activity and play: Does gender matter? *Adapted Physical Actively Quarterly* 22: 67–82.

Cantell, M.H. and Kooistra, L. (2002). Long-term outcomes of developmental coordination disorder. In S.A. Cermak and D. Larkin (eds) *Developmental Cordination Disorder*. Albany, NY: Delmar.

Cantell, M.H., Smyth, M.M. and Ahonen, T.P. (1994). Clumsiness in adolescence: Educational, motor, and social outcomes of motor delay detected at 5 years. *Adapted Physical Activity Quarterly* 11: 115–29.

Cermak, S.A., Gubbay, S.S. and Larkin, D. (2002). What is developmental coordination disorder? In S.A. Cermak and D. Larkin (eds) *Developmental Cordination Disorder*. Albany, NY: Delmar.

Chen, H.S., Tickle-Degnen, L. and Cermak, S. (2003). The treatment effectiveness of top-down approaches for children with developmental coordination disorder: A meta-analysis. *American Journal of Occupational Therapy* 21: 16–28.

Chu, S. (1998). Developmental dyspraxia 2: Evaluation and treatment. *British Journal of Therapy and Rehabilitation* 5(4): 176–80.

Crawford, S., Wilson, B. and Dewey, D. (2001). Identifying developmental coordination disorder: Consistency between tests. *Physical and Occupational Therapy in Pediatrics* 20(2/3): 29–50.

Davidson, T. and Williams, B. (2000). Occupational therapy for children with Developmental Coordination Disorder: A study of the effectiveness of a combined sensory integration and perceptual-motor intervention. *British Journal of Occupational Therapy* 63(10): 495–9.

Dewey, D. (2002). Subtypes of developmental coordination disorder. In S.A. Cermak and D. Larkin (eds) *Developmental Coordination Disorder*. Albany, NY: Delmar.

Dewey, D. and Kaplan, B.J. (1994). Subtyping of developmental motor deficits. *Developmental Neuropsychology* 7: 197–206.

Dewey, D. and Wilson, B.N. (2001). Developmental coordination disorder: What is it? In C. Missiuna (ed.) *Children with Developmental Coordination Disorder: Strategies for Success.* New York: Haworth Press.

Figg, J. and Elliott, J.G. (eds) (2003). Cognitive education. *Educational and Child Psychology* 20(2), themed edition.

Fletcher-Flinn, C., Elmes, H. and Strugnell, D. (1997). Visual-perceptual and phonological factors in the acquisition of literacy among children with congenital developmental coordination disorder. *Developmental Medicine and Child Neurology* 39: 158–66.

Gubbay, S. (1978). The management of developmental apraxia. *Developmental Medicine and Child Neurology* 20: 643–6.

Hellgren, L., Gillberg, C., Bagenholm, A. *et al.* (1994). Children with deficits in attention, motor control and perception (DAMP) almost grown up: General health at 16 years. *Developmental Medicine and Child Neurology* 35: 881–92.

Henderson, S.E. and Sugden, D.A. (1992). *The Movement Assessment Battery for Children.* San Antonio, TX: Psychological Corporation.

Henderson, S.E., Sugden, D.A. and Barnett, A.E. (2007) *The Movement Assessment Battery for Children,* Second edition. London: Pearson Education.

Howard, L. (1998). Dyspraxia: An update of current practice. *British Journal of Therapy and Rehabilitation* 5(3): 118–19.

Johnstone, B. and Garcia, L. (1994). Neuropsychological evaluation and academic implications for developmental coordination disorder: A case study. *Developmental Neuropsychology* 10: 369–75.

Junaid, K., Harris, S.R., Fulmer, A. *et al.* (2000). Teachers' use of the MABC Checklist to identify children with motor difficulties. *Pediatric Physical Therapy* 12: 158–63.

Kadesjo, B. and Gillberg, C. (1999). Developmental coordination disorder in Swedish 7-year-old children. *Journal of the American Academy of Child and Adolescent Psychiatry* 38: 820–8.

Kadesjo, B. and Gillberg, C. (2001). The comorbidity of ADHD in the general population of Swedish school-age children. *Journal of Child Psychology and Psychiatry* 42: 487–92.

Kaplan, B.J., Wilson, B.N., Dewey, D. *et al.* (1998). DCD may not be a discrete disorder. *Human Movement Science* 17: 471–90.

Kimball, J.G. (2002). Developmental coordination disorder from a sensory integration perspective. In S.A. Cermak and D. Larkin (eds) *Developmental Coordination Disorder.* Albany, NY: Delmar.

Kirby, A. (1999). *Dyspraxia: The Hidden Handicap.* London: Souvenir Press.

Kirby, A. and Drew, S. (2003). *Guide to Dyspraxia, and Developmental Coordination Disorders.* London: David Fulton.

Laszlo, J.I. and Bairstow, P.J. (1985). *Perceptual-Motor Behaviour: Developmental Assessment and Therapy.* London: Holt, Rinehart & Winston.

Laszlo, J.I., Bairstow, P.J. and Bartrip, J. (1988a). A new approach to treatment of perceptuo-motor dysfunction: Previously called clumsiness. *Support for Learning* 3: 35–40.

Laszlo, J.I., Bairstow, P.J., Bartrip, J. *et al.* (1988b). Clumsiness or perceptuo-motor dysfunction? In A.M. Colley and J.R. Beech (eds) *Cognition and Action in Skilled Behaviour* (pp. 293–309). Amsterdam: Elsevier Science Publishers.

Lewis, V. (2003). *Development and Disability,* Second Edition. Oxford: Blackwell.

Lingam, R., Hunt, L., Golding, J. *et al.* (2009). Prevalence of developmental coordination disorder using the DSM-IV at 7 years of age: A UK population-based study. *Pediatrics* 123(4): e693–700.

Livesy, D., Lum Mow, M., Toshack, T. *et al.* (2011). The relations between motor performance and peer relations in 9–12 year old children. *Child: Care, Health and Development* 37(4): 581–8.

Lord, R. and Hulme, C. (1987). Perceptual judgements of normal and clumsy children. *Developmental Medicine and Child Neurology* 29: 250–7.

Losse, A., Henderson, S.E., Elliman, D. *et al.* (1991). Clumsiness in children – do they grow out of it? A 10-year follow-up study. *Developmental Medicine and Child Neurology* 33: 55–68.

Macintyre, C. (2001). *Dyspraxia 5–11: A Practical Guide.* London: David Fulton.

Magalhães, L.C., Missiuna, C. and Wong, S. (2006). Terminology used in research reports of developmental coordination disorder. *Developmental Medicine and Child Neurology* 48: 937–41.

Mandich, A.D., Buckolz, E. and Polatajko, H.J. (2002). On the ability of children with developmental coordination disorder (DCD) to inhibit response initiation: The Simon effect. *Brain and Cognition* 50: 150–62.

Mandich, A.D., Buckolz, E. and Polatajko, H.J. (2003). Children with developmental coordination disorder (DCD) and their ability to disengage ongoing attentional focus: More on inhibitory function. *Brain and Cognition* 51: 346–56.

Mandich, A.D., Polatajko, H.J., Macnab, J.J. *et al.* (2001). Treatment of children with Developmental Coordination Disorders: What is the evidence? *Physical and Occupational Therapy in Pediatrics* 20(2/3): 51–68.

Martin, N.C., Piek, J.P. and Hay, D. (2006). DCD and ADHD: A genetic study of their shared aetiology. *Human Movement Science* 25(1): 110–24.

Miller, L.T., Missiuna, C., Macnab, J.J. *et al.* (2001). Clinical description of children with developmental coordination disorder. *Canadian Journal of Occupational Therapy* 68(1): 5–15.

Missiuna, C. and Polatajko, H.J. (1995). Developmental dyspraxia by any other name: Are they all just clumsy children? *American Journal of Occupational Therapy* 49: 619–28.

Missiuna, C. and Pollock, N. (1995). Beyond the norms: Need for multiple sources of data in the assessment of children. *Physical and Occupational Therapy in Pediatrics* 15: 57–71.

Missiuna, C., Pollock, N., Egan, M. *et al.* (2008). Enabling occupation through facilitating the diagnosis of Developmental Coordination Disorder. *Canadian Journal of Occupational Therapy* 75(1): 26–34.

Newnham, C. and McKenzie, B.E. (1993). Cross-modal transfer of sequential visual and haptic shape information by clumsy children. *Perception* 22: 1061–73.

Pennington, B.F. (2009). *Diagnosing Learning Disorders: A Neuropsychological Framework,* Second edition. New York: Guilford Press.

Peters, J.M., Barnett, A.L. and Henderson, S.E. (2001). Clumsiness, dyspraxia and developmental coordination disorder: How do health and educational professionals in the UK define the terms? *Child: Care, Health and Development* 27: 399–412.

Piek, J.P., Baynam, G.B. and Barrett, N.C. (2006). The relationship between fine and gross motor ability, self-perceptions and self-worth in children and adolescents. *Human Movement Science* 25(1): 65–75.

Pless, M. and Carlsson, M. (2000). Effects of motor skill intervention on developmental coordination disorder: A meta-analysis. *Adapted Physical Activity Quarterly* 17(4): 381–401.

Polatajko, H.J. and Cantin, N. (2006). Developmental coordination disorder (dyspraxia): An overview of the state of the art. *Seminars in Pediatric Neurology* 12: 250–8.

Polatajko, H.J., Fox, A.M. and Missiuna, C. (1995a). An international consensus on children with developmental coordination disorder. *Canadian Journal of Occupational Therapy* 62: 3–6.

Polatajko, H.J., Macnab, J.J., Anstett, B. *et al.* (1995b). A clinical trial of the process-oriented treatment approach for children with Developmental Coordination Disorder. *Developmental Medicine and Child Neurology* 37: 310–19.

Polatajko, H.J., Mandich, A.D., Miller, L.T. *et al.* (2001a). Cognitive orientation to daily occupational performance (CO-OP): Part II – the evidence. *Physical and Occupational Therapy in Paediatrics* 20(2/3): 83–106.

Polatajko, H.J., Mandich, A.D., Missiuna, C. *et al.* (2001b). Cognitive orientation to daily occupational performance (CO-OP): Part III – the protocol in brief. *Physical and Occupational Therapy in Paediatrics* 20(2/3): 107–23.

Portwood, M.M. (1999). *Developmental Dyspraxia: Identification and Intervention.* London: David Fulton.

Ramus, F., Pidgeon, E. and Frith, U. (2003). Motor control and phonology in dyslexic children. *Journal of Child Psychology and Psychiatry* 44: 712–22.

Rasmussen, P. and Gillberg, C. (2000). Natural outcome of ADHD with DCD at age 22 years: A controlled, longitudinal, community-based study. *Journal of the American Academy of Child and Adolescent Psychiatry* 39: 1424–31.

Ripley, K., Daines, R. and Barrett, J. (1999). *Dyspraxia: A Guide for Teachers and Parents.* London: David Fulton.

Rösblad, B. (2002). Visual perception in children with developmental coordination disorder. In S.A. Cermak and D. Larkin (eds) *Developmental Coordination Disorder.* Albany, NY: Delmar.

Schoemaker, M.M. and Kalverboer, A.F. (1994). Social and affective problems of children who are clumsy: How early do they begin? *Adapted Physical Activity Quarterly* 11: 130–40.

Schoemaker, M.M., Smits-Engelsman, B.C.M. and Jongmans, M.J. (2003). Psychometric properties of the Movement Assessment Battery for Children Checklist as a screening instrument for children with a developmental coordination disorder. *British Journal of Educational Psychology* 73: 425–41.

Short, H. and Crawford, J. (1984). Last to be chosen: The awkward child. *Pivot* 2: 32–6.

Sims, K., Henderson, S.E., Hulme, C. *et al.* (1996a). The remediation of clumsiness: An evaluation of Laszlo's kinaesthetic approach (part one). *Developmental Medicine and Child Neurology* 38: 976–87.

Sims, K., Henderson, S.E., Morton, J. *et al.* (1996b). The remediation of clumsiness: Is kinaesthesis the answer? (part two). *Developmental Medicine and Child Neurology* 38: 988–97.

Smyth, T.R. (1991). Abnormal clumsiness in children: A programming defect? *Child: Care, Health and Development* 17: 283–94.

Smyth, T.R. and Anderson, H.I. (2000). Coping with clumsiness in the school playground: Social and physical play in children with coordination impairments. *British Journal of Developmental Psychology* 18: 389–413.

Steinman, K.J., Mostofsky, S.H. and Denckla, M.B. (2010). Towards a narrower, more pragmatic view of developmental dyspraxia. *Journal of Child Neurology* 25(1): 71–81.

Stephenson, E., McKay, C. and Chesson, R. (1991). The identification and treatment of motor/learning difficulties: Parents' perceptions and the role of the therapist. *Child: Care, Health and Development* 17: 91–113.

Sugden, D.A. (2006). *Leeds Consensus Statement.* Leeds: University of Leeds. Downloadable on: http://www.dcd-uk.org/images/LeedsConsensus06.pdf.

Sugden, D.A. (2007). Current approaches to intervention in children with developmental coordination disorder. *Developmental Medicine and Child Neurology* 49: 467–71.

Sugden, D.A. and Chambers, M.E. (2003). Intervention in children with Developmental Coordination Disorder: The role of parents and teachers. *British Journal of Educational Psychology* 73: 545–61.

van Dellen, T. and Geuze, K.H. (1988). Motor response programming in clumsy children. *Journal of Child Psychology and Psychiatry* 29: 489–500.

Williams, H.G. (2002). Motor control in children with developmental coordination disorder. In S.A. Cermak and D. Larkin (eds) *Developmental Coordination Disorder*. Albany, NY: Delmar.

Wilson, B.N., Kaplan, B.J., Crawford, S.G. *et al.* (2000). Reliability and validity of a parent questionnaire on childhood motor skills. *American Journal of Occupational Therapy* 54: 484–93.

Wilson, P.H. (2005). Practitioner review: Approaches to assessment and treatment of children with DCD. *Journal of Child Psychology and Psychiatry* 46(8): 806–23.

Wilson, P.H. and McKenzie, B.E. (1998). Information processing deficits associated with developmental co-ordination disorder: A meta-analysis of research findings. *Journal of Child Psychology and Psychiatry* 39: 829–40.

World Health Organization (1992). *International Statistical Classification of Diseases and Related Health Problems*, Tenth Edition, vol. 1 ICD-10. Geneva: World Health Organization.

Zoia, S., Barnett, A., Wilson, P. *et al.* (2006). Developmental coordination disorder: Current issues. *Child: Care, Health, and Development*, 32(6): 613–18.

Author index

Subject index